T0317604

SPATIAL AGENT-BASED SIMULATION MODELING IN PUBLIC HEALTH

Wiley Series in Modeling and Simulation

Mission Statement

The *Wiley Series in Modeling and Simulation* provides an interdisciplinary and global approach to the numerous real-world applications of modeling and simulation (M&S) that are vital to business professionals, researchers, policymakers, program managers, and academics alike. Written by recognized international experts in the field, the books present the best practices in the applications of M&S as well as bridge the gap between innovative and scientifically sound approaches to solving real-world problems and the underlying technical language of M&S research. The series successfully expands the way readers view and approach problem solving in addition to the design, implementation, and evaluation of interventions to change behavior. Featuring broad coverage of theory, concepts, and approaches along with clear, intuitive, and insightful illustrations of the applications, the Series contains books within five main topical areas: Public and Population Health; Training and Education; Operations Research, Logistics, Supply Chains, and Transportation; Homeland Security, Emergency Management, and Risk Analysis; and Interoperability, Composability, and Formalism.

Advisory Editors ● Public and Population Health
Peter S. Hovmand, Washington University in St. Louis
Bruce Y. Lee, University of Pittsburgh

Founding Series Editors
Joshua G. Behr, Old Dominion University
Rafael Diaz, Old Dominion University

Homeland Security, Emergency Management, and Risk Analysis

Forthcoming Titles
Zedda ● *Risk and Stability of Banking Systems*

Interoperability, Composability, and Formalism

Operations Research, Logistics, Supply Chains, and Transportation

Public and Population Health

Arifin, Madey, and Collins ● *Spatial Agent-Based Simulation Modeling in Public Health: Design, Implementation, and Applications for Malaria Epidemiology*

Forthcoming Titles

Hovmand ● *Modeling Social Determinants of Health*
Kim and Hammon ● *Modeling and Simulation for Social Epidemiology and Public Health*

Training and Education

Combs, Sokolowski, and Banks ● *The Digital Patient: Advancing Healthcare, Research, and Education*

Forthcoming Titles

Tolk and Ören ● *The Profession of Modeling and Simulation*

SPATIAL AGENT-BASED SIMULATION MODELING IN PUBLIC HEALTH

Design, Implementation, and Applications for Malaria Epidemiology

S. M. NIAZ ARIFIN

Department of Computer Science and Engineering
University of Notre Dame
IN, USA

GREGORY R. MADEY

Department of Computer Science and Engineering
University of Notre Dame
IN, USA

FRANK H. COLLINS

Department of Biological Sciences
University of Notre Dame
IN, USA

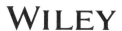

Library of Congress Cataloging-in-Publication Data:

Arifin, S.M. Niaz, author.
    Spatial agent-based simulation modeling in public health : design, implementation, and applications for malaria epidemiology / S.M. Niaz Arifin, Gregory R. Madey, Frank H. Collins.
        p. ; cm.
    Includes bibliographical references and index.
    ISBN 978-1-118-96435-4 (hardback)
    I. Madey, Gregory Richard, author. II. Collins, Frank H., author. III. Title.
    [DNLM: 1. Malaria–epidemiology. 2. Computer Simulation. 3. Geographic Information Systems. 4. Models, Theoretical. 5. Spatial Analysis. WC 755.1]
    RA644.M2
    614.5′32090285–dc23
                                        2015033121

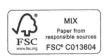

To my parents:

Engineer S. M. Golam Mostofa

B.Sc. Engg. (Civil), FIE (B), PGD (CS)
My Father and Guide

Professor Parvin Akhter Jahan

M.A. (Economics), B.A. (Honors)
My Mother and Best Friend

and my wife:
Rumana Reaz Arifin

B.S., M.S.
My Soulmate

and my sister:
Mafruhatul Jannat

Ph.D., M.S., B.S.
We Grew up Together

— S. M. Niaz Arifin

CONTENTS

LIST OF CONTRIBUTORS

Philip A. Eckhoff Research Scientist, Principal Investigator, Institute for Disease Modeling (IDM), Intellectual Ventures Management, LLC (IV), Bellevue, WA, USA

Edward A. Wenger, Sr. Research Manager, Institute for Disease Modeling (IDM), Intellectual Ventures Management, LLC (IV), Bellevue, WA, USA

LIST OF FIGURES

LIST OF TABLES

PREFACE

In today's scientific world, *computational science* is considered the *third pillar* of scientific inquiry, along with the two traditional pillars of theory and experimentation. Although science is still carried out as an ongoing interplay between theory and experimentation, the increased scale and complexity of both have compelled computational science to be an integral aspect of almost every type of scientific research.

Typically, computational science uses computer simulations (to construct computational models) and quantitative analysis techniques in order to analyze and solve scientific problems. In particular, *modeling & simulation* (*M&S*) techniques are being increasingly used to model complex systems, which in general exhibit complex properties such as heterogeneity, dynamic interactions, emergence, learning, and adaptation. With the ever-widening availability of computing resources, the increasing pool of human computational experts and due to its unconstrained applicability across academic discipline boundaries, the importance of M&S continues to grow at a remarkable rate.

Agent-based modeling and simulation (*ABMS*) is a class of M&S techniques for simulating the actions and interactions of autonomous agents with a view to assessing their effects on the simulated system as a whole. Having its roots from the investigation of complex systems, complex adaptive systems, artificial intelligence, and computer science, ABMS combines elements of game theory, complex systems, emergence, computational sociology, multiagent systems, and evolutionary programming. The suite of models developed using ABMS, known as *agent-based models* (*ABMs*), have applications in diverse real-world problems and have become increasingly popular as a modeling approach in almost all branches of science and engineering.

In public health research, epidemics and infectious disease dynamics modeling can be termed as a *signature success* of ABMS. Uses of M&S in public health include synthesizing knowledge from disparate disciplines, filling the gaps in existing knowledge, conducting cost-benefit trade-off studies, and generating hypotheses. As such, an increasing number of U.S. universities are incorporating systems science and M&S into their curricula and research programs through the schools of public health and other health-related academic departments.

A major objective of this book is to present a practical and useful introduction to the important facets of a sufficiently complex M&S project that largely involved the evolution of a complex ABM. The ABM was developed by experts from multiple academic disciplines. Thus, major portions of the contents of this book materialized as a result of interdisciplinary, collaborative research efforts concerning ABMS (from Computer Science and Engineering) and malaria epidemiology (from Biological Sciences) at the University of Notre Dame [547].

Malaria is one of the oldest and deadliest infectious diseases in humans, and the control of malaria represents one of the greatest public health challenges of the twenty-first century. According to the latest estimates (released in December 2014), the World Health Organization (WHO) reported about 198 million cases of malaria in 2013 and an estimated 584,000 deaths, with half of the world's population (about 3.3 billion) being at risk [567]. Human malaria is transmitted only by female mosquitoes of the genus *Anopheles*, which are regarded as the primary vectors for transmission.

The ABMs presented in this book were developed by following a conceptual, biological core model of *Anopheles gambiae* (*An. gambiae* for short) for malaria epidemiology. The notion of this core model plays a central role in the long development process of multiple versions of the ABMs, as well as in conducting such crucial steps as model verification, validation, and replication. Evolution of the core model has been guided by relevant biological features concerning *An. gambiae*, which were iteratively refined and incrementally added to the existing pool of model features. Subsequently, the ABMs were updated to reflect the changes.

OUTLINE OF CHAPTERS

Chapter 1 of this book introduces the reader to its major components, presents a brief introduction to malaria and ABMs, and lists our specific contributions. Chapters 2 and 3 present general introductions to malaria and ABMs. Their purpose is to collectively serve as a concise background for readers who are less familiar with the disease and its epidemiological aspects, and why ABMs are particularly useful in modeling diseases like malaria.

Chapter 4 thoroughly describes the biological core model of *An. gambiae*. After defining some relevant terms of interest, it addresses several important features of the mosquito life cycle, including development in different life-cycle stages, aquatic habitats, oviposition, vector senescence, and density- and age-dependent mortality rates. It also discusses some of the key features, characteristics, and limitations of the core model.

Chapter 5 discusses the design and implementation of a simplified, fixed version of the ABM. Since the ABM is developed in the *Java* object-oriented programming

(OOP) language, we present some relevant OOP terminology. We then describe the architecture of the ABM and present class diagrams to elaborate the agents and their environments. In order to capture the major daily events of a typical simulation in a standard fashion, a new type of descriptive diagram, called the *Event–Action–List* (*EAL*) diagram, is presented. The chapter also describes the mosquito population dynamics and some of the other characteristics and features of the ABM, including processing steps ordering, initialization, and simulation assumptions.

Chapter 6 presents a spatial extension of the ABM. In general, an ABM can be applied to a domain *with* or *without* an explicit representation of *space*. However, analysis of spatial relationships is fundamental to epidemiology research, as demonstrated by several recent studies. In some cases, an explicit spatial representation may be desired for certain aspects of the ABM to be modeled more realistically. For example, in a malaria ABM, some frequent events performed by the mosquito agents such as obtaining a successful blood meal (host-seeking) or finding an aquatic habitat to lay eggs (oviposition) can be *spatially* modeled in the landscape in which the agents move. These aspects are also affected by the underlying spatial heterogeneity, which defines the spatial distribution of resources and directly affects the mosquito population in the ABM. In Chapter 6, we describe the modeling aspects of the spatial ABM, the mosquito agents and their spatial movement, the landscapes, and the resource-seeking events. We also describe a custom-built landscape generator tool that is used to generate landscapes with desired characteristics for the spatial ABM and present results concerning the effects of varying landscape patterns, the relative size and density of the aquatic habitats, the overall capacity of the system, and the effects of spatial heterogeneity of the landscapes.

Chapters 7–9 describe the techniques and results of verification, validation, and replication of the ABMs, which in general deal with the measurement and assessment of accuracy of M&S research. They also present the results of examining the impact of two malaria control interventions, namely, larval source management (LSM) and insecticide-treated nets (ITNs). We investigate the effects of LSM and ITNs, applied both in isolation and in combination, on the mosquito agent populations. We compare our results to those reported by previously published malaria models and recommend guidelines for future ABM modelers, summarizing the insights and experiences gained from our work of replicating earlier studies.

Chapter 10 presents a landscape epidemiology modeling framework that integrates a Geographic information system (GIS) with the spatial ABM. The idea of integrating GIS with ABMs is not new, and several studies in multiple domains (e.g., urban land-use change, military mobile communications) have shown such integration. GIS and spatial statistical methods have also been extensively used in entomological and epidemiological studies. In particular, for malaria as a disease, GIS applications have been used for measuring the distribution of mosquito species, their habitats, the control and management of the disease, and so on. However, with the exception of the individual-based model named *EMOD* (which is presented in Chapter 11), no *ABM-based malaria study* has yet shown how to effectively integrate an ABM with GIS and other geospatial features and thereby harness the full power of GIS.

There is also a *vacuum of knowledge* in building robust integration frameworks that can guide the use of geospatial features (related to malaria transmission) as model inputs, as opposed to simply use these features as cartographic outputs from the models (as done by most previous studies). In Chapter 10, we show how to effectively integrate simulation outputs from our spatial ABM with a GIS. For a study area in Kenya, we construct different landscape scenarios and perform spatial analyses on the simulation results. Results indicate that the integration of epidemiological simulation-based outputs with spatial analyses techniques within a single modeling framework can be a valuable tool for conducting a variety of disease control activities such as exploring new biological insights, monitoring the changes of key disease transmission indices and epidemiological landscapes, and guiding resource allocation for further investigation.

Lastly, Chapter 11 presents the advanced individual-based model named *EMOD*, which is contributed as a guest chapter from the Institute for Disease Modeling (IDM) [536]. EMOD, which stands for *Epidemiological Modeling*, represents a suite of detailed, geographically specific, and mechanistic stochastic simulations of disease (including malaria) transmission through the use of complex software modeling. Chapter 11 showcases two important epidemiological scenarios in Africa with geospatial maps coupled with the model's outputs.

At the end, we conclude with a fully functional computer source code of a specific version of the spatial ABM is presented in the Book Companion Site and a software module called P-SAM (Post-Simulation Analysis Module) that we developed to analyze and visualize the postsimulation outputs of ABMs.

INTENDED AUDIENCE

This book is intended for students, individuals, and research groups who intend to learn and use the problem-solving methodology of M&S, particularly using the ABMS techniques. It can serve as a practical resource for students with a science or engineering background at the senior undergraduate or graduate level and other professionals interested, in general, in simulation modeling, epidemiology, public health, and bioinformatics. Although some familiarity with the basic notions of M&S, biology, and/or epidemiology may be helpful, no advanced background in these disciplines is necessary. Most of the core materials are accompanied by introductory details to important topics, definitions of relevant terms, and copious references. We use Java™ [264] as our programming environment of choice in developing the spatial simulation models. A reasonable level of computer programming skills is helpful, but not mandatory, to comprehend the results and discussions presented in Chapters 6, 8, and 9.

On the one hand, M&S researchers (including students and modelers) can benefit from the book's description of the core conceptual model (Chapter 4) followed by the implementation details of the ABMs (Chapter 5), the extension of the nonspatial ABM into a spatial ABM (Chapter 6), and the model verification, validation, and replication issues (Chapters 7–9). The transformation of mental images of a conceptual model (which often resides amorphously only in modelers' brains and may vastly differ among individual modelers due to countless ambiguities) into a computational, verifiable entity (an ABM) may help new modelers to comprehend the overall modeling life cycle.

On the other hand, this book can also prove useful to a wide range of other individuals from intellectuals and academics to professionals. Due to the multidisciplinary nature of the reported research that spans several academic disciplines including, ABMS, bioinformatics, malaria epidemiology, spatial models, and GIS, it can have broad implications and can be valuable to infectious disease dynamics researchers, malaria control managers (e.g., from ministries of health of malaria-endemic countries), and other public health policy makers and funding bodies. For example, sections describing the impact of malaria control interventions (in Chapters 9 and 10) can provide valuable biological insights to malaria modelers, as well as to policy makers and funding agencies concerning the disease's control and elimination efforts.

The last two chapters are especially relevant for specific user groups. The landscape epidemiology modeling framework presented in Chapter 10, which integrates a GIS with the spatial ABM (described in Chapter 6), showcases an ideal methodological framework and a useful application of the ABMs by taking the *virtual, simulated* world of agents one step closer to the *real, malarious* world of mosquitoes. Chapter 11, through the use of another advanced individual-based model, shows how knowledge from diverse but interconnected disciplines such as M&S, epidemiology, and GIS can be meaningfully combined to derive insights and analyze the implications for malaria eradication.

S. M. NIAZ ARIFIN
Notre Dame, Indiana
June, 2015

ACKNOWLEDGMENTS

We would like to thank Drs. Philip A. Eckhoff and Edward A. Wenger for their contributions on the EMOD model. Thanks also to our colleagues Ms. Rumana Reaz Arifin and Dr. Dilkushi de Alwis Pitts (from the University of Notre Dame) and Dr. M. Sohel Rahman and Ms. Sara Nowreen (from Bangladesh University of Engineering & Technology) for their support with GIS and spatial analyses; Drs. Ying Zhou, Gregory J. Davis, and James E. Gentile for their early contributions to the core model, the ABMs, and some of the verification and validation works; Drs. Ryan C. Kennedy, Kelly E. Lane-deGraaf, Agustin Fuentes, and Hope Hollocher for their collaboration; and Dr. Paul Brenner for his support at the High Performance Computing Group of the Center for Research Computing (CRC) at the University of Notre Dame.

We would also like to thank Drs. Joshua G. Behr and Rafael Diaz, Editors for the *Wiley Series in Modeling and Simulation*, for their initial encouragement and responses. Thanks also to Ms. Natalie K. Meyers at the Hesburgh Libraries at the University of Notre Dame for her help with the copyright management issues. We also express our appreciation for the help and support provided by Ms. Susanne Steitz-Filler, Senior Editor, Ms. Sari Friedman, Editorial Program Coordinator, and Ms. Roshna Mohan, Project Editor (Professional Practice and Learning) at Wiley.

The preparation and development of this book have consumed substantial amounts of time which, to a large extent, has been at the expense of time we would otherwise have shared with our families. We would therefore like to express our heartfelt gratitude to our families for their patience and support.

LIST OF ABBREVIATIONS

ABMs	Agent-based model(s)
ABMS	Agent-based modeling and simulation
ACT	Artemisinin-combination therapy
ADS	Agent-directed simulation
AH	Aquatic habitat
AI	Artificial intelligence
API	Application programming interface
ASMR	Age-specific mortality rate
ATT	Average travel time
CC	Creative Commons
CHC	Combined habitat capacity
CI	Cyberinfrastructure; confidence interval
DAG	Directed acyclic graph
DDT	Dichlorodiphenyltrichloroethane
DES	Discrete event simulation
DGPS	Differential global positioning system
DMR	Daily mortality rate
EAL	Event-Action-List
EIR	Entomological inoculation rate
EMOD	Epidemiological modeling
ESD	Effective shortest distance
FA	Failure avoidance
GIS	Geographic information system
GMMs	Genetically modified mosquitoes
GPS	Global positioning system

GUI	Graphical user interface
HC	Habitat capacity
HMR	Hourly mortality rate
IBM	Individual-based model
IDM	Institute for disease modeling
IOD	Inter-object distance
IRS	Indoor residual spraying
ITNs	Insecticide-treated nets
IVM	Integrated vector management
JAR	Java archive (File format)
JRE	Java runtime environment
LLINs	Long-lasting insecticide-treated nets
LSM	Larval source management
M&S	Modeling & simulation
MDA	Mass drug administration
MPI	Message passing interface
MSAT	Mass screening and treatment
OA	Open access
ODE	Ordinary differential equation
ODEL	One-day-old equivalent larval population
OOP	Object-oriented programming
OSS	Open source software
PR	Percent reduction
PRNG	Pseudo-random number generator
P-SAM	Postsimulation Analysis Module
QA	Quality assurance
R&R	Replication & reproducibility
RBM	Roll back malaria
SIT	Sterile insect technique
SQA	Simulation quality assurance
SR	Source reduction
TBV	Transmission-blocking vaccine
UI	User interface
UML	Unified modeling language
VA	Vector abundance
VBD	Vector-borne disease
V&V	Verification & validation
VV&A	Verification, validation, and accreditation
VecNet	Vector-borne disease network
WHO	World Health Organization
WNV	West Nile virus
XML	Extensible markup language

1

INTRODUCTION

1.1 OVERVIEW

In recent years, modeling and simulation (M&S) paradigms are being increasingly used as an efficient tool to model complex systems, which often exhibit complex properties such as emergence, learning, adaptation, heterogeneity, and dynamic interactions. With the ever-widening availability of computing resources, the increasing pool of human computational experts, and due to its unconstrained applicability across academic discipline boundaries, the importance of M&S continues to grow at a remarkable rate. M&S draws from academic disciplines such as computer science, mathematics, operational research, engineering, statistics, and physics, and covers a broad set of application areas such as biology, public health, commerce, defense, logistics, manufacturing, supply chains, and transportation [525]. Typical roles of M&S studies include forecasting, sensitivity analysis, comparison of control policy options, education and training, engineering design, performance evaluation, prototyping and concept evaluation, risk and safety assessment, and uncertainty reduction in decision-making [67].

Agent-based modeling and simulation (ABMS) is an M&S technique for simulating the actions and interactions of autonomous agents with a view to assessing their effects on the simulated system as a whole. Having its roots in the investigation of complex systems, complex adaptive systems, and artificial life, ABMS has evolved as

Spatial Agent-Based Simulation Modeling in Public Health:
Design, Implementation, and Applications for Malaria Epidemiology, First Edition.
S. M. Niaz Arifin, Gregory R. Madey and Frank H. Collins.
© 2016 John Wiley & Sons, Inc. Published 2016 by John Wiley & Sons, Inc.

a natural response to meet the needs of complex systems modeling [525]. The suite of models developed using ABMS, known as *agent-based models (ABMs)*, have applications in diverse real-world problems and have become increasingly popular as a modeling approach in social sciences and public health research problems.[1] To this end, the advances in epidemics and infectious disease dynamics research made possible through the use of ABMs can be termed as one of its signature successes [321].

This book primarily concerns spatial agent-based simulation modeling in public health. In particular, it presents the design, implementation, and applications of spatial ABMs for malaria, which is one of the largest causes of global human mortality and morbidity. The ABMs simulate the life cycle and the population dynamics of the malaria-transmitting mosquito vector *Anopheles gambiae* (*An. gambiae* for short),[2] from a biological core model.[3]

Figure 1.1 depicts the major components of the book. Logical connections between the components and the chapters are indicated, which may serve as visual cues for the readers. Chapters 2 and 3 present some general background of malaria and ABMs, and discuss the applicability of ABMs in malaria epidemiology research, which, in turn, broadly falls under the realm of computational biology. Chapters 4–6 describe the biological core model and the ABMs (including the spatial ABMs), and form the core of the book. Chapters 7–9 discuss the verification, validation, and replication issues of the ABMs. Chapter 10 presents a landscape epidemiology modeling framework that integrates the simulation outputs from the spatial ABMs with a geographic information system (GIS). Finally, Chapter 11 presents another spatial ABM – the *epidemiological modeling EMOD* individual-based model (IBM).[4,5] Note that some chapters may overlap into multiple components (see Fig. 1.1). All components of the book share the global/public health implications.

The remainder of this chapter provides a brief introduction to malaria and ABMs. We conclude this chapter by listing our specific contributions, and by providing a roadmap for the remainder of this book.

---

[1]In general, we distinguish between the usage of the two terms "ABMS" and "ABMs". ABMS (singular term) collectively denotes the M&S modeling approach, paradigm, methodology, and/or technology of *ABMS*; ABM (singular term) and ABMs (plural term, note the lowercase "s"), on the other hand, denote the class of computational *agent-based model(s)* that are developed using the ABMS technology. For further usage notation of ABM and ABMs, see Footnote 3.

[2]In epidemiology, a *vector* is an agent (person, animal, or microorganism) that carries and transmits an infectious pathogen into another living organism. Throughout this book, the two terms "mosquito" and "vector" are used interchangeably.

[3]Several language-specific implementations of the biological core model have been developed by individual researchers within our research group over the recent years. For this book, the plural term "ABMs" collectively refers to these implementations (which are compared solely for verification and validation (V&V) purposes, as described in Chapter 8). The singular term "ABM", where applicable, refers to the particular implementation developed by the authors.

[4]Chapter 11 is contributed as a guest chapter by Philip A. Eckhoff and Edward A. Wenger from the Institute for Disease Modeling (IDM) [536].

[5]IBMs, which are frequently used within the field of ecology, refer to a specific subclass of ABMs within which individuals may be simpler than fully autonomous agents. See Section 3.5.2 for examples of other malaria IBMs.

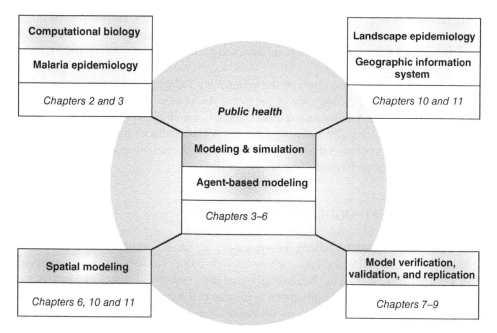

Figure 1.1   Book components. Logical connections between the major components and the chapters are indicated. This book primarily concerns modeling & simulation (M&S), specifically agent-based modeling (ABM), in public health (malaria epidemiology). Chapters 2 and 3 present some general background of malaria and agent-based models (ABMs) and discuss the applicability of ABMs in malaria epidemiology research, which, in turn, broadly falls under the realm of computational biology. Chapters 4–6 describe the biological core model, the agent-based models (ABMs), and the spatial ABMs, and form the core of the book. Chapters 7–9 discuss the verification, validation, and replication issues of the ABMs. Chapter 10 presents a landscape epidemiology modeling framework, and Chapter 11 presents the *EMOD* individual-based model. Note that some chapters may overlap into multiple components. All components of the book share the global/public health implications.

1.2   MALARIA

Malaria is one of the oldest and deadliest infectious diseases in humans. According to the latest estimates (released in December 2014), the World Health Organization (WHO) reported about 198 million cases of malaria in 2013 and an estimated 584,000 deaths [568]. Half of the world's population (about 3.3 billion) is at risk of malaria [568]. The population of sub-Saharan Africa, which accounts for 80% of the globally estimated annual deaths, experiences the highest burden of the disease, with a child dying every minute [568]. As highland malaria re-emerged in several African countries in the recent decades [443], the control of malaria represents one of the greatest global public health challenges of the twenty-first century.

Malaria is a complex disease. Being global in nature, it imposes a staggering burden on the public health. A variety of geographical, environmental, vector, host, and parasite factors determine its local and global characteristics. Different population groups in malaria-infected areas face different risks with regard to the disease. These groups range from pregnant women, infants, and young children to diversified groups such as travelers and migrants.

Caused by protozoan parasites of the genus *Plasmodium*, human malaria is transmitted only by female mosquitoes of the genus *Anopheles*. The group of *Anopheles* species known as the *Anopheles gambiae* complex, which refers to eight very closely related and morphologically indistinguishable species, includes the two most important malaria vectors in sub-Saharan Africa and the most efficient malaria vectors in the world: *An. gambiae* and *Anopheles coluzzii*.

1.3 AGENT-BASED MODELING OF MALARIA

An agent-based model (ABM) is typically an object-oriented, discrete-event, rule-based, stochastic, and often spatially explicit model for dynamic computational M&S [9, 72, 256].[6] ABMs are increasingly used to represent and investigate multiscale complex systems and have applications in diverse real-world problems.

An ABM consists of a collection of autonomous decision-making entities called *agents* [72]. By employing a set of rules, agents can individually assess the environment and may make decisions. Appropriate behaviors for the system may then be executed by the agents. ABMs possess inherent abilities to capture important modeling aspects such as space, geometry, and structure, which collectively facilitate the ability of modelers to express, represent, and test their hypotheses.

ABMs of malaria can play important roles in quantifying the effects of malaria-control interventions and in answering other interesting research questions. For example, ABMs can assist malaria control managers and policy makers in selecting appropriate combinations of interventions to interrupt transmission and in setting response timelines and expectations of impact. They can also be useful for testing how differences in multiple transmission settings can lead to different results when the same interventions are applied in two different populations and/or geographical locations. As *predictive tools*, ABMs can help to identify the appropriate set of existing and/or new interventions that are likely to be synergistic, and when they can be deployed to achieve the best results. Since ABMs are mostly computer-based simulations, they are *only approximations of* reality; however, they do provide a highly refined and structured way of synthesizing information, testing ideas, or exploring insights.

1.4 CONTRIBUTIONS

This book presents the following contributions:

- Developing a biological core model of *An. gambiae* mosquitoes for malaria epidemiology

---

[6]Although in most cases, a typical ABM often uses a subset of these features.

- Implementing ABMs by following the core model specifications
- Modeling and developing a spatial extension of the ABM
- Performing verification, validation, and replication tasks of the ABMs
- Developing a landscape generator tool (*VectorLand*) for the spatial ABM
- Examining the impact of vector control interventions
- Developing a landscape epidemiology modeling framework that integrates simulation outputs from the spatial ABM with a GIS
- Describing features and results from another advanced individual-based model (contributed as a guest chapter).

1.5   ORGANIZATION

This book is organized as follows. In Chapter 2, we present a brief history of malaria, including its historic perspectives and its early connections in relation to human history. We discuss a global view of its epidemiology, geographic distribution, transmission, risk mapping, and some of its major control measures. Chapter 3 provides a general background about ABMs and discusses the applicability of ABMs in malaria modeling. Chapter 4 thoroughly describes the biological core model of *An. gambiae*. Chapters 5 and 6 discuss the design and implementation of the ABMs, the spatial ABM, and a custom-built landscape generator tool. Chapters 7–9 describe the verification, validation, and replication issues of the ABMs, which, in general, deal with the measurement and assessment of accuracy of M&S research. They also present the results of examining the impact of two vector control interventions, applied both in isolation and in combination. Chapter 10 presents a landscape epidemiology modeling framework that integrates a GIS with the spatial ABM. Lastly, Chapter 11 presents the *EMOD* individual-based model and showcases two important epidemiological scenarios in Africa with geospatial maps coupled with the model's outputs.

At the end, we conclude with some supplementary information. Appendix A describes the theoretical background on the temperature-regulated rules and equations used in the core model (described in Chapter 4), Appendix B depicts a general flowchart for an implementation of the ABM, Appendix C presents some additional materials for Chapter 10, and Appendix D describes a software module called P-SAM (postsimulation analysis module) that we developed to analyze and visualize the postsimulation outputs of ABMs. A fully functional computer source code of a specific version of the spatial ABM is presented in the Book Companion Site.

2

MALARIA: A BRIEF HISTORY

2.1 OVERVIEW

This chapter provides a brief history of malaria. We describe some historic perspectives and early connections of the disease in relation to human history, including its naming, origins, early efforts of control and treatment, and key discoveries. Then, we present a global view of its epidemiology.[1] We also discuss its geographic distribution, transmission, and risk mapping efforts. At the end, this chapter provides a concise description of malaria control, elimination, and eradication efforts, and some of the current state-of-the-science research to combat the disease burden.

2.2 MALARIA IN HUMAN HISTORY

As a widespread and potentially lethal human infectious disease, at its peak, malaria infested every continent except Antarctica [97, 129]. The history of malaria predates humanity and stretches from its prehistoric origin as a disease in the primates of Africa through to the twenty-first century [480]. Human malaria likely originated in Africa

---

[1]The detailed life cycle of malaria-transmitting mosquitoes is presented in Chapter 4, in relation to the biological core model.

Spatial Agent-Based Simulation Modeling in Public Health:
Design, Implementation, and Applications for Malaria Epidemiology, First Edition.
S. M. Niaz Arifin, Gregory R. Madey and Frank H. Collins.
© 2016 John Wiley & Sons, Inc. Published 2016 by John Wiley & Sons, Inc.

and coevolved with its hosts, mosquitoes and nonhuman primates. Malaria has always been part of the rising and decline of nations, of wars, and of upheavals [381].

Human malaria results from encounters between *Anopheles* mosquitoes, *Plasmodium* parasites, and humans. Molecular methods have confirmed the presence of the malaria parasite in ancient Egyptian mummy tissues from about 4000 years ago [382]. From the Indus valley in northern India, Vedic (about 3500–2800 years ago) and Brahmanic (about 2800–1900 years ago) scriptures contain many references to fevers, some of which are said almost certainly to concern malaria [84]. The symptoms of malarial fever were also described in a Sanskrit medical treatise named *Susruta*. References to malarial conditions have been quoted from Sumerian and Egyptian texts dating from 3500 to 4000 years ago [159, 475]. Malaria seems to have been known in China for almost 5000 years. The *Nei Ching* (The Canon of Medicine) from 4700 years ago and several other references to the periodic fevers of malaria are found throughout recorded history beginning in 2700 B.C.E. in China [97, 381]. Malaria became widely recognized in ancient Greece by the fourth century B.C.E. and is implicated in the decline of many city-state populations, as evident from extensive references to it in the literature by Hippocrates and Pericles [420]. A number of early Roman writers attributed malarial diseases to the swamps. The infamous *Roman fever* refers to a particularly deadly strain of malaria that affected the Roman Campagna and the city of Rome throughout various epochs in history, an epidemic of which during the fifth century C.E. may have contributed to the fall of the Roman empire [97, 468].

2.2.1   The Malarial Path: Ancient Origins

The Ethiopian region in Africa is thought to be the cradle of malaria [85]. The *Anopheles* vector species existed in that region and also in the temperate climates long before the first hominids [84]. Humans may have originally caught the deadly malaria parasite *Plasmodium* from gorillas [319].

In the *Old World*, where epidemics had a major impact on ancient civilizations, the disease probably spread up the Nile valley to the Mediterranean shores and Mesopotamia, to the Indian peninsula and to China [84, 480]. From these main centers, malaria invaded a large part of the globe [84].

By the beginning of the Christian era, malaria was widespread around the shores of the Mediterranean, in southern Europe, across the Arabian Peninsula, and in Central, South, and Southeast Asia, China, Manchuria, Korea, and Japan [97]. Malaria probably began to spread into northern Europe in the Dark and Middle Ages.

The arrival of Europeans and West Africans in the *New World* at the end of the fifteenth century C.E. introduced the malaria parasite for the first time into the Americas [97, 140]. In the beginning, the malarious heartlands of the Americas were in the Caribbean and parts of Central and South America. Accompanying the economic growth of the Southern States of North America based on slaves brought from West Africa, malaria took firm hold across the North American continent, and by around 1850 C.E. prevailed through the tropical, subtropical, and temperate regions of the two American continents [97]. The impressive extent of early human travel encompassed huge movements of people across continents. As the mobile human host traveled and dispersed, the disease also spread globally.

2.2.2 Naming and Key Discoveries

The term malaria originated from the Italian *mala* (meaning "bad") and *aria* (meaning "air"). Since ancient times, malaria was linked with poisonous vapors of swamps or stagnant water on the ground. This probable relationship gave the two most frequently used names to the disease: *mal'aria* (later shortened to one word malaria), and *palud-isme* [535]. It was also termed as *jungle fever, marsh fever, paludal fever,* or *swamp fever.* Depending on the location of affliction, the disease was also known as ague, paludisme, Wechselfieber, triasuchka, and so on [480].

The key discoveries regarding the *Plasmodium* parasite are attributed to travelers and expatriates (often army doctors) working in malarial areas [480]. The identification of the exact organism is attributed to the French army surgeon Charles Louis Alphonse Laveran, who, while working in a military hospital in Algeria, was the first to discover the parasites in the blood of a patient in 1880. Ronald Ross, a British army surgeon posted to India, demonstrated the mosquito-malaria relationship in an avian model in 1897. Giovanni Battista Grassi first recognized the anopheline transmission of human malaria in Italy in 1898.

2.2.3 Antimalarial Drugs

Antimalarial drugs have been used to prevent or cure malaria from ancient times. The Qinghao plant (*Artemisia annua*) was described in the medical treatise in ancient China during the second century B.C.E. (the active ingredient of Qinghao was isolated by Chinese scientists in 1971). Derivatives of Qinghao extract are collectively known as *artemisinins* and are considered today as some of the most effective antimalarial drugs, especially in combination with other medicines [535].

Following their arrival in the *New World*, Spanish Jesuit missionaries learned of a medicinal bark from indigenous Indian tribes in Peru. Known as the *Peruvian bark* or *Cinchona bark*, it was used for the treatment of fevers [480, 535]. The medicine from the bark is now known as the antimalarial *quinine.* Along with artemisinins, quinine is one of the most effective antimalarial drugs available today.

In 1934, *chloroquine* was discovered by a German named Hans Andersag and was finally recognized and established as an effective and safe antimalarial drug in 1946 by the British and U.S. scientists. In 1939, Paul Müller in Switzerland discovered the insecticidal property of dichlorodiphenyltrichloroethane (DDT). DDT was used for malaria control at the end of WWII after it had proven effective against malaria-carrying mosquitoes by British, Italian, and American scientists. However, although many other synthetic antimalarials were developed in the recent times, there is still no effective vaccine to protect against human malaria.

Malaria researchers have won multiple Nobel Prizes in Physiology or Medicine for their achievements, including Ross in 1902, Laveran in 1907, Wagner-Jauregg in 1927 (for his discovery of the therapeutic value of malaria inoculation), and Müller in 1948.

2.2.4 Prevention Measures

The use of innovative prevention measures for malaria dates back long before some of the key discoveries of the disease. The use of pyrethrum as an insecticide was known to the ancient Persians [480]. The drainage of swamps and the control of breeding sites were extensively used by Western colonists. Various other insecticides including larvicidal oil, Paris green, pyrethrum spray, and DDT were advocated by the World Health Organization (WHO) [568]. The use of bed nets have long been regarded as one of the most effective tools for personal protection.

In 1955, the WHO started to conduct major eradication efforts on house spraying with residual insecticides, antimalarial drug treatment, and surveillance. The eradication campaign was carried out in four successive steps of preparation, attack, consolidation, and maintenance, bringing enormous success in many regions of the world. Unfortunately, it was eventually abandoned due to several factors, including the emergence of drug resistance, widespread resistance to available insecticides, wars, massive population movements, difficulties in obtaining sustained funding from donor countries, and lack of community participation. [535, 568].

2.3 MALARIA EPIDEMIOLOGY: A GLOBAL VIEW

A global view of malaria epidemiology is described here. For a comprehensive discussion, see, for example, [388, 480].

The epidemiology of malaria transmission and the severity of the disease vary greatly across geographical locations and within populations. Despite its worldwide spread, malaria is a *focal* disease: the complex interactions among the human host, mosquito vector, malaria parasite, and the local environment affect discrete population groups in different ways. This high degree of heterogeneity is a major reason of the difficulties and challenges involved in designing effective and all-encompassing control strategies [388].

As stated before, human malaria results from encounters between *Anopheles* mosquitoes, *Plasmodium* parasites, and humans. The parasites are spread to human through the bites of infected *Anopheles* mosquitoes. Of about 3000 mosquito species, about 500 *Anopheles* species are recognized, while over 100 can transmit human malaria [480, 568]. Among these, about three dozen are considered important malaria vectors.

Anopheles have mean life spans of 5–12 days (in the tropics), flight ranges of several hundred meters, and are active from sunset to sunrise. Nocturnal biting can have one to three peaks. Females seek blood meals indoors (endophagic) or outdoors (exophagic), on humans (anthropophilic) or mammals (zoophilic), and rest indoors (endophilic) or outdoors (exophilic).

The breeding sites (habitats) of *Anopheles* can include many types such as ponds, canals, fields, lagoons, wells, and drains [517]. Other forms of habitats include natural swamps, cultivated swamps, river fringes, puddles, open drains, burrow pits (boreholes), and so on [380]. Both the mosquito densities and the risk of receiving infective bites decrease with increasing distance from the breeding sites. Human activities such as irrigation projects and deforestation have a profound impact on breeding sites. Malaria habitats are usually grouped by *strata*, some examples of which include rain forests, highlands, oases, islands, coastlines, cities, and so on [517].

2.3.1 The Malaria Parasite

Four *Plasmodium* species cause human malaria: *Plasmodium falciparum*, *Plasmodium vivax*, *Plasmodium malariae*, and *Plasmodium ovale*. *P. falciparum* and *P. vivax* are the most common. *P. falciparum*, being the most deadly, accounts for 80% infections and about 90% of malarial deaths [362]. In recent years, some human cases of malaria have also occurred with the species *Plasmodium knowlesi* (a nonhuman primate species) in certain forested areas of Southeast Asia [568].

The malaria parasite *Plasmodium* relies on two hosts (the female *Anopheles* mosquito and humans) to complete its life cycle. The parasite is transmitted through the bite of an infected *Anopheles* mosquito to a human host, within which it undergoes many asexual replicative stages. One blood stage form (gametocyte) is transferred to the mosquito when the mosquito bites an infected human host. Once inside the mosquito, the parasite replication cycle is completed. The life cycle of the malaria parasite, summarized from the Centers for Disease Control and Prevention (CDC) [105], is shown in Fig. 2.1 and is briefly outlined below:

- During a blood meal, a malaria-infected female *Anopheles* mosquito inoculates sporozoites into the human host.
- Sporozoites infect liver cells and mature into schizonts, which rupture and release new morphological stages of the parasite called merozoites.
- Merozoites emerge from the liver, infect red blood cells, and rapidly replicate.
- Some merozoites in red blood cells develop into a sexual form known as gametocytes.
- The gametocytes (male and female) are ingested by an *Anopheles* mosquito during a blood meal.
- The parasites' multiplication in the mosquito is known as the *sporogonic cycle*; in the mosquito's digestive system, the gametes combine to form zygotes.
- The zygotes go through several developmental stages to form sporozoites.
- The sporozoites migrate to the salivary glands of the mosquito.
- Inoculation of the sporozoites into a new human host perpetuates the malaria life cycle.

The immunological status of an infected person greatly affects the severity of malarial illness. Partial immunity can develop over time through repeated infection; without recurrent infection, immunity is relatively short-lived [388].

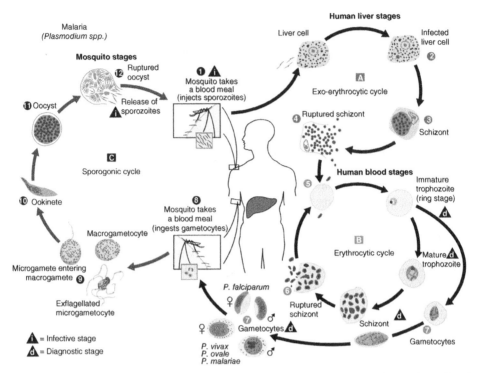

Figure 2.1   Life cycle of the malaria parasite. Adapted from the Center for Disease Control and Prevention (CDC) [333].

2.3.2   Geographic Distribution

Although primarily a disease of the tropics, malaria is also found in many temperate regions of the world, including parts of the Middle East and Asia [568]. Outbreaks are rare in temperate climates and in regions where environmental conditions are unfavorable. *P. vivax* is the most widely distributed and the most common in temperate regions; *P. falciparum*, being clinically the most dangerous, is the most widespread in sub-Saharan Africa and in the tropics; *P. ovale* is most frequently found in Africa but is also found at low frequencies in much of Asia and the Pacific; *P. malariae* has the same geographic range as *P. falciparum*, although it is much less prevalent [388].

2.3.3   Types of Transmission

The type of malaria transmission in a particular area is classified in a number of ways. Based on endemicity and stability, two of the most common are epidemic and endemic: *epidemic* malaria has a sudden rise in the number of cases in a defined population, and *endemic* malaria is characterized by a relatively constant and measurable incidence of cases over a number of years. Great variation in the intensity of transmission between and within malaria endemic regions further categorized them as *holoendemic* (regions of intense year-round transmission), *hyperendemic* (regions with seasonal transmission), *mesoendemic* (regions with some transmission), and *hypoendemic* (regions with limited transmission) [388]. The level of endemicity in a region can be quantified by determining the percentage of children with enlarged spleens and malaria parasites in their blood [363, 369].

2.3.4 Risk Mapping and Forecasting

Malaria risk mapping is an extremely useful tool to map the geographical distribution of the disease's spread or the populations at risk [68, 432, 517]. Risk mapping helps in identifying vulnerable areas by comparing past and present situations. The more recent research field of *landscape epidemiology* allows us to study the patterns, processes, and risk factors of malaria (and other diseases) across time and space. It describes how the spatiotemporal dynamics of human, mosquito, and pathogen populations interact within a permissive environment to enable malaria transmission [450]. Numerous recent tools have been developed using geographic information systems (GISs), global positioning systems (GPS), remote sensing, and spatial statistics for risk mapping.[2] For malaria forecasting, some of the same tools are used to measure the environmental variables (such as rainfall, surface water, ambient temperature, and vegetation) that influence malaria transmission. Data with high spatial and temporal resolution are required for accurate surveillance and forecasting.

Some of the recent malaria risk mapping projects include the Mapping Malaria Risk in Africa (MARA) collaboration [339] and the Malaria Atlas Project (MAP) [537]. The MARA project was set up as a pan-African enterprise in 1996 to provide an accurate atlas of malaria risk for sub-Saharan Africa, based on assembling malaria prevalence data from published and gray literature. Currently, MARA is an open-access and user-friendly Internet-based platform to extract and display malaria prevalence data. The MAP project provides a plethora of geographical maps on dominant malaria vectors, their spatial distribution, estimated human populations at risk, and so on, organized by geographical regions. The MAP team has assembled a spatial database on linked information based on medical intelligence and satellite-derived climate data, and the largest ever archive of community-based estimates of malaria parasite prevalence.

2.4 MALARIA CONTROL

Historically, malaria control efforts relied on proven antimalarial drugs, insecticides, and environmental sanitation. An overview of recent vector-control tools for malaria control can be found in [524]. Major control measures include the following:

Drugs: Antimalarial drugs are used to prevent the onset of disease, to treat clinical cases in individuals, and to prevent transmission within populations. Some drugs, including chloroquine and quinine, kill the parasite within red blood cells,

[2]In Chapter 10, we present a landscape epidemiology modeling framework for risk mapping of several malaria-related outputs.

while others, such as doxycycline and primaquine, prevent the release of parasites within red blood cells [388]. However, the emergence and spread of drug-resistant strains of *Plasmodium* parasites raised concerns about the use and efficacy of available antimalarial drugs.

Larval source management (LSM): LSM, also known as source reduction, is one of the oldest tools in the fight against malaria. LSM refers to the management of larval development sites (aquatic habitats) in order to restrict the completion of immature stages of mosquito development. Recent studies have indicated that LSM can be successfully used for malaria control in African transmission settings [28, 115, 181, 570, 574]. It is particularly effective in areas where malaria transmission has been aided by human activities such as irrigation, public works, and construction projects. In areas with moderate and focal malaria transmission, where larval habitats are accessible and well defined, LSM is also cost-effective compared to other interventions [570]. LSM can be further classified into (1) habitat modification, (2) habitat manipulation, (3) biological control, and (4) larviciding [181]. *Habitat modification* refers to permanent change of land and water, including landscaping, drainage of surface water, land reclamation and filling, coverage of large water storage containers, and wells. *Habitat manipulation* is a recurrent activity that includes measures such as flushing, drain clearance, shading. *Biological control* of mosquitoes refers to the introduction of natural enemies such as predatory fish, parasites, or disease organisms into aquatic habitats. *Larviciding* is the regular application of chemical or biological insecticides to aquatic habitats. Insecticides available for larval control have different modes of action, including surface films, synthetic organic chemicals, and microbials. Chemical larvicides include petroleum oils (e.g., Paris green), pesticides (e.g., temephos), and so on. Biological methods employ larvivorous fishes, toxin-producing bacteria, and so on.

Insecticide-treated nets (ITNs): ITNs, particularly the long-lasting insecticidal nets (LLINs), are considered among the most effective vector control strategies currently in use [77, 231, 574]. Bed nets (ITNs and LLINs) primarily work by reducing human-mosquito contact. ITNs can offer direct personal protection to users as well as indirect, community protection to nonusers through insecticidal and/or repellent effects. Scale-up applications of ITNs are advocated to combat against the major malaria vectors (including *An. gambiae*) in Africa [231]. Other contact reduction methods include protective clothing, insect repellents, mosquito coils, and so on.

Indoor residual spraying (IRS): IRS is the process of spraying the interior (walls and other surfaces) of dwellings with an insecticide to kill mosquitoes. IRS is particularly effective for endophilic mosquitoes that rest inside houses after taking a blood meal. IRS kills and/or repels mosquitoes, preventing the transmission of malaria. Several pesticides have historically been used for IRS, the first and most well-known being DDT. IRS with DDT was the principal method by which malaria was eradicated or greatly reduced in many countries in the world during the Global Malaria Eradication Campaign (1955–1969) [105].

Vaccines: Although much recent research has focused toward developing malaria vaccines, there is currently no effective malaria vaccine on the market. Barriers to the development of an effective malaria vaccine include the lack of enough human and financial resources and the technical complexities of developing any vaccine against malaria parasites [105]. These complexities involve the genetically complex life cycle of malaria parasites, poor understanding of the complex immune response to malaria infection, partial acquired immunity, and so on. Status of recent global malaria vaccine research projects can be found in the WHO Rainbow Table [569].

The last decade (2000–2010) of worldwide malaria control efforts has seen an unprecedented increase in the coverage of some of the established frontline vector control tools (including LSM, ITNs, and IRS). However, these control measures alone are not sufficient to break the malaria transmission cycle in the most intensely endemic parts of Africa and the Pacific [284, 504]. Thus, in addition to the time-tested existing tools, new and novel intervention tactics and strategies in the form of new drugs, vaccines, insecticides, improved surveillance methods, and so on are also being investigated [216]. Some of the recent promising approaches include genetically engineered mosquitoes through sterile insect technique (SIT) or Release of Insects Carrying a Dominant Lethal (RIDL) [297, 434], fungal biopesticides [228, 229], the development of genetically modified mosquitoes (GMMs) or transgenic mosquitoes [340], transmission blocking vaccines (TBVs) [96], and so on. Renewed emphasis on older tools such as the use of spatial repellents in order to prevent contact between human and mosquito is also being explored [2].

In malaria control research, two related terms to combat the disease are also widely used: elimination and eradication. *Elimination* entails reducing to zero the incidence of locally acquired malaria infection in a specific geographic area as a result of deliberate efforts, with continued measures in place to prevent re-establishment of transmission [155]. *Eradication* is the permanent reduction to zero of the global incidence of infection caused by *Plasmodium* parasites as a result of deliberate efforts, so that intervention measures are no longer needed [155].

In most settings, achieving malaria elimination will require interventions that target mosquitoes outside of human habitations. Thus, existing and new interventions must be combined into integrated packages that control mosquitoes at multiple points in the continuum from egg to adult by targeting the key environmental resources (e.g., larval habitats, resting sites) upon which they rely to complete their life cycle [543, 565].

Recently, a growing number of countries have adopted malaria elimination as a goal. Many regional and global organizations have set specific objectives regarding elimination. The African Union's 2007 Africa Malaria Elimination Campaign, the recent declaration by Bill & Melinda Gates Foundation reinstating global eradication as a long-term objective [65], the Global Malaria Action Plan launched by the Roll Back Malaria (RBM) partnership [456] – all have reinforced goals of local elimination in some settings, as well as global eradication as a feasible long-term vision.

3

AGENT-BASED MODELING AND MALARIA

3.1 OVERVIEW

This chapter provides a general background on agent-based models (ABMs).[1] We discuss the major components of an ABM, its history, example applications, advantages, and limitations. With regard to malaria modeling, we present a literature review of malaria models by broadly categorizing these as either *mathematical* or *agent-based* and highlight the spatial dimension of some of these models.

3.2 AGENT-BASED MODELS (ABMS)

As mentioned in Chapter 1, ABMs are a class of computational model developed using the M&S technique known as agent-based modeling and simulation (ABMS). An ABM simulates the actions and interactions of autonomous agents with a view to assessing their effects on the simulated system as a whole. It allows direct representation of individual entities and their interactions in a system. ABMs have applications in diverse real-world problems and have become increasingly popular as a modeling approach

---

[1]Some excellent tutorials on ABMs can be found in Bonabeau [72], Gilbert [199], Macal and North [324], and De Marchi and Page [144].

Spatial Agent-Based Simulation Modeling in Public Health:
Design, Implementation, and Applications for Malaria Epidemiology, First Edition.
S. M. Niaz Arifin, Gregory R. Madey and Frank H. Collins.
© 2016 John Wiley & Sons, Inc. Published 2016 by John Wiley & Sons, Inc.

in most branches of science and engineering. The modeling technique, ABMS, has its roots in the investigation of complex systems, complex adaptive systems, artificial intelligence, and computer science, and combines elements of game theory, emergence, computational sociology, multiagent systems, and evolutionary programming.

The three major components of an ABM are agents, environment, and rules [171]. Agents can be individual or collective entities (such as organizations or groups). Each agent represents an actor in the simulated (virtual) *environment* in which they interact with other agents. Employing a set of rules, agents individually assess the environment and make decisions. As a whole, the set of agents, the environment, and the rules, with their clearly defined boundaries, inputs, and outputs, composes the *system* of the ABM [525]. These components are described as follows.

3.2.1   Agents

An ABM typically consists of one or more sets/types of agents (e.g., mosquitoes, parasites, and humans in a malaria model). Each agent is an autonomous, self-directed entity that can function independently of other agents and the environment [525]. Agents typically have certain essential characteristics:[2]

- An agent is a *self-contained, modular,* and *uniquely identifiable* individual; each agent is a discrete object in the simulation; the modularity requirement implies that an agent has a boundary.
- An agent is *autonomous* and *self-directed* and can function independently in its environment and in its interactions with other agents.
- Agents have *attributes* that allow them to be distinguished from and recognized by other agents; attributes can be static, not changeable during the simulation (e.g., name or id), or dynamic, changeable as the simulation progresses (e.g., age or life-cycle stage); agents' attributes and data are typically stored as their internal states, which can be represented by discrete or continuous variables.
- An agent has *behaviors* that relate information sensed by the agent to its decisions and actions; this information is obtained through interactions with other agents and with the environment; an agent's behavior can be specified by simple rules or abstract models (e.g., neural networks, genetic programs) that map inputs to agents to behaviors.
- An agent has a *state* that varies over time and represents the essential variables associated with the agent's current situation; the state consists of a set or subset of its attributes; an agent's behaviors are conditioned on its state; thus, the richer the set of an agent's possible states, the richer the set of behaviors that an agent can have.
- An agent is a *social* entity having dynamic interactions (e.g., communication, movement, competition/contention for space and resource) with other agents that

---

[2]See, for example, the excellent tutorial by Macal and North for a description of the essential characteristics for agents [324].

influence its behavior; these interactions may involve agent protocols and can lead to self-organizing emergent phenomena observable at the global scale.

In addition, agents may also have the following characteristics [324]:

- An agent may be *adaptive*, for example, by having rules or other abstract mechanisms that modify its behaviors; based on its accumulated experiences, an agent may have the ability to learn (which requires some form of memory) and adapt its behaviors; sophisticated ABMs sometimes incorporate neural networks, evolutionary algorithms, or other learning techniques to allow realistic learning and adaptation; agents may also be capable of evolving, allowing unanticipated behaviors to emerge.

- An agent may be *goal-directed* with respect to its behaviors and be able to adjust its responses for future interactions.

- Agents may be *heterogeneous*; ABMs often consider the full range of agent diversity across a population; agent characteristics and behaviors may vary in several aspects, including the extent, sophistication, amount of information needed for decision-making, and extent of memory of past events.

3.2.2 Environment

The agents' environment represents the virtual, simulated world in which they exist. The environment can be thought of as a medium on which agents operate and with which they interact. A typical environment may consist of the set of global variables and/or other computational structures that collectively define the agents' behaviors and interactions. Thus, the state of an ABM is the collective states of all the agents along with the state of the environment [324].

The ABM's environment is often described by its *topology*, which defines how agents are connected to each other and to their environment. For example, a landscape in which agents move to find resources can be naturally modeled as a lattice environment topology of resource-bearing sites for the agents. Topologies can be as simple as an abstract nonspatial 'soup' model (in which agents have no location) [37, 324], Euclidean spaces (in which agents roam in two-, three-, or higher dimensional spaces), and so on, or as complex as cellular automata (e.g., Conway's *Game of Life* [192] or Epstein and Axtell's *Sugarscape* model [171]), spatial grid or network of nodes (e.g., the *Epidemiological Modeling* (*EMOD*) individual-based model [160, 536]), geographic information system (GIS) (e.g., our landscape epidemiology modeling framework presented in Chapter 10), and so on.

The topology may also define the general concept of an agent's *neighborhood* in ABMs in which the agent spaces are well defined in the model [324]. Typical neighborhoods include the *von Neumann* and *Moore* neighborhood.[3,4] On a two-dimensional

---

[3]The notion of neighborhoods originated from *cellular automata* and *graph theory*; the number of neighbors usually do not include the central/focal cell.

[4]For our ABMs of malaria, we use the *Moore* neighborhood with a 2D Euclidean space in Chapter 6 and with a GIS space in Chapter 10.

square lattice, the von Neumann neighborhood comprises the four cells orthogonally surrounding a central cell, and the Moore neighborhood comprises the eight cells surrounding a central cell. More advanced ABMs can include topology and connectivity that may change over time.

3.2.3   Rules

In an ABM, the agents' behaviors are modeled by *rules* that define how agents behave in response to changes in the environment, and toward the set of agent objectives. These rules also define a set of agent *relationships*: each relationship governs how each agent interacts with, and is connected to, other agents and its environment [525].

Rules couple the agents with their environment. Both the agents and the environment can have their own set of rules, which can be operated between agent-environment level, environment-environment level, or agent-agent level. For example, an agent-environment level rule for movement may instruct an agent to look around as far as it can, find the site richest in resource, go there, and grab the resource. An environment-environment level rule for site-resource update may treat the rate of resource change at a particular site as a function of resource levels at neighboring sites, where the neighborhood is predefined according to some criteria. Finally, agent-agent level rules may include how a male agent mates with a female agent, how one type of agents (e.g., predator) interact with another type (e.g., prey), and so on.

Everything associated with an agent is either an agent attribute or an agent method that operates on the agent. Agent methods include behaviors that link the agent's situation with its action(s). For example, in our spatial ABM of malaria (described in Chapter 6), the resource-seeking behavior of a mosquito agent is modeled with random flights until the agents can perceive resources at close proximity, and directional flights when the resources can be found within a defined distance.

Once an agent's state variables are defined, its behavior can be represented as a state-determined automata or finite state machine, in which a state transition occurs whenever the agent interacts with another agent. Thus, all the interactions and changes of states are regulated by rules of behavior for the agents and the environment. Examples of agent behaviors include production or consumption of resources, communication to other agents and to the environment, and so on.

3.2.4   Software for ABMs

For developing ABMs, there are numerous free or commercially available software toolkits, integrated modeling environments, and multiagent programmable modeling environments. Some of the more popular ones include StarLogo [453], Swarm [531], NetLogo [561], RePast [452], and AnyLogic [15].

3.3   HISTORY AND APPLICATIONS

Although being developed as a relatively simple concept in the late 1940s, the idea of ABMs did not become widespread until the 1990s. Early developments of ABMs can be traced back to the theoretical self-replicating machine known as the von Neumann machine, who created the first of such devices later termed as *cellular automata*. Another advance was introduced by the mathematician John Conway with his well-known *Game of Life*, which operated by very simple rules in a virtual world in the form of a two-dimensional checkerboard. Some of the first conceptual ABMs were published during the 1970s and 1980s. These include Thomas Schelling's segregation model published in 1971 [479], Robert Axelrod's Prisoner's Dilemma model published in the early 1980s [32], and Craig Reynolds' flocking models published in the late 1980s [454], and so on.

The range of domains in which ABMs were applied started to grow rapidly during the 1990s and 2000s. The 1990s were especially notable for the expansion of ABMs within the social sciences, with the noteworthy effort of the large-scale ABM named *Sugarscape*, which was developed by Epstein and Axtell [171]. It simulated and explored the role of complex social phenomena such as seasonal migrations, pollution, sexual reproduction, combat, and transmission of disease.

ABMS applications span a broad continuum of research areas and academic disciplines. ABMs range from elegant, minimalist academic models to large-scale decision support systems [324]. Minimalist models are designed to capture only the most salient features of a system, while decision support models are designed to answer real-world policy questions and to serve large-scale applications.

Some of the applications, categorized under broad umbrella terms, are listed in Table 3.1, in which the second column lists the ABMs with corresponding references. References marked with *s denote reviews or surveys.

3.3.1   M&S Organizations

There are numerous professional associations, societies, and organizations that collaborate in M&S research in national and international levels. These organizations aim to advance the diverse field of basic and applied M&S research, arrange regular conferences and workshops, promote standards of scientific excellence in research and teaching, and publish research findings and results. Some of these organizations focus on particular disciplines. For example, the three organizations that collaborate internationally on the field of computational social science are the Computational Social Science Society of the Americas (CSSSA) [126], the European Social Simulation Association (ESSA) [175], and the Pacific Asian Association for Agent-Based Approach in Social Systems Science (PAAA) [415]. The OpenABM Consortium, which later grew into the Network for Computational Modeling for SocioEcological Science

TABLE 3.1   Applications of Agent-Based Models (ABMs)

Categories	ABMs
Public health, Biology, Infectious diseases, Epidemics	Infectious diseases (general) [50, 364, 430] Malaria [29, 38, 160, 222] Influenza [7, 94, 145, 172] Cancer [167, 442, 583] HIV [100] Tuberculosis [142, 486], [545]* Inflammation and fibrosis [81] Sleeping sickness [375] Pathogen transmission, host-pathogen systems [54, 306] Disease dynamics, outbreaks [74, 90, 174] Adaptive immune system [183] Cellular systems [3] Biomedical (cellular and molecular) research [121]
Commerce, Industry, Business, Enterprise	Stock market management [31] Software agents (shopbots and pricebots) [280] Supply chains management [269, 325, 523] Intelligent manufacturing [490], [489]* Credit risk analysis [581] Wholesale electricity market [520] Operational risk and organizational design [72]* Consumer purchasing behavior [386] Enterprise environments management [71]
Computing, Internet, Artificial life (using *ALife*), Decision support systems, Economics	Product development on the Internet [250] Robot control, robot manufacturing, computer graphics, entertainment, games, music, economics, Internet, information processing, industrial design, electronics, security, data mining, telecommunications, etc. [323]*, [291] Control systems [265] Social computing and social intelligence [550] Decision support systems [8, 11, 86, 185, 440] Economics [532] Finance [311]
Ecology	Ecology (general) [219] Predator–prey relationships (killer whales and sea lions/sea otters) [533] Land use [346]*, [99] Forest ecosystem management [387]
Environment, Infrastructures	Environmental health impact [511] Critical infrastructures modeling [158, 455]

(*continued overleaf*)

TABLE 3.1   (*continued*)

Categories	ABMs
Evacuation management	Escape panic and crowd evacuation [230, 238, 418, 451, 491, 584] Fire [492], urban evacuation [109] Evacuation needs of individuals with disabilities [117] Carnivals and street parades [53] Pedestrian movement and virtual crowds [52, 226, 478]
Natural disaster management	Hurricane evacuation [108, 154] Flood management [137] Earthquake and tsunami management [344]
Transport and travel	Transport logistics [135]* Travel behavior [426]*
Warfare	Bio-warfare [92] Engagement of forces on battlefield [368] or at sea [243]

(CoMSES Net) [393], is sponsored by the National Science Foundation (NSF) [379]. It is a scientific research coordination network to support and expand the development and use of computational modeling in the social and life sciences. Some of these organizations (e.g., OpenABM [393]) also provide open repositories for models and simulations, and valuable forums for collaboration, learning, and networking.

3.4   ADVANTAGES OF ABMS

ABMs offer several advantages over other modeling techniques. Some of these are briefly described as follows.

3.4.1   Emergence, Aggregation, and Complexity

Emergence, or self-organization, refers to the creation of some pattern or form from the bottom–up, and is often considered as a nonequilibrium and complex outcome [144]. Examples of such self-organized behavior include the flocking of birds, the schools of fish, the origin of life itself (in biology), the formation of crystals, stars, or planetary systems (in physics), the reaction-diffusion systems and molecular self-assembly (in chemistry), swarm intelligence, social networks, small-world networks, or scale-free networks (in network science), market economy (in economics), traffic flow, and so on.[5]

---

[5]Network science, as defined by the United States National Research Council [315], is the study of network representations of physical, biological, and social phenomena that leads to predictive models of these phenomena. It is an interdisciplinary field that studies complex networks such as telecommunication networks, computer networks, biological networks, cognitive and semantic networks, and social networks. The field draws on theories and methods including graph theory from mathematics, statistical mechanics from physics, data mining and information visualization from computer science, inferential modeling from statistics, and social structure from sociology.

ABMs allow modelers to link behavioral rules resulting from the interactions of individual agents to aggregate or complex patterns, and to capture the emergent phenomena at the macro or societal level [72, 144, 199]. The aggregation of the agents' individual behaviors can produce system-level outcomes (e.g., competition, cooperation) that are sometimes also referred to as generative or bottom-up [144]. Because of the interactions between the parts, the whole is often more than the sum of its parts. Thus, an emergent phenomenon can have properties that are decoupled from the properties of the part. ABMs can also show how small changes in agents' rules can have dramatic impacts on the group's collective behavior [72].

3.4.2 Heterogeneity

In a typical ABM, each agent can operate according to its own preferences or its own rules of action. The agents' heterogeneity spectrum can be vastly diverse, including their location, beliefs, information, preferences, ability, and also their learning rules, perspectives, mental models, behavioral repertoires, and cognitive framing [144]. The heterogeneity can be modeled to capture and calibrate the actual distributions for parameters of interest (e.g., income distributions, life expectancies, number of friends), allowing ABMs to help answering questions such as when does heterogeneity cancel out so that only the average outcome matters, or when do the actual distributions matter.

3.4.3 Learning and Adaptation

ABMs can simulate learning at both the individual and population levels. Learning can be modeled in several ways, including (1) *individual learning*, in which agents learn from their own experience; (2) *evolutionary learning*, in which the population of agents learns; and (3) *social learning*, in which some agents imitate or are taught by other agents [198]. For example, as described by Gilbert [199], the model of innovation networks is an adaptive learning model: the individual innovating firms learn how to make better products, and because poorly performing firms become bankrupt to be replaced by better start-ups, the sector as a whole can learn to improve its performance.

In complex adaptive ABMs, agents can also be adaptive in their actions and interactions with other agents. Usually, agents adapt by moving, imitating, and/or replicating [329]. Similar to learning, adaptation can occur at two levels: (1) the *individual* level, in which individual agents can learn through processes such as reinforcement, Bayesian updating, or the back-propagation of error in artificial neural networks; and (2) the *population* level, in which population of agents learn through evolutionary processes of selection, imitation, and social influence [329].

3.4.4 Flexibility in System Description

In most cases, ABMs offer the most natural way for describing and simulating a system composed of behavioral entities, making the models seem closer to reality [72]. This holds true for most of the example ABMs presented in Table 3.1, and is one of the major reasons for selecting an ABM as the first choice over other mathematical modeling techniques.

The flexibility of ABMs, which can be observed along multiple dimensions, comes from the ability to model several important factors such as (1) modeling individual behavior of each agent; (2) focusing on agents' activities (rather than processes) as a more natural way of describing the system being modeled; (3) connecting the domain experts by model verification, validation, and calibration processes; (4) applying stochasticity to agents' behavior in appropriate places; and (5) canceling stochasticity bias by performing model replication. Other flexibility factors include the ability to provide a natural framework for tuning complexity features such as agent behavior, degree of rationality, ability to learn and evolve, rules of interactions, levels of agent description, and aggregation [72].

3.4.5 Inclusion of Multiple Spaces

ABMs provide numerous choices to the modeler to select the agents' environment by offering several *topologies* (e.g., abstract nonspatial soup model, Euclidean spaces, cellular automata), as described in Section 3.2.2. They also permit the inclusion of multiple types of spaces (e.g., geographic, social, network) simultaneously at multiple levels of resolution or granularity. For example, our landscape epidemiology modeling framework (see Chapter 10) simultaneously includes a spatial model and a geographic space, the resolution/granularity of which can be varied according to the study area being modeled.

Spatial heterogeneity is one of the most important factors in modeling complex systems. As shown by applied statistical politics models, complex social networks, and social interactions models, *space matters*: people tend to segregate by race, income, religion, and other characteristics, and an individual's behavior depends partly on that of people around them [79, 207, 258]. The capability of ABMs to simultaneously include multiple types of spaces makes them a natural choice to model complex systems.

3.4.6 Limitations of ABMs

There are several issues and limitations related to the general application of ABMs to different branches of sciences, many of which have been pointed out in the recent literature. For example, Galán *et al.* list some errors and artifacts typically associated with ABMs [188]. In the social sciences in particular, Epstein lists some limitations and fallacies of ABMs, including the fallacies of individualism [170]. Some of the issues and limitations of ABMs are described as follows:

Universality: In general, both the purpose of a model and the nature of a system being modeled make any single modeling paradigm inadequate to be generally applicable. As different models demand different domain-specific knowledge and levels of expertise, there is perhaps no single method or tool that can be termed as universally applicable. In addition, the existence of closed-form, equation-based solutions to many simplistic problems may render other modeling paradigms preferable over an ABM [33]. Thus, as is the case with any other modeling paradigm, the "one size fits all" prescription does not apply well with ABMs. Although ABMs have been tremendously successful in areas such as epidemiology, power/energy markets, and combat simulation, they tend to become comparatively less effective in certain other domains, especially the social, political, and economic sciences [72, 101, 170]. For example, the very nature of the systems modeled with ABMs in the social sciences often involve human agents with potentially subrational/irrational behavior, subjective choices, and complex psychology, making the modeling task challenging for ABMs to quantify, calibrate, and justify these *soft factors* [72].

Computational Demands: Due to the requirement of finer granularity of information, ABMs tend to require more data than other approaches such as differential equations or other equation-based models [72, 121, 383]. Thus, relatively high computational costs are involved in modeling a system with an ABM. In addition, ABMs are usually slower to run when compared to other modeling techniques. As correctly pointed out by Bonabeau, since by definition an ABM looks at a system not at the aggregate level but at the level of its constituent units, the lower level description sometimes involves describing the individual behavior of potentially *too many* constituent units, and simulating the behavior of all these units can be extremely computation intensive and time-consuming [72]. For example, the anatomic scale biological ABM developed by Cockrell *et al.* [121] requires each simulated cell to store information regarding its function and current state in *in silico* data structures (in reality, this information is stored in the form of DNA or RNA of the biological cells). As the ABM approaches an anatomic scale, it requires billions of cells to be simulated simultaneously, which soon becomes problematic for two major reasons: (1) cycling through billions of cells on a single processor can take a significant amount of time and (2) anatomic scale simulations require large amounts of system memory.

Scalability: In addition to the computational demands issue described above, with growing complexity and increasing number of simulated entities, the scalability of a simulation environment becomes a crucial measure of its ability to cope with the complexity of the modeled system. Complex models may require the capability to simultaneously simulate billions or more complex deliberative agents. While ABMS as a methodology has received much attention from the research community in the past, scalability and thus industrial applicability of ABMS has often been neglected, with only a small number of research efforts explicitly focusing on the area of scalable ABMs [425]. As rightly noted by Law, scalability issues are not completely solved just because a system is executed on a distributed computing architecture [308]. The speed and scalability of most ABMS software systems are considerably limited as they are designed for serial von Neumann computer architectures. Although recent ABM toolkits lower some of these barriers by making developed models more accessible, customizable, and scalable, they cannot alleviate the barriers completely [121]. To this end, the recent development and use of data-parallel algorithms on Graphics Processing Units (GPUs) seem to be promising directions for ABMs [146, 157, 322, 553].

Assessment of Accuracy and Acceptability: In its modeling life cycle, the development of an ABM usually requires several critical and time-consuming steps such as verification and validation (V&V), replication and reproducibility (R&R), accreditation, quality assurance (QA), and certification. As we discuss and show in Chapters 7–9, without properly conducting these steps, there can be little trust in the insights and predictions provided by a simulation study.

In addition, other issues such as the need for computer programming efficiency (ABMs demand knowledge/skill of programming languages), reusability, rigorous data analysis (the search spaces are usually much bigger for parameter analysis, calibration, etc.), and extensive result analysis (due to the finer granularity and massive data requirement) can diminish the general applicability of ABMs.

3.4.7   ABMs vs Mathematical Models

In many domains, ABMs compete with mathematical (e.g., equation-based) approaches that identify system variables and evaluate or integrate sets of equations relating to these variables. Excellent discussions on comparing ABMs to various types of mathematical models can be found in [199, 422, 446].

ABMs rely on the power of computers to explore system dynamics that is otherwise out of the reach of traditional mathematical models, which usually include differential equation-based models [36, 171]. In the past, the majority of theories in ecology evolved from simple differential equations (e.g., the predator-prey equations, also known as the Lotka-Volterra equations) in which a single variable represented population sizes. Solutions of these were then mathematically analyzed, and/or compared to population sizes from field or laboratory observations. Although these models greatly influenced ecological theories, their aggregated form was particularly difficult to relate to observational biology. In addition, their application to complex natural systems with *spatially* and *temporally* varying environmental factors led to models that were not analytically tractable, and must be investigated numerically [220].

According to Gros [220], one of the first factors in designing these mathematical models was to determine whether the key features of the problem under consideration required a *discrete* or *continuous* formulation. For example, in population biology, a *discrete* model may use matrices or systems of nonlinear difference equations in order to compare populations with discrete life stages, whereas a *continuous* model may use systems of differential equations with overlapping generations. A second factor concerned whether to include or ignore stochastic elements. A third factor was dealing with spatial aspects: whether to ignore them by assuming homogeneous mixing, or include them using various available mechanisms such as discrete patches, discrete lattices, and partial differential equations.

However, all of the above approaches involve state variables, which represent a form of *aggregation*. As a result, some factors of the real-world problem that affect individual actions can only be dealt with in a highly aggregated manner in traditional mathematical models. As described earlier, ABMs offer the powerful capability to analyze these aggregated variables and to observe them as a function of the actions and interactions of the agents. In addition to describing the basic processes that control the actions of agents, ABMs can also aggregate these to determine the resultant macro descriptors that arise at higher levels of model organization. Thus, as correctly pointed out by Gilbert [199], ABMs often offer a better modeling alternative to some of the other types of mathematical models.

3.4.8 Applicability of ABMs for Malaria Modeling

In this section, we discuss the general applicability of ABMs for malaria modeling. Although computer-based simulation studies (including ABMs) are not a substitute for reality, they do provide a highly refined and structured way of synthesizing information and testing ideas. In particular, they provide a useful tool for testing how differences in transmission can lead to different results when the same interventions are applied in two different populations. In the history of malaria research, several examples show how vector control measures such as indoor spraying of insecticides, larval control, and environmental management have helped control or eradicate malaria in areas of marginal or unstable transmission. However, a valuable lesson gained in that is the strategies to effectively control malaria in one ecological setting may not be appropriate in another [57]. It is difficult to predict where successful approaches will emerge, and there is every indication that integrated approaches will be needed for effective and sustainable control. Thus, simply having a new antimalarial drug, an effective malaria vaccine, or a new way to kill mosquitoes is still a long way and many years from the achievement of effective malaria control. These challenges warrant for detailed modeling of almost every aspect associated with the disease.

As mentioned earlier, ABMs have increasingly become popular and useful as tools to represent complex systems as they allow the construction of model frameworks to include substantial details and reality. In modeling malaria (and epidemiology in general), ABMs are particularly useful for the following reasons:

Treatment of Space: Treatment of space in ABMs differs fundamentally from that in traditional mathematical models (see Section 3.5.3). Usually, ordinary differential equation models have no spatial component, and all agents interact in time but not in space. Some partial differential equation models include a physical space, but the state variables that represent agent populations are still continuous. On the other hand, in ABMs, agents are usually distributed over a two-dimensional space lattice (or other forms of space). As we show in Chapters 5 and 6, our ABM provides a flexible framework to incorporate a spatial extension that can capture the spatial properties of both the mosquito agents and their environments.

Compartmentalization: In mathematical epidemiology, the society being modeled is often divided into homogeneous subpopulations called *compartments*. Each compartment represents a subpopulation in which members are not distinguishable from each other. Homogeneity is assumed within each subpopulation and/or species. For example, to model malaria infectivity, McKenzie *et al.* divided the host and vector populations into *infected*, *infectious*, and *susceptible* compartments [355, 357]. In these models, as the compartments are homogeneous, individuals within each compartment cannot have *any* variation. ABMs, by contrast, permit substantial variation within a compartment by allowing agents to possess and display heterogeneous behavior, and hence are free from this limitation. As a result, important phenomena such as immunological memory and persistence of genetic traits can emerge naturally within the system dynamics.

Adaptation: In an ABM, individual traits of an agent can adapt as a result of interaction with other agents and components of the environment. In the real world, selection pressures operate in evolutionary time to alter the distribution of traits in populations. ABMs offer a natural way to model such phenomena. This can be especially helpful for certain aspects of malaria modeling, for example, to model insecticide resistance and genetic variations within a mosquito population.

3.5 MALARIA MODELS: A REVIEW

Since major portions of the contents of this book deal with spatial ABMS for malaria epidemiology, a discussion on the early and recent malaria models is warranted. In this section, we briefly introduce some of these models by broadly categorizing them as either *mathematical* or *agent-based*. Then, based on the representation of the *spatial* dimension in the models, we also classify some of these into nonspatial and spatial categories. Note that the criteria for this classification do not include other model-specific features (e.g., use of a GIS), and hence models falling under different categories may share some common features.

Models from both of the mathematical and agent-based categories have played important roles in answering important biological research questions for malaria control. Some of these questions include quantifying the effects of malaria-control interventions, selecting appropriate combinations of interventions to interrupt transmission, setting response time lines and expectations of impact, and so on. Some of the models also helped to elucidate whether different interventions are likely to be synergistic, and when they should be deployed in combination to achieve optimal effects. Thus, models have become an indispensable tool for thinking carefully and quantitatively about the dynamics of malaria control and elimination.

Note that some of the malaria models may encompass major components from both of these categories. For example, the discrete-event simulation model developed by McKenzie *et al.* was further advanced by embedding a differential-equation model (see the following discussion) [355, 357].

3.5.1   Mathematical Models of Malaria

Mathematical modeling, being predominantly deterministic and differential equation-based, has been used to provide an explicit framework for understanding malaria transmission dynamics in human population for over 100 years [337]. Also known as population-based models, these models often use top-down approaches that describe the dynamics of populations as a whole, usually by means of differential equations [178]. A thorough literature survey, describing some important mathematical models, their underlying features, and their specific contributions in the understanding of malaria spread and transmission, can be found in [337]. Key conclusions of several mathematical models of malaria with emphasis on their relevance for control can be found in [300].

Mathematical malaria modeling dates back to the early pioneering models of Ronald Ross who developed the first mathematical model (now known as the classical "Ross model") for understanding malaria transmission [459]. He demonstrated the life cycle of the malaria parasite in mosquito, and in the early 1900s published a series of papers using mathematical functions to study malaria transmission.

In the 1950s, Macdonald developed a reformulated model that identified mosquito vector longevity as the single most important variable in the force of transmission, and combined Ross's more famous differential equation model with epidemiological and entomological field data [326, 328]. Since then, the Ross-Macdonald theory has played a central role in the development of research on mosquito-borne pathogen transmission and the development of strategies for mosquito-borne disease prevention [30, 225, 300, 463, 498].

Molineaux and Gramiccia presented a well-known malaria model developed during the Garki project for the planning and management of malaria control [371]. The study was carried out in the Garki district of northern Nigeria in 1969–1976 by a joint research team of the WHO and the Government of Nigeria. With a focus on the epidemiology and control of malaria in the African savanna, the model comprehensively studied the effects of a residual spraying campaign and mass drug administration (MDA) on malaria transmission. The specific objectives of the project included an epidemiological study of malaria in the lowland savanna (concentrating on the measurements and relationships of entomological, parasitological, and other variables), to measure the effects of house-spraying with propoxur (to control the vectors *Anopheles gambiae* and *Anopheles arabiensis*) alone or in combination with MDA, and to construct and test a mathematical model of the transmission of malaria to compare various control strategies in terms of their expected effects.

Janssen and Martens described an epidemiological dynamics model of malaria that simulated the adaptation of mosquitoes and parasites to available pesticides and drugs [262]. To address the evolutionary character of the development of resistance, they coupled genetic algorithms with the model to simulate the evolving processes within the mosquito and parasite populations. Their results suggested that adequate use of insecticides and drugs may reduce malaria occurrence in low endemicity areas, with increased efforts in the event of a climate change. However, in high endemicity areas, the use of insecticides and drugs may lead to an increase in malaria incidence due to enhanced resistance development in the mosquito and parasite populations.

Craig *et al.* described a simple numerical, fuzzy logic-based modeling approach of the distribution of stable malaria transmission in sub-Saharan Africa based upon biological constraints of climatic suitability on parasite and vector development [130]. Using GIS software and large global data sets including climate, population, satellite imagery, and topography, the model defined the geographic regions as *perennial* (where conditions were always suitable for transmission), *seasonal* (where conditions became suitable for a short season every year), *epidemic* (where long-term variations in climate rendered conditions suitable for transmission on an irregular basis with a potential of epidemic malaria), and *malaria-free*. To examine the pattern of mean climate as it relates to different epidemiological settings, the model extracted and used monthly rainfall and temperature data from the climate data surfaces for 20 different sites. The model compared well with contemporary field data and historical "expert opinion" maps, excepting small-scale ecological anomalies. It provided a numerical basis for further refinement and prediction of the impact of climate change on transmission. Together with population, morbidity, and mortality data, the model provided a fundamental tool for strategic control of malaria.

Hay *et al.* presented a first-order autoregressive model to analyze the potential effects of climate change on highland malaria [233, 234]. Using the model and meteorological data obtained from a global gridded data set of monthly terrestrial surface climate for the 1901–1995 period, they investigated long-term meteorological trends in four high-altitude sites in East Africa, where increases in malaria have been reported in the past two decades. They showed that temperature, rainfall, vapor pressure, and the number of months suitable for *Plasmodium falciparum* transmission had not changed significantly during the past century or during the period of reported malaria resurgence, and concluded that the claimed associations between local malaria resurgences and regional climate changes were overly simplistic.

Killeen *et al.* presented a kinetic model of mosquito foraging for aquatic habitats and vertebrate hosts that allowed estimation of malaria transmission intensity by defining the availability of these resources as the rate at which individual mosquitoes encountered and used them [287]. The model analyzed the individual and combined effects (predicted proportional impact) of four environmental interventions at 80% coverage levels: water management, larvicide application, physical domestic protection, and zooprophylaxis (the diversion of host-seeking mosquitoes from human beings to animals), and presented an integrated program combining all of these interventions.

Hoshen and Morse described a weather-driven dynamic mathematical malaria model that output new infections in the human host and was able to capture the gross spatial dynamics of malaria transmission across the African continent [247]. The model used the ERA-40 weather reanalysis-climate data set, which provided daily estimates of a range of potentially significant weather variables for the whole globe, and was the reference data for the *DEMETER* (Development of a European Multimodel Ensemble system for seasonal to inTERannual prediction) multimodel system

[150]. By numerical evaluations of the model in both time and space, they showed that the model qualitatively reconstructed the prevalence of infection across Africa.

Menach *et al.* described a malaria epidemiology model on heterogeneous landscapes that incorporated a detailed description of the gonotrophic cycle into models for mosquito infection dynamics [360]. Spatial heterogeneity was abstractly incorporated by subdividing the landscape into finite number of patches in an array grid, where the location and state (e.g., fed, unfed, gravid, infective) of the mosquito could be identified in each patch. They argued that since mosquitoes commute between blood meal hosts and water bodies (aquatic habitats), heterogeneity in human biting reflected the underlying spatial heterogeneity in the distribution and suitability of larval habitat as well as inherent differences in the attractiveness, suitability, and distribution of blood meal hosts. The model demonstrated that oviposition was an important factor explaining heterogeneous biting and vector distribution in a landscape with a heterogeneous distribution of larval habitat. Since adult female mosquitoes tended to aggregate around oviposition places (thereby increasing the risk of malaria regardless of the suitability of the habitat for larval development), an aquatic habitat might be unsuitable for adult mosquito emergence but simultaneously could be a source for human malaria.

Chitnis *et al.* presented a linear difference equation model and a deterministic dynamical systems model to describe the dynamics of malaria in a mosquito population interacting with a heterogeneous population of humans, and used them for exploring the impact of combinations of two vector control interventions – insecticide-treated nets (ITNs) and indoor residual spraying (IRS) [113, 115]. They also described a periodically forced difference equation model that captured the effects of seasonality and allowed the mosquitoes to feed on a heterogeneous population of hosts [114]. An open-source version of the full model, named *OpenMalaria*, is available online [394].

Yakob and Yan used a mathematical model to analyze the effects of integrating larval source management (LSM) and ITNs on reducing malaria transmission, applied separately and in combination [574]. They argued that attacking multiple points in the transmission cycle might yield synergistic benefits and improve upon current single-tool interventions based on the use of ITNs.

In recent years, several mathematical malaria models have also focused on the likely impact of climate change on malaria transmission. For example, Martens *et al.* described an integrated linked-system mathematical climate assessment model to study the effects of projected changes in temperature and precipitation on mosquito and parasite characteristics and their potential impact on malaria risk [342, 343]. Using the Integrated Model to Assess the Greenhouse Effect (*IMAGE*), they assessed the sensitivity of the biological activity and geographic distribution of the malaria mosquitoes and parasite to climatic influences (e.g., temperature, precipitation) [461]. The model simulated the cause–effect chain with respect to climate change, and consisted of a number of independent, interlinked, and integrated submodels, each of which represented a separate component of the climate system (e.g., a world energy/economy model, land-use change model, atmospheric chemistry model). They concluded that the simulated changes in malaria risk must be interpreted on the basis of local environmental conditions, the effects of socioeconomic developments, and malaria control programs or capabilities, and that increased risk of malaria due to climate change might seriously affect human health in the next century. The study also showed that the transmission potential of malaria as a vector-borne disease was very sensitive to climate changes on the periphery of the endemic areas and at higher altitudes within these areas, and the health impact would be most pronounced in populations living in the less economically developed temperate areas in which endemicity was low or absent.

Another climate malaria model assessed the impact of climate change on potential malaria transmission using the Modeling Framework for the Health Impact ASsessment of Man-Induced Atmospheric changes (*MIASMA*) model [341]. Main features of the model included continental-scale estimates regarding the distribution of 18 main malaria vectors, species-specific relationships between temperature and transmission dynamics, and a more realistic approach regarding malaria endemicity to explore changes in populations at various degrees of malaria risk (e.g., risk of epidemics vs year-round transmission). In this model, global estimates of the potential impact of climate change on malaria transmission were calculated based on future climate scenarios produced by the *HadCM2* and *HadCM3* global climate models [254]. The model showed that at the borders of malaria transmission, the changes in average length of the transmission season might be important. The simulations also showed that in most high endemic regions, an increase in seasonal transmission occurred at the expense of year-round transmission. Although strongly varying between the climate change scenarios, this implied that the malaria situation in these regions moved toward unstable malaria. They concluded that estimates of future populations at risk of malaria would differ significantly between regions and between climate scenarios. The results, though not to be treated as predictions of the future, showed trajectories of possible changes in malaria risk with the given assumptions.

3.5.2 Agent-Based Models (ABMs) of Malaria

In this section, we provide a brief description of several malaria ABMs. Some of these models are sometimes also termed as discrete event simulation (DES) models, individual-based models (IBMs), and so on. A DES model performs the operation of a system as a discrete (as opposed to continuous) sequence of events in time [49]. IBMs, which are frequently used within the field of ecology, refer to a specific subclass of ABMs within which individuals may be simpler than fully autonomous agents [219]. Most of these models have been extensively used to model the behavior of individual mosquitoes, including interactions within agents and to their environment. These interactions, involving a large number of agents, provide the opportunities to explore interesting emerging phenomena, such as population-level characteristics.

McKenzie *et al.* developed a DES model using a single time-line variable to represent the *P. falciparum* life cycle in individual hosts and vectors within interacting host and vector populations [357]. This work was further advanced by embedding a differential-equation model of parasite-immune system interactions within each of the individual humans represented in the discrete event model, and by examining the effects of human population turnover, parasite diversity, recombination, and gameto-cyte production on the dynamics of malaria [355]. The integrated approach provided a framework for investigating relationships between pathogen dynamics within an individual host as well as within interacting host and vector populations.

Depinay *et al.* presented an IBM of African malaria vectors that incorporated knowledge of the mechanisms underlying *Anopheles* population dynamics and their relations to the environment [148]. The model, being the first to integrate both biological and environmental factors of malaria vector population dynamics, incorporated basic biological requirements for *Anopheles* development. It represented the life cycle of each individual mosquito through four stages: three immature aquatic stages (egg, larva, and pupa), and the mature stage, a flying adult. Using local environmental data as input, it considered five basic factors: temperature, moisture (in the form of precipitation and relative humidity), nutrient competition, predation or death by disease, and dispersal. Results showed that the model could reproduce some broad, diverse patterns found in the field, allowing detailed analyses and explanations of vector population dynamics.

Gu and Novak used an ABM to explore the impact of source reduction (SR, which is a type of LSM) under various intervention scenarios [222], and the impact of ITNs under various levels of diversion and coverage of the bed nets [221].[6] They represented mosquito resource-seeking as a two-stage process: *random flight* when the resource was not within the mosquito's perception range and *directional flight* to the resource when it was detected. For comparison, they designed three scenarios of targeted and nontargeted SR to eliminate all aquatic habitats within certain distances of human habitations. The SR study showed that the elimination of habitats within 100, 200, and 300 m of surrounding houses caused 13, 91, and 94% reductions in malaria incidence, respectively, compared with 3, 19, and 44%, respectively, for the corresponding conventional scenarios. They reported two major findings: first, SR might not require coverage of extensive areas: coverage of up to 300 m surrounding houses could lead to interruption of the gonotrophic cycle and significant reductions in malaria transmission. Second, distance to the nearest houses could be the primary measure for habitat targeting and might serve as an operational indicator in the field. In the ITNs study, they modeled the responses of individual mosquitoes to ITNs by a series of parameters: coverage, repellence (diversion), mortality (insecticide effect of bed nets), and personal protection (of net users from being bitten). Results showed that the application of ITNs could give rise to varying impacts on population-level metrics, which depended on parameter values governing interactions of mosquitoes and treated nets at the individual level. In their simulation results, the most significant factor in determining effectiveness was the killing effectiveness (mortality) of the ITNs. They also showed that strong excito-repellent effect of impregnated nets might lead to higher risk exposure to nonusers of bed nets.

Griffin *et al.* described an individual-based model for *P. falciparum* transmission in an African context incorporating the three major vector species (*An. gambiae* sensu

---

[6]In Chapter 9, we investigate the effects of LSM and ITNs using our spatial ABM, and compare our results to those reported by Gu and Novak [221, 222].

stricto, *An. arabiensis*, and *Anopheles funestus*) with parameters obtained by fitting to parasite prevalence data from 34 transmission settings across Africa [218]. The model investigated the effects of applying different combinations of long-lasting insecticide-treated nets (LLINs), IRS, artemisinin-combination therapy (ACT), mass screening and treatment (MSAT), and vaccines [218]. It used six representative settings with varying transmission intensities summarized by the annual entomological inoculation rates (EIRs), vector-species combinations, and patterns of seasonality. The results showed that interventions using existing tools could result in major reductions in *P. falciparum* malaria transmission and the associated disease burden in Africa, and the combined interventions could result in substantial declines in malaria prevalence across a wide range of transmission settings.

Eckhoff presented a cohort-based vector simulation model named *EMOD* that included mosquito population dynamics, effects of weather, and impacts of multiple simultaneous interventions [160].[7] It demonstrated the effects of increasing coverage of interventions with perfect IRS, combining IRS and ITNs, and combining larval control (using larvicides) and space spraying, with a focus on local elimination of malaria. Mosquito population behaviors (e.g., anthropophily, indoor feeding) were also included to study their effect upon the efficacy of vector control-based elimination campaigns.

3.5.3   The *Spatial* Dimension of Malaria Models

Since this book particularly focuses on spatial ABMs, the *spatial* dimension of malaria models is worth discussing. Considering the spatial dimension, malaria models can also be classified as nonspatial and spatial. This classification is based on the form of the environment's *spatial* representation embedded within the models, and some instances may overlap with those from both categories of *mathematical* and *agent-based* models (as described above).

The *nonspatial* malaria models do not model space explicitly. These models usually represent space abstractly using, for example, an abstract *point* space, a lattice of *point* spaces, a patch-based abstract landscape, and a shared abstract environment with an observed aggregate. To model various features, they usually assume various statistical distributions such as a certain probability of successful completion of a specific event. Although some models in this category may include space in various nontrivial forms, agents in these models do not possess explicit spatial attributes, and the choices made by the agents as well as the effects of actions performed by them do not involve the use of any spatial feature. Examples of these models include the DES model presented by McKenzie *et al.* [355, 357], the model presented by Janssen and Martens that simulates the adaptation of mosquitoes and parasites to available pesticides and drugs [262], the

---

[7]*EMOD* is developed and maintained by the Institute for Disease Modeling (IDM) at the Intellectual Ventures Laboratory [536]. It represents a suite of detailed, geographically specific, and mechanistic stochastic simulations of disease (including malaria) transmission through the use of complex software modeling. In Chapter 11, the *EMOD* model is presented with two important epidemiological scenarios in Africa with geospatial maps coupled with the model's outputs.

IBM presented by Depinay *et al.* [148], the patch-based transmission dynamics model presented by Menach *et al.* [360], and so on.

On the other hand, the *spatial* malaria models explicitly model space. In these models, the agents and/or their environments have explicit spatial coordinates. These models include the ABMs of Gu and Novak [221, 222], the *EMOD* individual-based model [160], our spatial ABM (described in Chapter 6), and so on.

Comparison of various characteristics and features of some malaria models (as described above) with our spatial ABM is worth noting.[8] In Table 3.2, we present a summary of comparing relevant model features from two mathematical models [114, 574] and two ABMs [160, 221]. These models include the *EMOD* model and the *OpenMalaria* model.[9] Note that the compared features of different models reflect the reported facts and characteristics of the respective models (as can be found in the cited references listed in Table 3.2), and hence do not necessarily imply inherent limitations of a particular model.

In Table 3.2, each row represents a specific model feature, and each column represents a specific malaria model. Features marked with *s are either modeled with improvements/extensions, or may be treated as new (not modeled earlier by other studies) in our spatial ABM. Text in the cells represent whether the feature is implemented/available in the model, including simple yes/no, or other comments. "N/A" means *not applicable* or *not available*. "Dynamic" means the feature or parameter can be changed dynamically for individual simulation runs. Time-step resolution indicates the most fine-grained time resolution (e.g., models reported as *hourly* are also capable of reporting events on a *daily* basis). For some features, we specify whether the model implements variability of the feature (e.g., variability in daily temperature), and note the default value used in the model in parentheses. For fecundity, N indicates a normal distribution with *mean* and *standard deviation*. Daily mortality and age-dependent mortality refer to mortality of mosquitoes. "LE" denotes life expectancy.

3.6 SUMMARY

Agent-based modeling is a promising tool to model complex systems, which often exhibit complex properties such as emergence, learning, adaptation, heterogeneity, and dynamic interactions. For modelers, ABMs are particularly useful as they offer a bridge in minimizing the gaps between the *micro* and *macro* level aspects of modeling. ABMs are one of the most vibrant and important areas of research and development to have emerged in information technology in recent times [320], and hold out the promise of a revolutionary advance in social science theory [48].

In this chapter, we presented a general introduction to ABMs. We discussed the three major components of an ABM (agents, environment, and rules), its history and application domains, and its advantages and limitations. We also discussed the general applicability of ABMs for malaria modeling.

---

[8]The spatial ABM is presented in Chapter 6.
[9]Note that Chapter 11 presents the *EMOD* model, which is contributed as a guest chapter from the IDM [536].

TABLE 3.2   Malaria Models: A Comparison of Features

Model Feature	Malaria Models				
	Gu & Novak [221, 222]	Yakob & Yan [574]	EMOD [160]	OpenMalaria [115]	Our Spatial ABM
Model type	Agent-based	Mathematical	Agent-based	Mathematical	Agent-based
Spatial representation(s)	Landscape-based	N/A	Point, nodes, GIS (see Chapter 11)	Abstract	Point, GIS (see Chapters 6 and 10)
Automation of landscape generation (e.g., using separate tools)*	No	N/A	Yes	N/A	Yes (see Chapter 6)
Boundary type of landscape*	Absorbing	N/A	Reflecting	N/A	Nonabsorbing
Average of multiple simulations*	No	No	Yes	Yes	Yes
Time-step resolution	Daily	Daily	Daily	Daily	Hourly
Age-specific mortality	No	No	Yes	Yes	Yes (see Chapter 4)
Daily mortality rate (immature stages)	Fixed (0.2)	Fixed (0.15)	Age-specific	Age-specific	Age-specific (for larvae)
Daily mortality rate (adult stages)	Fixed (0.2)	Fixed (0.15)	Adult LE of 10 days	Age-specific	Age-specific
Fecundity (eggs/oviposition)	Fixed (80)	N/A	Fixed (100)	N/A	$N(170, 30)$
Variability in daily temperature	No	No	Yes	Yes	Yes (25 °C)
Length of individual simulation run	200 or 300 days	N/A	Dynamic	Dynamic	Dynamic (1 year)
Interventions modeled	LSM, ITNs	LSM, ITNs	IRS, ITNs, larvicides, space spraying, etc.	ITNs, IRS, etc.	LSM, ITNs
Time-step of intervention application	Day 100 for LSM, day 150 for ITNs	N/A	Dynamic	Dynamic	Day 100
Explores combined interventions	No	Yes	Yes	Yes	Yes
Variability in human populations	No	Yes	Yes	Yes	Yes
Coverage scheme used for ITNs*	Proportion of households with bed nets	Proportion of populations sleeping under bed nets	Proportion of populations sleeping under bed nets	Proportion of populations sleeping under bed nets	Partial and complete coverage (see Methods)
Comparison of coverage schemes for ITNs*	No	No	No	No	Yes

* The compared features of different models reflect the reported characteristics of the respective models (as listed in the cited references), and hence do not necessarily imply inherent limitations of a particular model.

We then compared ABMs to mathematical models, presented a literature review of malaria models by broadly categorizing them as either *mathematical* or *agent-based*, and compared features of our ABM with those of some of the other malaria models discussed in this chapter. The *spatial dimension* of malaria models was also highlighted.

Considering the advantages offered by an ABM, its ability to handle emergent phenomena is what drives the other benefits. To summarize, using an ABM is more convenient when the interactions between the agents are complex, nonstationary, and nonlinear, the space is crucial, and the population and topology are heterogeneous, all of which, in general, hold true for malaria modeling.

In the following chapters, we first thoroughly describe the biological core model of the malaria-transmitting mosquitoes (Chapter 4), and then present the design and implementation of our ABM (Chapter 5) and its spatial extension (Chapter 6).

4

THE BIOLOGICAL CORE MODEL

4.1 OVERVIEW

In this chapter, we describe the conceptual biological core model (hereafter referred to as the core model) of the population dynamics of *Anopheles gambiae*.[1,2,3] Several versions of the core model evolved in the multiyear development process. The earlier versions mostly dealt with exploratory features and have been previously described elsewhere [25, 26, 28, 587]. The version described in this chapter reflects the most recent updates as presented in [29], in an attempt to enrich the models with features that reflect the population dynamics of *An. gambiae* in a more comprehensive way. A summary of major improvements incorporated in the version presented here is given in Table 4.1.

An. gambiae is the major vector of malaria in much of sub-Saharan Africa. Due to its pivotal role in malaria transmission, modeling its population dynamics can assist in finding factors in the mosquito life cycle that can be targeted to decrease malaria transmission to a lower level. The *An. gambiae* complex, a closely related group of eight

---

[1] Major components of the core model have been developed as parts of dissertation research of several graduate students (including SMNA) supervised by GRM and FHC, and other simulation projects performed in the course *Computer Simulation*, taught over Fall 2009 and Spring 2010 at the University of Notre Dame. We would like to thank our colleagues Ying Zhou, Gregory J. Davis, and James E. Gentile for their early contributions to the core model, and all students who actively contributed to the development process.

[2] The agent-based implementations derived from the core model are described in Chapters 5–6.

[3] Portions of the text and figures presented in this chapter appeared in Arifin *et al.* [29].

Spatial Agent-Based Simulation Modeling in Public Health:
Design, Implementation, and Applications for Malaria Epidemiology, First Edition.
S. M. Niaz Arifin, Gregory R. Madey and Frank H. Collins.

TABLE 4.1   Summary of Updated Features in the Core Model

Feature	Previous Versions	Current Version
Time-step resolution	Daily	Hourly
Host seeking and oviposition	Anytime	Only at night
Stage transitions	Anytime	Only during permitted time windows
Egg development time	Constant	Temperature-dependent; consists of egg incubation and hatching times

named mosquito species found primarily in Africa, includes three nominal species, *An. gambiae, Anopheles coluzzii*, and *Anopheles arabiensis* that are among the most efficient malaria vectors known. The model described here has been designed specifically around the mosquito *An. gambiae*. While the respective ecologies and involvement in malaria transmission among other members of the *An. gambiae* complex differ in important ways, this model could effectively apply to all three and even to many of the several dozen other major malaria vectors in the world.

The core model addresses several important features of the *An. gambiae* life cycle, including the development and mortality rates in different stages, the aquatic habitats, oviposition and so on.[4] Another important feature, vector senescence, is adopted to account for the age-dependent aspects of the mosquito biology, and implemented using density- and age-dependent larval and adult mortality rates.

The organization of this chapter is as follows: in the remainder of this section, we define some terms that are relevant to the core model. Sections 4.2 and 4.3 describe the aquatic and adult stages of the *An. gambiae* mosquito life cycle, respectively.[5] Section 4.4 discusses the aquatic habitats and the process of oviposition. Sections 4.5 and 4.6 discuss the importance of incorporating senescence (biological aging) into vector mortality modeling and present the exact formulations used in the core model, respectively. Lastly, Section 4.7 discusses some of the key features, characteristics, and limitations of the core model, and Section 4.8 concludes.

4.1.1   Relevant Terms of Interest

Before discussing the life cycle stages and other major concepts of the biological model, we define some terms that are relevant to the model.

Parasite: The term *parasite* refers to any organism that lives in or on another organism without benefiting the host organism. Parasites are commonly referred to as pathogens, which are organisms that can cause disease.

---

[4]Throughout the book, we differentiate between the two terms 'stage' and 'state'. *Stage* refers to a distinct biological stage (time duration) in the mosquito life cycle. *State*, on the other hand, refers to the object-oriented programming (OOP) usage: the state of an object encompasses all of the (usually static) properties of the object plus the current (usually dynamic) values of each of these properties [75].

[5]Life cycle of the malaria parasite (*Plasmodium*) was briefly described in Section 2.3.1.

Malaria Parasite: Malaria parasites are microorganisms that belong to the genus *Plasmodium*. There are more than 100 species of *Plasmodium*, which can infect many animal species such as reptiles, birds, and various mammals. The malaria parasite requires specific human and mosquito tissues to complete its life cycle. Once inside a human, the parasite develops and multiplies, causing periodic bouts of flu-like symptoms, including fever, headache, and chills. The developing parasites destroy red blood cells, which may cause death by severe anemia as well as by the clogging of capillaries that supply the brain or other vital organs with blood (for other details, see Section 2.3).

Vector: In biology, the term *vector* refers to the carrier of a pathogen from one host to another. In epidemiology, a vector is an insect or any living carrier that transmits an infectious agent. Vectors are vehicles by which infections are transmitted from one host to another. A vector is not only required for part of the parasite's developmental cycle, but it also transmits the parasite directly to subsequent hosts. For this reason, a mosquito is treated as *vector* as well as a *host* for malaria transmission [347].[6]

***An. gambiae*:** Human malaria is transmitted only by females of the genus *Anopheles*. Female *Anopheles* mosquitoes are the primary (definitive) hosts and transmission vectors of the malaria parasite *P. falciparum*. *An. gambiae* is one of the best-known malaria vectors because of its predominant role in the transmission of the parasite (for other details, see Section 2.3).

The complete *An. gambiae* mosquito life cycle consists of aquatic and adult phases, as shown in Fig. 4.1. The *aquatic* phase (also known as the *immature* phase) consists of three aquatic stages: Egg (E), Larva (L), and Pupa (P). The *adult* phase consists of five adult stages: Immature Adult (IA), Mate Seeking (MS), Blood Meal Seeking (BMS), Blood Meal Digesting (BMD), and Gravid (G). The development and mortality rates in all eight stages of the life cycle are described in terms of the aquatic and adult mosquito populations. All symbols and parameters used in the core model are summarized in Table 4.2.

4.2 THE AQUATIC PHASE

Since malaria vectors are *poikilothermic*, the ambient temperature is a critical variable in the growth and development kinetics of *An. gambiae* [56, 148, 193].[7] Thus, development rates in most stages in the core model are temperature dependent.

Although the aquatic stages do not themselves transmit malaria, they play a major role in determining the form that diseases assume [347]. The course of development

[6]Not surprisingly, the term *vector* appears in many disciplines with *different* meanings, including mathematics, physics, computer science, and business. In this book, it is exclusively used to refer to malaria-transmitting mosquitoes.

[7]A *poikilotherm* is a plant or animal whose internal temperature varies along with that of the ambient environmental temperature. See Appendix A for a theoretical discussion on the temperature-regulated enzyme kinetics model for mosquito vectors used in this chapter.

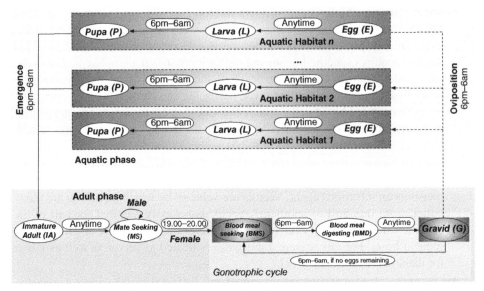

Figure 4.1   Life cycle of mosquitoes in the models. The *An. gambiae* mosquito life cycle consists of *aquatic* and *adult* phases. The *aquatic* phase consists of three aquatic stages: *Egg (E)*, *Larva (L)*, and *Pupa (P)*. The *adult* phase consists of five adult stages: *Immature Adult (IA)*, *Mate Seeking (MS)*, *Blood Meal Seeking (BMS)*, *Blood Meal Digesting (BMD)*, and *Gravid (G)*. Each oval represents a stage in the model. Permissible time transition windows (from one stage to another) are shown next to the corresponding stage transition arrows as rounded rectangles. Note that adult males, once reaching the *Mate Seeking* stage, remain forever in that stage until they die; adult females cycle through obtaining blood meals (in *Blood Meal Seeking* stage), developing eggs (in *Blood Meal Digesting* stage), and ovipositing the eggs (in *Gravid* stage) until they die. By Arifin *et al.* [28], used under a Creative Commons Attribution 4.0 International License.

during the aquatic stages (from a fertilized egg to a mature adult) is broadly the same in all mosquitoes. The aquatic stages are described as follows.

4.2.1   Egg (E)

Adult females lay 50–200 eggs per oviposition. Eggs are laid singly and directly on water and are unique in that they have floats on either side. Eggs are not resistant to drying; they hatch within 2–3 days in tropical temperatures, although hatching may take up to 2–3 weeks in colder climates [13].

In the core model, development in the *Egg* stage is comprised of two distinct components: *incubation* and *hatching*. Egg incubation depends on the ambient temperature and usually requires 1–2 days. It is governed by a linear function:

$$Incubation_{Egg}(T) = -0.9 \times T + 61 \qquad (4.1)$$

where T is the ambient temperature (°C) in the range $15 \leq T \leq 40$. As found in a recent study, *An. gambiae* egg hatching time distribution is strongly skewed to the right, with

TABLE 4.2   Symbols and parameters used in the core model and the ABMs. Parameters are listed in order of appearance in the text

Parameter	Description	Unit	Default Value
T	Ambient temperature	°C	30
$P_{FindHost}$	Probability of a female adult to find a human host	N/A	25%
$P_{FindBloodMeal}$	Probability of finding a blood meal	N/A	100%
$P_{FindHabitat}$	Probability of a female adult to find an aquatic habitat	N/A	25%
HC	Habitat capacity	N/A	1000
r	Combined seasonality factor	N/A	1.0
$Biomass$	Age-adjusted biomass in a habitat	N/A	Dynamic
N_{Eggs}	Number of eggs in a habitat	N/A	Dynamic
N_e	1-day-old equivalent larval population	N/A	Dynamic
N_{Pupae}	Number of pupae in a habitat	N/A	Dynamic
Age_{Cohort}	Common age of a cohort	Day	Dynamic
$N_{LarvaePerCohort}$	Number of larvae in an age cohort	N/A	Dynamic
gcn	Gonotrophic cycle number	N/A	Dynamic
$Eggs_{Max}$	Maximum number of eggs a female can lay	N/A	Dynamic
$N(170, 30)$	Normal distribution for fecundity in the first gonotrophic cycle	N/A	$mean = 170$, $s.d. = 30$
$Eggs_{Potential}$	Potential number of eggs a female is allowed to lay	N/A	Dynamic
w	Habitat sampling weight (within the *same* gonotrophic cycle)	N/A	1, 2, or 3
DMR	Daily mortality rate	Day^{-1}	0.1
HMR	Hourly mortality rate	Hour^{-1}	0.00438
α	Baseline DMR (for larvae and adults)	Day^{-1}	0.1
β	Exponential mortality increases with age	N/A	0.04
s	Degree of mortality deceleration	N/A	0.1

N/A means not applicable or not available. *Dynamic* means the parameter value can change within a simulation run.

89% of the eggs hatching during the second and third day after oviposition, 10% hatching during the next 4 days, and the remaining 1% hatching over the subsequent week [575]. The egg hatching time distribution is shown in Fig. 4.2.

4.2.2   Larva (L)

Larvae (Larva-singular) have a well-developed head with mouth brushes used for feeding, a large thorax, a segmented abdomen, and no legs. In contrast to other mosquitoes, *Anopheles* larvae lack a respiratory siphon and for this reason position themselves so that their body is parallel to the surface of the water [13]. Also being commonly called *wigglers* or *wrigglers*, they feed on algae, bacteria, and other microorganisms in the water surface microlayer, dive below the surface only when disturbed, and swim either by jerky movements of the entire body or through propulsion with the mouth brushes. During growth, the larvae molt shedding their exoskeleton, or skin, to allow for further growth [13]. The stages between molts are

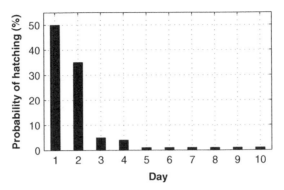

Figure 4.2   The egg hatching time distribution used in the core model. The *An. gambiae* egg hatching time distribution is strongly skewed to the right, with 89% of the eggs hatching during the second and third day after oviposition, 10% hatching during the next 4 days, and the remaining 1% hatching over the subsequent week [575]. The x-axis denotes hatching time (days), and the y-axis denotes the probability of hatching. By Arifin *et al.* [29], used under a Creative Commons Attribution 4.0 International License.

called *instars*.[8] Larvae develop through four instars, after which they metamorphose into pupae [13].

Larvae can be found in a wide range of habitats, but most species prefer clean, unpolluted water. Larvae of *Anopheles* mosquitoes have been found in fresh- or salt-water marshes, mangrove swamps, rice fields, grassy ditches, the edges of streams and rivers, and small, temporary rain pools. Many species prefer habitats with vegetation. Some breed in open, sunlit pools, while others are found only in shaded breeding sites in forests. A few species breed in tree holes or the leaf axils of some plants [13].

In the core model, development in the *Larva* stage primarily depends on temperature. To model the growth and development of larvae, the enzyme kinetics model used in Depinay *et al.* [148] is adopted (see Appendix A for details). Earlier formulation of the kinetics models can be found in [483, 488].

The mean larval development rate per hour at temperature T (in K), $r(T_K)$, is given by Eq. (4.2):

$$r(T_K) = \frac{\rho_{25\,°C} \times \dfrac{T}{298} \times e^{\frac{\Delta H_A^{\ddagger}}{R}\left(\frac{1}{298} - \frac{1}{T}\right)}}{1 + e^{\frac{\Delta H_L}{R} \times \left(\frac{1}{T_{\frac{1}{2}L}} - \frac{1}{T}\right)} + e^{\frac{\Delta H_H}{R} \times \left(\frac{1}{T_{\frac{1}{2}H}} - \frac{1}{T}\right)}} \tag{4.2}$$

where all parameters and their values are summarized in Table 4.3. Eq. (4.2) is derived on the basic assumption that poikilotherm (*An. gambiae* larvae in this case) development is regulated by a single control enzyme whose reaction rate determines the

---

[8]An *instar* is a developmental stage of the mosquito larva between each molt until sexual maturity is reached.

TABLE 4.3   Larval development parameters for *An. gambiae*

Parameter	Description	Unit/Dimension	Value used
$\rho_{25\,°C}$	Larval development rate per hour at 25°C, assuming that there is no temperature inactivation of the critical enzyme	Hour^{-1}	0.037
R	The universal gas constant	cal $\times$ K^{-1} $\times$ mol^{-1}	1.987
$\Delta H_A^{\neq}$	The enthalpy (change) of activation of the reaction catalyzed by the enzyme	cal $\times$ K^{-1} $\times$ mol^{-1}	15,684
ΔH_L	The enthalpy change associated with *low* temperature inactivation of the enzyme	cal $\times$ K^{-1} $\times$ mol^{-1}	−229,902
ΔH_H	The enthalpy change associated with *high* temperature inactivation of the enzyme	cal $\times$ K^{-1} $\times$ mol^{-1}	822,285
$T_{\frac{1}{2}L}$	The temperature where 50% of the enzyme is inactivated by *low* temperature	K	286.4
$T_{\frac{1}{2}H}$	The temperature where 50% of the enzyme is inactivated by *high* temperature	K	310.3

* The enzyme kinetics model and the values used are adopted from Depinay *et al.* [148]. K represents temperature in kelvins. $\rho_{25\,°C}$ relates the standard reference temperature (25 °C) at which most poikilotherms experience little low- or high-temperature enzyme inactivation.
Details about the enzyme kinetics model can be found in [483, 488].

development rate of the organism [148]. Substituting the parameters from Table 4.3 in Eq. (4.2), the mean larval development rate *per hour* at temperature T (°C), $r(T)$, is obtained as

$$r(T) = T \times 0.000305 - 0.003285 \qquad (4.3)$$

The cumulative larval development, CD_{larva}, is accumulated *per day* through days $0, 1, \ldots, n$:

$$CD_{larva} = \sum_{i=0}^{n} r(T)_i \times 24 \qquad (4.4)$$

To complete the larval development, a threshold is defined with a normal random variable N (to allow for 10% variability); thus, the larval development is completed (i.e., the pupation begins) when

$$CD_{larva} > 1 + N(0, 0.1)$$

4.2.3   Pupa (P)

The pupal stage is a resting, nonfeeding stage that turns the immature mosquito into an adult. Pupae (pupa - singular) are comma-shaped when viewed from the side, and are lighter than water (therefore can float at the surface). As with the larvae, pupae must come to the surface frequently to breathe, which they do through a pair of respiratory trumpets on the cephalothorax. After a few days as a pupa, the dorsal surface of the cephalothorax splits and the adult mosquito emerges [13]. They are also commonly called *tumblers*. The metamorphosis of the mosquito into an adult is completed within the pupal case. The adult mosquito splits the pupal case and emerges to the surface of the water, where it rests until its body can dry and harden. The duration from egg to adult varies considerably among species and is strongly influenced by ambient temperature. Mosquitoes can develop from egg to adult in as little as 5 days, but usually take 10–14 days in tropical conditions [13].

In the core model, development in the *Pupa* stage also depends on temperature and is modeled similarly as in $Incubation_{Egg}(T)$ following Eq. (4.1).

4.3 THE ADULT PHASE

Adult mosquitoes primarily have two objectives, to mate and to feed. They usually mate within a few days after emerging from the pupal stage. In most species, the males form large swarms, usually around dusk, and the females fly into the swarms to mate [12]. The males, after mating, seek out for nectar to feed on from plants and fruits. Females also feed on sugar sources for energy but usually require a blood meal for the development of eggs. After obtaining a full blood meal, the female will rest for a few days while the blood is digested and the eggs are developed. Once it hatches and oviposits the eggs, it searches for another blood meal. This process of blood-feeding, egg maturation, and oviposition is repeated several times throughout the life cycle until the female dies and is known as the *gonotrophic cycle*. Length of an adult's life cycle usually depends on several factors including sex of the mosquito, temperature, rainfall, humidity, and season of the year.

The five stages of the adult phase in the core model are described as follows.

4.3.1 Immature Adult (IA)

The *Immature Adult (IA)* stage contains the period (1–3 days, depending on temperature) after emergence and before the mosquito is sexually capable of mating. Development in this stage is governed by a linear function of temperature, derived from the adult development curves by Depinay *et al.* [148], as shown in Eq. (4.5):

$$Development_{IA}(T) = -2.67 \times T + 120 \qquad (4.5)$$

where T is the ambient temperature (°C) in the range $15 \leq T \leq 40$. Substituting T for 36, 27, and 18 °C in Eq. (4.5) yields the corresponding development times of 1, 2, and 3 days, respectively.

4.3.2 Mate Seeking (MS)

In the *Mate Seeking (MS)* stage, a pair of male and female mate. This stage is assumed instantaneous in the core model. After entering the MS stage from the IA stage, female adults are assumed to always find males for mating (before 7 pm, see Fig. 4.1). Male adults stay in the stage for the rest of their lives, while female adults enter the *BMS* stage at 7 pm.

4.3.3 Blood Meal Seeking (BMS)

In the *BMS* stage, female adults search for blood meals. Since *An. gambiae* has been observed to bite mostly throughout the night [194, 270, 410, 412, 465], the host-seeking activities are restricted within the time window of 6 pm to 6 am (i.e., from dusk to dawn). During each (*hourly*) time step, the probability of a female adult to encounter a human host, $P_{FindHost}$, is set as 25%. Once it finds a host, obtaining a blood meal is always assumed successful (i.e., $P_{FindBloodMeal}$ is set as 100%), and it immediately enters the BMD stage. If it cannot find a host, host seeking continues in the next time step, and so on, as long as the time window (from 6 pm to 6 am) permits.

   In general, mosquitoes seek their host in response to a combination of chemical and physical stimuli, including carbon dioxide plumes, body odors, warmth, and movement [388]. Anophelines feed most frequently at night and occasionally in the evening, or in shaded areas during the early morning. During a blood meal, the mosquito injects a minute amount of salivary fluid into the host to increase blood flow to the area. Thus, if the mosquito is infective, sporozoites are transmitted to the host via the salivary fluid.

4.3.4 Blood Meal Digesting (BMD)

Development in the *BMD* stage is also governed by a linear function of temperature, derived from the adult development curves by Depinay *et al.* [148], as shown in Eq. (4.6):

$$Development_{BMD}(T) = -1.23 \times T + 77 \tag{4.6}$$

where T is the ambient temperature (°C) in the range $15 \leq T \leq 40$. Depending on the temperature, Eq. (4.6) yields the corresponding development times of 1–2.5 days.

   The BMS stage is also termed as the *resting* stage, because the female simply rests for a few days while the blood is being digested and eggs are being developed. Some females seek out cool, humid areas of a house (e.g., walls, undersides of furniture), while others find dark spots outdoors near the ground.

4.3.5 Gravid (G)

In the *Gravid (G)* stage, a female mosquito lays its developed eggs in batches. Since *An. gambiae* mosquitoes are nocturnal in their oviposition activities [351, 389, 521], oviposition, like host seeking, is also restricted within the time window of 6 pm to 6 am in the core model. During each (*hourly*) time step, the probability of a female adult to sample a randomly selected aquatic habitat, $P_{FindHabitat}$, is set as 25%. If all eggs are not laid within the night, it rests until the next night to lay the remaining eggs. Once all the eggs are laid, and the time window (from 6 pm to 6 am) permits, it enters the *BMS* stage to search for another blood meal, thus starting a new gonotrophic cycle.

4.4   AQUATIC HABITATS AND OVIPOSITION

The aquatic habitats and the process of oviposition are described as follows.

4.4.1   Aquatic Habitats

The core model assumes simplistic, homogeneous aquatic habitats for all mosquitoes. All habitats are uniform in size and capacity, and the water temperature of the habitats is assumed the same as the air temperature. To account for the combined seasonality factor r, each aquatic habitat is set with a habitat capacity, HC, as a linear function of r:

$$HC = HC_{Baseline} \times r \qquad (4.7)$$

where $HC_{Baseline}$ represents the baseline habitat capacity. $r \in [0, 1)$ indicates capacity *below* the baseline (which may occur due to several seasonality/weather factors, for example, low precipitation), and $r > 1$ indicates capacity *above* the baseline (which may occur due to high precipitation, lack of sunlight, and so on). HC essentially represents the *density-dependent oviposition* mechanism by regulating an age-adjusted biomass (see Section 4.4.2) that the habitat can sustain.

4.4.2   Oviposition

Oviposition is the process by which gravid female mosquitoes lay new eggs. The oviposition behavior of *An. gambiae* gravid mosquitoes can be affected by a variety of factors, as demonstrated by several studies [118, 206, 244, 261, 302, 376, 521, 522]. For example, Koenraadt and Takken showed that *An. gambiae* s.l. females tend to avoid oviposition sites containing older instar larvae, and thus reduce the risk of predation of offspring (it is not fully understood, however, which physical or chemical cues female mosquitoes use for selection of sites optimal for the development of their offspring) [302]. Munga *et al.* compared oviposition choices of *An. gambiae* in rainwater conditioned with different numbers and densities of conspecific larvae and found that in the presence of different densities of larvae, more eggs were laid in rainwater that had the fewest or no larvae; in addition, the greatest number of eggs were laid in rainwater that contained the lowest concentration of larvae [376]. Other studies also showed that increased competition within the larval environment may have negative impacts on several aspects of the life cycle, including larval development rate, adult survivorship, adult body size, and fecundity [206, 261].

In the core model, all larvae are categorized into different age groups, or *cohorts*, according to the *common age* of the cohort. The model keeps track of the age-adjusted biomass *Biomass* in each aquatic habitat, which is defined as the sum of the eggs, pupae, and the *1-day-old equivalent larval population*, N_e (see Eq. (4.9)), in the habitat:

$$Biomass = N_{Eggs} + N_e + N_{Pupae} \qquad (4.8)$$

where N_{Eggs} and N_{Pupae} represent the number of eggs and pupae, respectively, in the selected habitat. N_e is computed by first multiplying the number of larvae in each age cohort ($N_{LarvaePerCohort}$) by the cohort's age (Age_{Cohort}, in days), and then summing up the values for all age cohorts:

$$N_e = \sum_{Age_{Cohort}=0}^{max} Age_{Cohort} \times N_{LarvaePerCohort} \qquad (4.9)$$

This, in turn, provides a *check and balance* mechanism for the model, since for each habitat, the habitat capacity *HC* may serve as a soft upper limit for the aquatic population (by limiting the larval density and *Biomass* of the habitat).

Since *An. gambiae* females have been reported to use multiple habitats for oviposition [107], the core model assumes that a *Gravid* female lays the developed eggs in multiple habitats (within the time window of 6 pm to 6 am), and its inclination to lay the remaining eggs successively increases as it visits more habitats. Due to several factors, *An. gambiae* fecundity can be affected to produce smaller egg-batch sizes [160, 245]. Thus, in successive gonotrophic cycles, the maximum number of eggs a female can lay, $Eggs_{Max}(gcn)$, is reduced by 20% from the previous cycle:

$$Eggs_{Max}(gcn) = \begin{cases} N(170, 30) & : gcn = 1 \\ 0.8 \times Eggs_{Max}(gcn - 1) & : gcn > 1 \end{cases} \qquad (4.10)$$

where *gcn* represents the gonotrophic cycle number, and $N(170, 30)$ represents the fecundity in the very first gonotrophic cycle, drawn from a normal distribution with *mean* = 170 and *standard deviation* = 30.

Successive oviposition attempts within the *same* gonotrophic cycle are distinguished by a habitat sampling weight, w. To account for the composite factors that arise from conspecific density and competition, the age-adjusted biomass (*Biomass*) is checked against the habitat capacity (*HC*) to determine the potential number of eggs, $Eggs_{Potential}(gcn, w)$, that a female is allowed to lay in a given habitat:

$$Eggs_{Potential}(gcn, w) = Eggs_{Max}(gcn) \times \left(1 - \frac{Biomass}{w * HC}\right) \qquad (4.11)$$

Once all the eggs are laid, the current gonotrophic cycle is completed, and the gravid female starts a new cycle by entering into the *BMS* stage (within the time window of 6 pm to 6 am).

4.5   SENESCENCE AND MORTALITY RATES

In this section, we discuss the importance of incorporating senescence (biological aging) into vector mortality modeling, present the basic mathematical formulation of the senescent mortality models, and the exact formulations used in the core model.

4.5.1   Senescence

In most epidemiology models, the mortality of the organisms being modeled plays a crucial role in shaping the model's characteristics. Daily mortality is the most important determinant of a mosquito's ability to transmit pathogens [518]. Senescence, or biological aging (also spelled *ageing*), is the gradual deterioration of function characteristic of most complex life-forms including the mosquito vectors.

In vector mortality modeling, most malaria transmission models traditionally assume *nonsenescent* (i.e., age-independent) mortality. However, nonsenescent mortality could only lead to approximate estimates and misleading predictions since they obscure the age-dependent aspects of the mosquito biology. It assumes an unrealistic, simplified view that the vector potential of all mosquitoes, regardless of their age, is the same. This, in turn, also affects other determinants of pathogen transmission (e.g., biting rate, host preference, vector competence, dispersal, resistance to insecticides).

Modeling senescence is important because the longer a mosquito lives, the more likely it is to encounter an infectious host, survive the incubation period, and transmit an infectious agent during subsequent feeding attempts. Thus, small changes in daily mortality can result in relatively large changes in the pathogen transmission cycle. Several recent studies have shown the impact of vector senescence on malaria transmission. For example, using large-scale laboratory life table techniques ($N > 100,000$), Styer *et al.* showed that mosquito mortality was low at young ages (less than 10 days old), steadily increased at middle ages, and decelerated at older ages [518]. Clements and Paterson analyzed the mortality and survival rates in wild populations of mosquitoes of 11 tropical species, and indicated that in most of these populations, the adult female mortality rates are age dependent [120]. Bellan developed a simple mathematical model of vector-borne disease transmission to assess how relaxing the classical assumption of constant mortality affects the predicted effectiveness of antivectorial interventions [59]. He showed that with constant mortality assumption, control of survival reduced the life expectancy of all mosquitoes by a large amount. With age dependence, however, the reduction in life expectancy was less dramatic and skewed toward younger age classes. By defining C^* as the *scaled vectorial capacity*, he showed that while reducing survival dramatically reduced the C^* contribution of older mosquitoes in a constant mortality model, this effect was less important in age-dependent models. The effectiveness of mosquito control when mosquitoes die at age-dependent rates was compared across different extrinsic incubation periods. Thus, the constant mortality model overestimated the effectiveness of reducing survival in controlling transmission. He concluded that future transmission models that examine antivectorial interventions should incorporate realistic age-dependent mortality rates.

Based on the above observations, *age-specific* mortality rates are used for the *Larva* stage, and for all the adult stages in the core model.

4.5.2   Mortality Models: Basic Mathematical Formulation

Standard age-dependent mortality models are based on age-specific mortality rate, $u(x)$, which is an instantaneous measure of mortality that can be estimated from empirical data with the approximation:

$$u(x) = -\ln p(x)$$

where $p(x)$ is the probability that an individual alive at age x survives to age $x + 1$.

The mortality patterns were well described by Benjamin Gompertz in 1825 in the famous *Gompertz mortality function* [210]. It is a sigmoid function for a time series, where growth is slowest at the start and end of a time period. According to the Gompertz function, the mortality rate increases with age in such a manner that its logarithm is directly proportional to age, and a *law of geometric progression* dominates the mortality after a certain age. Gompertz mortality model can be represented as

$$u(x) = a * e^{bx}$$

where $u(x)$ is the age-specific mortality rate, a is the baseline mortality rate, b is the senescent/aging component (the exponential mortality increase with age), and x is the age of the age cohort considered. In 1860, William Makeham extended the Gompertz model by adding an age-independent constant c [332]:

$$u(x) = a * e^{bx} + c$$

In a protected environment where external causes of death are rare (e.g., due to improved laboratory conditions, low mortality countries), the age-independent mortality component is often negligible.

Based on these, Styer *et al.* defined the *logistic mortality model* as the following [518]:

$$u(x) = \frac{a * e^{bx}}{1 + \left(\frac{a*s}{b}\right)(e^{bx} - 1)}$$

where s is the degree of mortality deceleration.

4.6   MORTALITY IN THE CORE MODEL

Based on the age-dependent mortality models discussed in Section 4.5.2, we use age-specific mortality functions to compute the *daily* mortality rates (DMRs) and *hourly* mortality rates (HMRs) for the larva stage and for all the adult stages in the core model.

4.6.1   Aquatic (Immature) Mortality Rates

Since in general, *An. gambiae* egg and pupa survival are not density dependent, the
DMRs of egg and pupa stages are set as an empirical constant of 10%, yielding the
HMR of 0.00438:

$$1 - (1 - 0.1)^{\frac{1}{24}} = 0.00438$$

Larvae mortality rate is affected by a variety of factors, which include the age of
larvae [120, 136, 148, 160, 413], the density-dependent effects arising from predation, cannibalism, resource competition in the larval population [56, 148, 302], habitat
capacity, and weather factors such as rainfall [148, 160, 414].

The effects of predation and cannibalism on larvae mortality have been investigated
by several studies. For example, Koenraadt and Takken explored the occurrence of
predation and cannibalism within and between members of the *An. gambiae* complex,
assessing the effects of larval food availability and the presence of older instars on the
development of younger instars [302]. The study showed that older larvae of the *An.
gambiae* complex are able to prey on younger larvae of conspecifics (cannibalism) as
well as on larvae of closely related species (predation). Biotic factors such as the presence of predators, parasites, and pathogens in and around the aquatic habitats affected
the survival and growth of *An. gambiae* s.l. larvae.

Koenraadt *et al.* analyzed the impact of the presence of a fourth-instar larva (*An.
gambiae* Giles s.s. or *An. arabiensis* Patton), the quantity of food, and the available
space on the survival and development of freshly hatched larvae by constructing two
proportional hazard models [301]. Results suggested that cannibalism and predation
occurred readily. Limitation in space significantly increased mortality of larvae,
whereas a limitation of food reduced larval development rate but did not affect
mortality. They concluded that inter- and intraspecific interactions among larvae of the
An. gambiae complex strongly affected survival and development and that the quantity
of food and the available space were important determinants of the outcome of these
interactions. Studies on inter- and intraspecific competition showed that competition
might result in reduced larval development rate, lower larval survival, smaller adult
size, lower fecundity, and a distorted sex ratio [301]. Over time, these effects might
even lead to the replacement of one species by another. Increasing densities of *An.
gambiae* negatively affected larval survival, development rate, and adult size. Some
aquatic habitats of *An. gambiae* might dry up within a few days, and this transient
nature might lead to inter- and intraspecific competition for food and space [301].

In the core model, we incorporate the effects of predation and cannibalism in an
aquatic habitat using the notion of the age-adjusted *1-day-old equivalent larval population* N_e (see Eq. (4.9)). The DMR for the larva stage is computed on a *per-cohort*
basis using the cohort's age Age_{Cohort} (in days), N_e, and the habitat capacity *HC*:

$$DMR_{Larva}(Age_{Cohort}) = \alpha \times e^{\frac{N_e}{Age_{Cohort} \times HC}}$$

$$HMR_{Larva}(Age_{Cohort}) = 1 - (1 - DMR_{Larva}(Age_{Cohort}))^{\frac{1}{24}}$$

where α represents the baseline DMR (set as an empirical constant of 10%), and $HMR_{Larva}(Age_{Cohort})$ represents the corresponding HMR of the larvae cohort.

As mentioned before, larvae mortality is also affected by rainfall (precipitation). Paaijmans *et al.* explored the effect of natural rainfall as a density-independent factor on flushing, ejection, and mortality of larvae of *An. gambiae* under ambient conditions in western Kenya [414]. Their results showed that precipitation flushed, ejected, and killed a significant proportion of larvae of *An. gambiae* in different stages of development. Young larvae (L1 instar stage) experienced the highest flushing, ejection, and mortality, while the oldest larvae (L4 instar stage) were better suited to withstand the effects of rainfall. This study demonstrated that immature populations of malaria mosquitoes suffered high losses during rainfall events. Thus, rainfall has a profound effect on the productivity of mosquito breeding sites and, as a result, on malaria transmission.

The effect of rainfall is incorporated in the core model through the combined seasonality factor, r, which can linearly modify the habitat capacity HC (see Eq. (4.7)). Thus, low and high rainfall can be modeled using $r \in [0, 1)$ and $r > 1$, respectively.

4.6.2   Adult Mortality Rates

For the adult stages, DMRs are calculated using a modified version of the logistic mortality model in which the age-dependent component of mortality increases exponentially with age [518]. Newly emergent adults have the baseline DMR of α (10%). However, as mosquitoes age, the age-specific mortality rate for each age cohort is calculated as

$$DMR_{Adult}(Age) = \frac{\alpha \times e^{Age \times \beta}}{1 + \frac{\alpha \times s}{\beta}(e^{Age \times \beta} - 1)}$$

$$HMR_{Adult}(Age) = 1 - (1 - DMR_{Adult}(Age))^{\frac{1}{24}}$$

where α is the baseline DMR (10%), β is the exponential mortality increase with age (0.04), s is the degree of mortality deceleration (0.1), and Age_{Cohort} is the common age of the adult cohort.

Note that while many of the coefficients and parameters described above are specified as constant values (e.g., $P_{FindHost} = 25\%$), these values can be calibrated (tuned) to reflect specific modeling scenarios as needed.

4.7   DISCUSSION

Some of the key features, characteristics, and limitations of the core model are highlighted as follows.

4.7.1   An Extendible Framework for Other Anopheline Species

Although the model has been designed specifically around the mosquito *An. gambiae*, a wider range of other anopheline species with different behaviors or biology can also be incorporated into the model. For example, in the current model, the host-seeking mosquitoes are assumed to be uniformly anthropophilic, and alternative hosts for blood-feeding (e.g., cattle) are not modeled. By modifying the host-seeking assumptions in the BMS stage, the zoophilic behavior of other species can be easily modeled.

4.7.2   Weather, Seasonality, and Other Factors

As mentioned before, abundances of most anopheline species are profoundly affected by a variety of factors including weather (e.g., temperature, rainfall, humidity, seasonality cycles) and habitat (e.g., habitat size, surface area, habitat characteristics). In order to adapt other species, some of these factors also need to be included with finer details. The model currently captures the effect of all weather variables using a single factor of combined seasonality r (see Eq. (4.7)), which can be adjusted in different models with different seasonality settings (e.g., to model one rainy season vs year-round transmission). Although the current model does not explicitly include various habitat and other factors, it provides an excellent framework for such extensions in the future.

4.7.3   Mortality Rates

The core model implements density- and age-dependent larval mortality and age-dependent adult mortality rates. Density- and age-dependent larval mortality incorporates the combined effects arising from the age of larvae and other important factors in the larval population that include predation, cannibalism, resource competition, and so on. By keeping track of the 1-day-old equivalent larval population and the age-adjusted biomass in an aquatic habitat, the model provides a *check and balance* mechanism to regulate the habitat's capacity and to maintain a soft upper limit for the aquatic population. Age-dependent adult mortality (vector senescence) allows the model to capture the age-dependent aspects of the mosquito biology and thus provides a more realistic foundation to examine, in the future, other important determinants of the pathogen transmission cycle (e.g., biting rate, host preference, vector competence, dispersal, resistance to insecticides), which have been reported to be affected by vector senescence [120, 245, 518].

4.8   SUMMARY

In this chapter, we presented a conceptual entomological model of the population dynamics of *An. gambiae*, which we call the *core model*. After defining a few relevant terms of interest, we described the three aquatic stages and the five adult stages in the life cycle of the mosquito vector *An. gambiae*, and discussed the modeling aspects of aquatic habitats and oviposition. To detail vector mortality modeling, we discussed the importance of incorporating senescence into mortality, the basic mathematical formulation of mortality models, and the exact formulations of age-specific mortality rates, as adopted in the core model.

The notion of the conceptual core model presented in this chapter plays a central role in the long development process of multiple versions of the ABMs, as well as in conducting such crucial steps as model verification, validation, and replication. In the next chapter, we describe the agent-based models (ABMs) that are designed from the specification of this core model.

5

THE AGENT-BASED MODEL (ABM)

5.1 OVERVIEW

In this chapter, we describe the design and implementation of the agent-based model (ABM), which is built according to the specification of the biological core model described in Chapter 4. As mentioned before, the ABM simulates the life cycle of the mosquito vector *Anopheles gambiae* by tracking attributes relevant to the vector population dynamics for each individual mosquito.[1] It is developed using the Java [264] object-oriented programming (OOP) language in the Eclipse Software Development Kit (SDK, Version: 3.5.2, freely available from [534]). Some of the model features (e.g., random number generators, probability distributions) are implemented using the Repast (Recursive Porous Agent Simulation) Toolkit, [452], which is a software framework for agent-based simulations created by the Social Sciences Computing Services at the University of Chicago [510]. Repast provides an integrated library of classes for creating, running, displaying, and collecting data from an agent-based simulation. The Java implementation, being highly portable, provides some key advantages.

---

[1] As we mentioned in Chapter 1, several language-specific ABM implementations have been developed (from the same biological core model described in Chapter 4) by individual researchers within our research group over the recent years. This chapter describes a simplified, fixed version of the ABM. A fully functional computer source code of a specific version of the spatial ABM is presented in the Book Companion Site.

Spatial Agent-Based Simulation Modeling in Public Health:
Design, Implementation, and Applications for Malaria Epidemiology, First Edition.
S. M. Niaz Arifin, Gregory R. Madey and Frank H. Collins.
© 2016 John Wiley & Sons, Inc. Published 2016 by John Wiley & Sons, Inc.

For example, Repast provides built-in graphical visualization tools allowing the agents to be readily inspected. This aids in the debugging process, and the results can also be shared rapidly in graphical form. Programming in Java is more efficient and results in less error-prone code.

The organization of this chapter is as follows: Section 5.2 describes the basic architecture of the ABM, including its agents, environments, and major class diagrams. It also presents a new type of diagram called the event-action- list (EAL) diagram. Section 5.3 describes the population dynamics of the mosquito agents, which is governed by the key operations performed at each simulated day. It also discusses other assumptions of the ABM and the simulation runs, and the ordering of key processing steps performed in a single time step in the ABM. Section 5.5 concludes.

5.2   MODEL ARCHITECTURE

In this section, we describe the architecture of the ABM, the agents, and the environments. The class diagrams are represented in the UML notation [546].[2] Since the ABM is developed in OOP, we first revisit some basic OOP terminologies that are relevant to the points of discussion.

5.2.1   Object-Oriented Programming (OOP) Terminology

Object-Oriented Programming (OOP): Object-oriented programming (OOP) is a programming paradigm based on the concept of *objects*. The fundamental principles of OOP include abstraction, encapsulation, inheritance, and polymorphism.[3]

Object: Objects are simplified representations of their real-world counterparts. In OOP, an object is a self-contained module (software unit or data structure) that contains data in the form of *attributes* (also known as *fields*). The relevant codes to create, access, and modify these attributes are called *methods* (also known as *procedures*). A distinguishing feature of objects is that an object's procedures can access and often modify the attributes of the object with which they are associated. An object stores its state in attributes and exposes its behavior through methods. Methods operate on an object's internal state and serve as the primary mechanism for object-to-object communication.

Class: A class is a blueprint or prototype from which objects are created or instantiated. A class defines the state and behavior of a real-world object using its attributes and methods, respectively. A class is depicted as a three-section

---

[2]The unified modeling language (UML) [546] is a general-purpose visual modeling language in the field of software engineering; it provides a standard visual way for specifying, constructing and documenting the design artifacts of a system.

[3]There are many excellent books covering the concepts, methods, and applications of object-oriented programming, modeling, analysis, and design. Some of the more popular ones include Booch [75], Rumbaugh *et al.* [464], Gamma *et al.* [191], Jacobson [259], Pressman [441], and so on.

rectangle: the top section includes its name, the middle section includes its attributes, and the bottom section includes its methods.

Instance: An instance is a specific realization of any object. In other words, an object is an instance of a class; objects are created from classes by special methods called constructors.

Composition: Composition provides a way for an object to contain references to other objects. With composition, references to the constituent objects become fields of the containing object. *Recursive composition* is a special type of composition using which objects can be composited recursively (e.g., may contain other objects of the same type). The relationship between the composite and the component can be thought of as a semantic *has-a* relationship, as the composite object takes ownership of the component. Composition is depicted as a filled diamond and a solid line. An optional notation of *multiplicity* is often added at each end of the line to indicate the multiplicity of instances of the class (i.e., the number of objects that participate in the composition). For example, the multiplicity notation 1..* indicates "one or more instances" of a class.

Inheritance: Inheritance provides a powerful and natural mechanism for organizing and structuring objects. It enables new classes to receive or inherit the attributes and methods of existing classes. A class that is derived from another class is called a *subclass* (also known as *derived class*, *extended class*, or *child class*). The class from which the subclass is derived is called a *superclass* (also known as *base class* or *parent class*). The inheritance relationships form a hierarchy of classes, in which each inheritance can be thought of as a semantic *is-a* relationship. Thus, a subclass *is-a* more specific instance of a superclass. Inheritance is depicted as an empty triangle and a solid line.

In the ABM, *An. gambiae* mosquitoes are the only dynamic agents. However, the ABM also has provision to include human beings as agents. The version described in this chapter and the accompanying source code (presented in the Book Companion Site) implement humans as static agents (in an agentlist, see later). In the future, when the human and parasite dynamics models are fully implemented, the human agents will be dynamic as well.

The *Simulation* class instance creates all other required class instances, initiates and runs the simulations, keeps track of the global and simulated timer variables, instantiates the required random number generators and the initial mosquito agents, and logs outputs to time-stamped output text files. It contains references to one or more instances of the *Environment* class. The agents are instances of the *Agent* class, can be in different states (instances of the *State* class), and are connected to their environments by instances of the *AgentList* class. Each instance of the *State* class represents a distinct biological stage in the mosquito life cycle (see Chapter 4). In some simulations, mosquito control interventions (instances of the *Intervention* class) can be applied on specific environments (see Chapter 9 for the details of modeling malaria control interventions). A simplified model architecture class diagram is shown in Fig. 5.1.

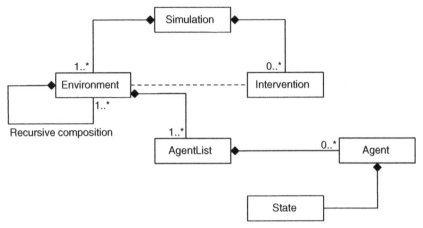

Figure 5.1 A simplified class diagram of the model architecture in the ABM. Attributes and methods are omitted for simplicity.

5.2.2 Agents

A new *An. gambiae* mosquito agent begins its life cycle in the aquatic phase as an *Egg (E)* and then proceed through the *Larva (L)* and *Pupa (P)* stages.[4] When the aquatic phase completes, the agent emerges as an adult mosquito into the adult phase and advances through the five adult stages of *Immature Adult (IA)*, *Mate Seeking (MS)*, *Blood Meal Seeking (BMS)*, *Blood Meal Digesting (BMD)*, and *Gravid (G)* (see Fig. 4.1). When a female adult mosquito agent enters the BMS stage, it searches for a human blood meal. After successful blood-feeding, it rests in the BMD stage, develops its eggs, and then enters the G stage to lay the eggs. Then, it returns back to the BMS stage, thus initiating a new gonotrophic cycle. A male adult mosquito, after reaching the MS stage, stays in this stage for the rest of its life. The stage transitions (from one stage to another), development rates, and mortality rates are governed by the rules as described in the core model (see Chapter 4).

Agents have their own attributes, methods, hierarchy, and internal states. Each *MosquitoAgent* class instance is inherited as a subclass of an *Agent* superclass instance. The major attributes of an *Agent* class instance include age, state, environment, spatial location, and so on. The major attributes of a *MosquitoAgent* class instance include id (identifier), sex (gender), available eggs, egg batch identifier, agent move per day counter, and so on. A simplified class diagram for the agents is shown in Fig. 5.2. Attributes and methods that are added for the spatial extension (described in Chapter 6) are marked in gray.

---

[4]As mentioned in Footnote 4 in Chapter 4, we differentiate between the usage of the two terms *stage* and *state*: *stage* refers to a distinct biological stage (time duration) in the mosquito life cycle; (see Chapter 4); *state*, on the other hand, refers to the static and dynamic properties and values of any computational object (e.g., a mosquito agent object).

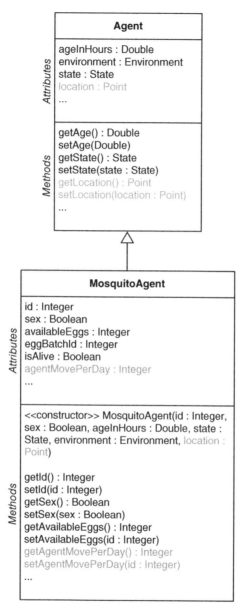

Figure 5.2 A simplified class diagram for the agents in the ABM. Each *MosquitoAgent* class instance is inherited as a subclass of an *Agent* superclass instance. The *get* and *set* methods are used to access and modify the corresponding attributes, respectively. Attributes and methods that are added for the spatial extension are marked in gray.

5.2.3 Environments

A generic *Environment* class can be inherited as a *MosquitoEnvironment* class, which can be further specialized as either an *AquaticEnvironment* or a *HumanEnvironment* class. An *AquaticEnvironment* class instance represents an aquatic habitat with specific habitat capacity for the mosquito agents (see Section 4.4.1). A *HumanEnvironment* class instance represents a house with specific number of persons residing in the house. A simplified class diagram for the environments is shown in Fig. 5.3. Attributes and methods that are added for the spatial extension (described in Chapter 6) are marked in gray.

The mosquito agents, depending on their life-cycle phases (aquatic or adult), are tied to different environments via instances of the *AgentList* class. An *AgentList* class is inherited as either the *AquaticAgentList* or *AdultAgentList* class. An *Aquatic-AgentList* instance contains aquatic mosquito agents for a specific *AquaticEnvironment* instance, and an *AdultAgentList* instance contains adult mosquito agents for a specific *MosquitoEnvironment* instance. The *AgentList* class instances facilitate the addition of new mosquito agents, placing newly emerged mosquito agents from the aquatic to the adult phase, and removal of dead mosquito agents, as described later. It also provides easy access to various cohort-based operations such as the total counts of agents filtered by a particular criterion (e.g., all female adult agents or all pupae). A simplified class diagram for the agentlists is shown in Fig. 5.4. The *get* and *set* methods are used to access and modify the corresponding attributes, respectively. Note that the *HumanEnvironment* class does not have an explicit agentlist, since at a given point in time, the set of mosquitoes or humans in a particular house need not be identified separately.

As we will see in Chapter 10, the above approach promotes an efficient way for our landscape modeling framework to be seamlessly coupled with real-world landscape scenarios (e.g., from a GIS): following a grid-based approach, a large landscape can be easily subdivided into desired objects of aquatic and human environments.

5.2.4 Event-Action-List Diagram

In order to capture the major daily events of a simulation in a standard, canonical manner, we propose and present a new type of diagram, called the EAL diagram. It depicts the simulation *events* (occurring on a daily basis), the corresponding *actions* triggered by those events, and the *list(s)* of agents (data structures) affected by them.

In an EAL diagram, each *event* represents a *biological* phenomenon, and the corresponding *action* represents the programmatic task(s) performed by the simulation. Optionally, some *list(s)* of agents may be modified as a direct result of the performed *action*. Thus, an EAL diagram summarizes the daily events of the simulation model by listing all major events, actions, and lists. For example, when the simulation is started, it needs to create initial adult mosquito agents. The biological phenomenon "*create initial adults*", termed as an event, is realized by the (simulation) action "*add agents*"; this event-action pair affects the *list of adult agents* in the simulation. An EAL diagram for the ABM is shown in Fig. 5.5.

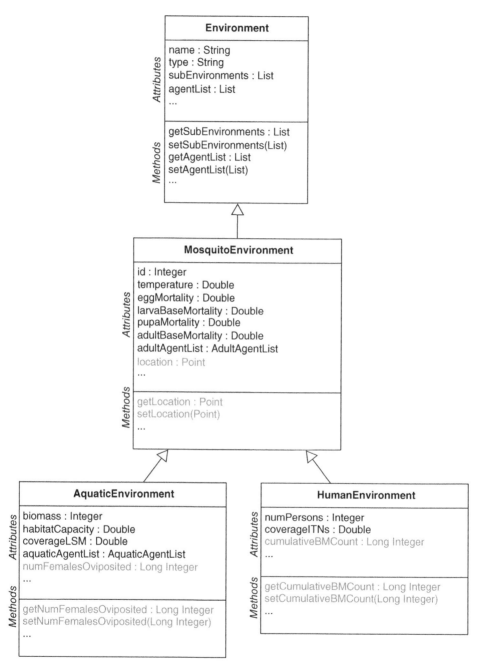

Figure 5.3   A simplified class diagram for the environments in the ABM. A generic *Environment* class can be inherited as a *MosquitoEnvironment* class, which can be further specialized as either an *AquaticEnvironment* or a *HumanEnvironment* class. The *get* and *set* methods are used to access and modify the corresponding attributes, respectively. Attributes and methods that are added for the spatial extension are marked in gray.

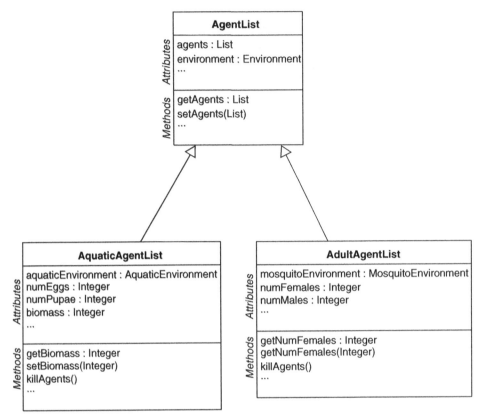

Figure 5.4   A simplified class diagram for the agentlists in the ABM. Agentlists bind different sets of mosquito agents to their corresponding environments depending on their life-cycle phases. A generic *AgentList* class instance can be inherited as either an *AquaticAgentList* or an *AdultAgentList* class instance. An *AquaticAgentList* instance contains aquatic mosquito agents for a specific *AquaticEnvironment* instance and an *AdultAgentList* instance contains adult mosquito agents for a specific *MosquitoEnvironment* instance. The *get* and *set* methods are used to access and modify the corresponding attributes, respectively.

5.3   MOSQUITO POPULATION DYNAMICS

In the ABM, mosquito populations are dynamic in nature. The population dynamics is governed by three key operations performed at each simulated day: creating new mosquito agents, updating adult and immature mosquito agents, and killing adult and immature mosquito agents. These key operations reflect the population dynamics as described in the core model (see Chapter 4). These are described as follows:

- Creating new mosquito agents: Initially, 1000 new adult mosquito agents are randomly placed in the mosquito environment. During the course of a simulation run, a *Gravid* female agent visits different aquatic environments and try to lay eggs (oviposit) in batches. For each aquatic habitat *H*, successive oviposition

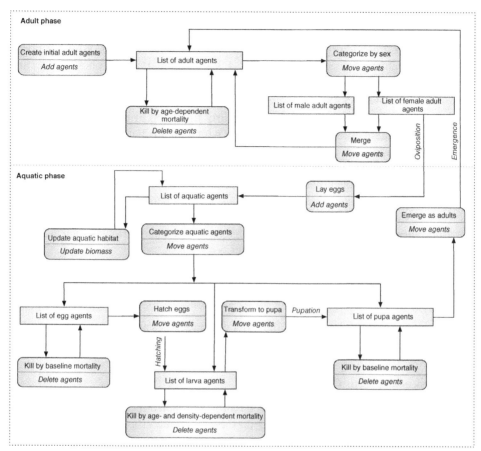

Figure 5.5   An event-action-list (EAL) diagram for the ABM. Each *squashed rectangle* represents an event-action pair, in which the *event* is denoted at the upper half, and the *action* is denoted at the lower half. Each *rectangle* represents the *list(s)* (data structures) of agents affected by the event-action pair. Used from Arifin *et al.* [20] under a Creative Commons Attribution 4.0 International License.

attempts within the same gonotrophic cycle are distinguished by a habitat sampling weight w. The age-adjusted biomass (*Biomass*) in habitat H accounts for the density-dependent *1-day-old equivalent larval population* (N_e), and provides a *check and balance* mechanism for habitat H by serving as a soft upper limit for the aquatic population in H. The potential and actual numbers of eggs the female can lay ($Eggs_{potential}$ and $Eggs_{laid}$, respectively) in H are then calculated, and new mosquito agents are created in the form of eggs into the simulation.

- Killing adult mosquito agents: To kill the adult mosquito agents, we use a modified version of the logistic mortality model in which the age-dependent component of mortality increases exponentially with age (see Section 4.6.2). Newly emergent adult agents have a baseline daily mortality rate of α. For each adult age cohort, agents are killed with the daily mortality rate of $DMR_{Adult}(Age)$.

- Killing immature mosquito agents: Eggs and pupae are killed with a constant mortality rate α of 10%. Larvae mortality rate depends on both the age and the *1-day-old equivalent larval population*, N_e (see Section 4.6.1). Within a given aquatic habitat, N_e is computed by Eq. 4.9. For each larva age cohort, agents are killed with the rate of $DMR_{Larva}(Age_{Cohort})$, which is calculated using N_e as well as the habitat capacity HC.

- Updating mosquito agents: For each hourly time step in a simulation, existing mosquito agent objects are updated along with their attributes in a recursive manner. The simulation object first updates all independent global variables and then calls the update functions of all its environments. Each environment first updates its attributes and agentlists and then recursively calls the update functions of all its subenvironments. An agentlist updates itself by performing list-specific operations such as arranging its agents into cohorts and calculating cohort-specific mortality rates. Finally, the mosquito agents update their attributes such as states, available eggs, and egg batch identifiers.

5.4 MODEL FEATURES

In this section, we describe some of the other characteristics and features of the ABM, including the processing steps ordering, initialization, and assumptions.

5.4.1 Processing Steps Ordering

The ordering of the key operations or processing steps performed in a single time step in the ABM has important implications on the model output as well as model accuracy. These steps are shown in Fig. 5.6: during each time step of a simulation run, the ABM collects, saves, and prints output data (mosquito abundance, model parameters, etc.) to time-stamped output files, kills larva and adult mosquito agents according to age-specific mortality rates, and kills egg and pupa mosquito agents with fixed mortality rates; it then updates the age, state duration, and state transition for all agents (adults and aquatic). Since some of these processing steps are interdependent, it naturally leads to many possible *dependency relationships*, which can ensure the interdependence accuracy. Preservation of the dependency relationships is important to ensure the correctness of the model's output, since alteration of these may drastically change the simulation results.

To illustrate the importance of the dependency relationships, the ordering of processing steps can also be viewed as a *directed acyclic graph (DAG)*, and hence, a topological sort can be performed on it.[5] A topological sort can be viewed as an ordering of vertices along a horizontal line so that all directed edges go from left to right. Every DAG will have one and possibly more topological sorts. Figure 5.7 depicts two possible topological sorts of the model's processing steps performed in a single time step of a

---

[5]In graph theory, a *topological sort* (or *topological ordering*) of a directed acyclic graph $G = (V, E)$ is a linear ordering of all its vertices such that if G contains an edge (u, v), then u appears before v in the ordering [127], p. 549.

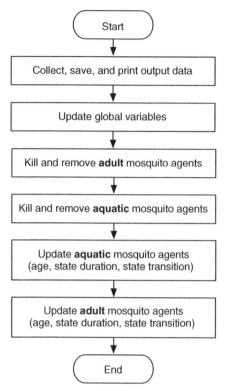

Figure 5.6   The ordering of the key processing steps performed in a single time step of a simulation run. The *dependency relationships* between the processing steps are crucial to ensure the correctness of the model's output. By Arifin *et al.* [23], copyright by ACM.

simulation run: Figure 5.7a shows the interdependent steps performed in a single time step of a simulation run are connected by directed dashed lines; Figure 5.7b and c show two possible ordering that preserve the dependency relationships of all the major processing steps. By topological sort, Fig. 5.7c can be rearranged so that all directed edges go from left to right, as in Fig. 5.7b.

5.4.2   Model Assumptions

The ABM represents a theoretical (as opposed to field-based) model. We assume the presence of only one mosquito vector, *An. gambiae.* The mosquito life cycle dynamics is emphasized, and the parasite life cycle and the malaria transmission cycle are not yet included. Mosquitoes senesce and their probability of death increases with age. The influence of habitat size, surface area, solar insulation, and other related factors, which may influence habitat capacity, is not modeled explicitly. Daily temperature, variations in which can affect our model's output, is fixed at 30 °C (but can be varied to represent warmer or colder climates). Seasonality and other weather/climate parameters (except daily temperature) are not included. In aquatic habitats, survival of eggs and pupae is not influenced by the aquatic mosquito density (hence, the mortality rates in the egg and

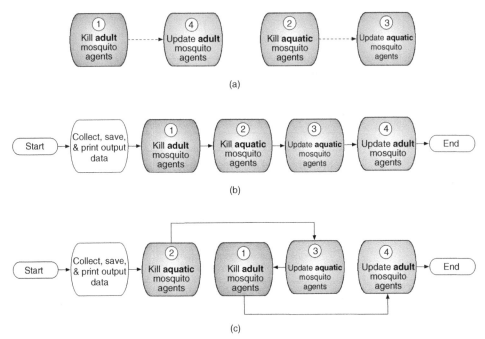

Figure 5.7 Dependency relationships in processing steps ordering can be viewed as a *directed acyclic graph (DAG)*. (a) The interdependent steps performed in a single time step of a simulation run are connected by directed dashed lines. (b) and (c) Two possible ordering that preserve the dependency relationships of all the major processing steps. By *topological sort*, (c) can be arranged so that all directed edges go from left to right, as in (b).

pupa stages are treated as constants). Female adults, once entering the mate-seeking stage, are always assumed to successfully find males to mate with (in the next time step). For egg maturation, a single blood meal is assumed sufficient. The mortality rate of female adults is assumed independent of their malaria infectivity states. Female fecundity is assumed normally distributed with mean of 170 and standard deviation of 30. The human population is modeled as static, that is, humans do not move in space. All humans are assumed to be identical.

For host-seeking, we do not model alternative hosts for blood-feeding (e.g., cattle), and the only blood meal sources are humans in the houses. Time is modeled with hourly (instead of daily) time steps since this approach provides much more flexibility in modeling certain agent behaviors (e.g., host-seeking to start at a particular hour at night). Female adult mosquito abundance is treated as the primary output of the model.[6] Each aquatic habitat is set with a capacity (*HC*, with default 1000), which serves two purposes: (1) it limits the number of eggs a female mosquito may oviposit in an aquatic habitat (thus determining soft limits on larval density of the habitat) and (2) it is used to model a gravid female's inclination to avoid less suitable (e.g., overcrowded) habitats. Unlike other studies [221, 222], *HC* is not treated as a hard limit.

---

[6]Other spatial outputs are reported in Chapter 10.

When no intervention is in action, the mosquito population is governed by the combined capacities of all aquatic habitats and the density-dependent oviposition mechanism, which limits the potential number of eggs that a female mosquito may preferentially lay in an aquatic habitat, considering both the associated *HC* and the biomass already present in the habitat.

In addition, the model makes the following assumptions:

- The male-female ratio of newly laid eggs is assumed to be 50 : 50.
- In the *MS* stage, a female always finds a male mosquito to mate (within the first time step it seeks to mate).
- In the *BMS* stage, a female always finds a blood meal (either immediately after mating or after completing oviposition of an egg batch).

5.4.3 Simulations

Although the ABM is implemented as computer simulations in multiple programming languages (Java and C++) to compare language-specific dependencies as well as verification and validation (V&V) features, the source code of the spatial extension (presented in the Book Companion Site) is written in Java.[7] Each simulation starts with a prespecified initial number of eggs as agents, typically consisting of a 50 : 50 male-female ratio. Other input parameters include prespecified numbers of aquatic habitats with adjustable habitat capacities, hourly temperature profiles, habitat capacity profiles, and so on. For parameter sweep experiments and other modeling scenarios, each simulation is replicated at least 50 times to eliminate any biases introduced by different sources of randomness and stochasticity, the behavior uncertainties of the agents' actions, states, and so on.[8] With around 25,000 adult agents and one million aquatic agents in the system, a sample simulation run takes about an hour to output 1-year results data on a 2.4 GHz Intel Core 2 Duo computer with 2 GB of memory.

5.5 SUMMARY

In this chapter, we presented the design and implementation details of a simplified, fixed version of the ABM, which was built according to the specification of the biological core model described in Chapter 4. We described the agents, environments, and major class diagrams for the ABM, its features, initialization settings, and other assumptions. We also demonstrated the use of a new type of diagram called the EAL diagram.

The ABM described in this chapter is mostly *nonspatial* (except for the additional spatial attributes and methods in the class diagrams presented in Section 5.2, which were clearly marked). In the next chapter, we present its *spatial* extension.

---

[7] See Chapter 8 for results and discussion on V&V.
[8] See Chapter 9 for results and discussion on the importance of replication.

6

THE SPATIAL ABM

6.1 OVERVIEW

In the previous chapter, we described the agent-based model (ABM) of *Anopheles gambiae* mosquitoes, which was derived from the biological core model presented in Chapter 4. The ABM, as mentioned before, was largely nonspatial. In this chapter, we describe its spatial extension (hereafter called the *spatial ABM*).[1]

Analyses of spatial relationships are fundamental to epidemiology research. To this end, spatial statistical methods, geospatial methods, geostatistics, and more recent technologies such as geographic information system (GIS) and global positioning system (GPS) have been extensively used in public health and epidemiology studies [83, 88, 119, 132, 134, 204, 232, 293, 316, 350, 367, 380, 484, 540, 551].[2] For example, in a large-scale longitudinal study of malaria, in a $70 \, km^2$ area in western Kenya, Hightower *et al.* applied spatial analysis and examined spatial hypotheses for a malaria field study to produce maps with highly accurate locational information for all of the geographic features of interest [242]. In the discipline of *landscape epidemiology* (also known as

---

[1]Portions of this chapter appeared in Arifin *et al.* [25] and [26], and as a stand-alone chapter in Zhang [582, Chapter 14].
[2]See Section 10.2 for a review of GIS and spatial statistical methods in the fields of public health and epidemiology, with a special focus on malaria.

Spatial Agent-Based Simulation Modeling in Public Health:
Design, Implementation, and Applications for Malaria Epidemiology, First Edition.
S. M. Niaz Arifin, Gregory R. Madey and Frank H. Collins.
© 2016 John Wiley & Sons, Inc. Published 2016 by John Wiley & Sons, Inc.

spatial epidemiology, medical geography, geographical epidemiology, or health geomatics), the notion of *spatial heterogeneity* is considered as one of the most important factors for an effective representation of the environment being modeled.[3] In most cases, the probability of disease transmission significantly declines with distance from an infected host. Thus, the spatial locations of pathogens, hosts, and vectors are fundamentally important to disease dynamics, as reported by numerous research studies [408]. For example, Benavides *et al.* showed that the spread of infectious diseases in wildlife populations is influenced by patterns of between-host contacts: the habitat *hotspots* (places attracting a large numbers of individuals or social groups) can significantly alter contact patterns and, hence, disease propagation [60].

Place, space, disease, and human health are correlated in intricate ways, and these relationships are well known for many decades [303]. Some of these relationships are expressed in terms of spatial heterogeneity, which is generally ascribed to a landscape or to a population. It refers to the uneven distribution of various concentrations of each species and resource type within an area.

Like most other human diseases, the dynamics of malaria can be subject to substantial local variations that result from spatial factors. Thus, representation of space can be crucial in malaria modeling [204, 221, 222, 242, 303, 360]. The prevailing large within-site spatial variations in the abundance and temporal dynamics of malaria vector populations indicate that the risk of parasite transmission differs among sites [257]. Several studies have reported large spatiotemporal variations in commonly used assessment metrics such as mosquito density, sporozoite rate, and entomological inoculation rate (EIR) [6, 149, 156, 317, 499]. Such variations may arise from several factors, including the weather and climate, the locations of aquatic habitats and blood meal events, characteristics of the mosquito species.

An ABM can be applied to a domain *with* or *without* an explicit representation of space. In some cases, however, an explicit spatial representation may be required for certain aspects of the ABM to be modeled more realistically. In addition, some of the more frequent modeling events may *by nature* require spatial attributes. For example, in a spatial ABM of malaria, events like obtaining a successful blood meal (host-seeking) or finding an aquatic habitat to lay eggs (oviposition) can be modeled by utilizing the distribution of corresponding resources in the landscape. As we mentioned in Section 3.5.3, other published malaria models can also be classified into nonspatial and spatial models, considering the form of the spatial representation embedded within the models (this classification may overlap with both categories of mathematical and ABMs).

In our ABMs, spatial heterogeneity defines the spatial distribution of resources in landscapes and controls how easily adult female mosquitoes may find these resources (which are necessary to complete their gonotrophic cycle).[4] Thus, it has profound impact on the mosquito populations [25, 26].

---

[3]See Chapter 10 in which we present a landscape epidemiology modeling framework that integrates a GIS with the spatial ABM of malaria (described in this chapter).

[4]Recall from Chapter 4 that the *gonotrophic cycle* refers to the cycle of blood-feeding, egg maturation, and oviposition by a female mosquito in its life cycle until it dies.

As mentioned in Chapter 3, an ABM's *environment* or *space* is often described by its *topology*, which can be represented in various ways such as an abstract (nonspatial) "soup" model, 2-*D* or 3-*D* Euclidean spaces, cellular automata, spatial grid or network of nodes, and GIS.[5] For example, Bian categorizes *grid* and *patch* as the two fundamentally different data models to represent space [64]. A grid consists of a finite number of regular cells. In the patch model, space is partitioned according to landscape features (e.g., patches, corridors, and nodes). Within malaria models, environments may represent simulated mosquito worlds, simulated aquatic habitats (for the mosquito agents), simulated houses (for the human agents), and so on. In our spatial ABM, we represent space with a landscape-based approach, where each landscape comprises discrete and finite-sized cells (grids).

Since the nonspatial ABM (described in Chapter 5) did not have any explicit spatial representation, its resource-seeking events were modeled with separate probability distributions, which accounted for the additional search and travel times incurred by the mosquito agents [26]. For example, oviposition was probability based: during each simulated hour, a gravid female tried to find an aquatic habitat with 25% probability of success. As long as the female agent had remaining eggs to lay, it was allowed to make at most three attempts per 12 hours (i.e., each night), which translated to 25% chance of finding an aquatic habitat per hour. To model this behavior, uniform statistical distributions generated by the Repast pseudorandom numbers generator library [452] were used. All simulation events (described in Chapter 5) occurred without any spatial context. A spatial model, however, provides opportunities to model these events by connecting them with the corresponding locations of resources in the landscape. This concept can be generalized for most resource-seeking events.

In both the nonspatial and the spatial models, all mosquito agents are represented individually. However, the agents in the spatial extension presented in this chapter also possess explicit spatial information. We show how the previous model and the current spatial model yield consistent results with identical parameter settings (whenever applicable). We also show how spatial heterogeneity affects some results of the spatial model.

The organization of this chapter is as follows: In Section 6.2, we define some relevant terms for the spatial ABM and then describe the spatial ABM in detail, including the mosquito agents, the spatial movements, and the landscapes. It also presents our landscape generator software tools, which are used to facilitate the specification of parameters and to generate appropriate landscapes for the spatial ABM. Section 6.3 presents different clustering schemes to generate landscapes in which the resources are clustered according to specific strategies. Section 6.4 describes agents' flight heuristics in the form of flowcharts. Section 6.5 discusses simulation results that include the effects of varying the landscape patterns, the relative size and density of the aquatic habitats, and the overall capacity of the system. Section 6.6 demonstrates the effects of spatial heterogeneity of the landscapes by considering the resource density and Section 6.7 concludes.

---

[5]In this chapter, in the context of ABMs and agents, the terms "environment", "space", and "landscape" are used interchangeably.

6.2   THE SPATIAL ABM

In this section, we define some relevant terms for the spatial ABM and then discuss the spatial ABM in detail.

6.2.1   Definition of Terms

In the following, we describe some terms of interest that are used throughout the rest of this chapter.[6]

- *Average Travel Time (ATT)*: For a given landscape, the average travel time (*ATT*) is defined as the average time (hours) taken by an adult female mosquito agent to successfully find a resource (of a particular resource type). In this study, though we do not explicitly measure *ATT*, it reflects a statistically expected measure in our spatial analyses (as described later).
- *Biomass*: The biomass of an aquatic habitat (see Section 4.4) is the sum of the number of eggs $Eggs_{habitat}$, the 1-day-old equivalent larval population N_e, and the number of pupae $Pupae_{habitat}$, as described in Eq. (4.8):

$$Biomass = N_{Eggs} + N_e + N_{Pupae}$$

- *Combined Habitat Capacity (CHC)*: The combined habitat capacity *CHC* is the sum of the habitat capacities (*HCs*) of all aquatic habitats in a landscape (recall from Section 4.4 that the habitat capacity *HC* is a soft limit on the aquatic mosquito population that the aquatic habitat can sustain); since the combined aquatic population, controlled by *HC* in each aquatic habitat, eventually limits the overall mosquito abundance, *CHC* effectively represents the overall capacity of the landscape (in terms of the mosquito population).
- *Inter-Object Distance (IOD)*: This parameter controls the average linear distance between resources in a landscape.[7]
- *Oviposition*: As described in Section 4.4, oviposition is the process by which gravid female agents lay new eggs; referring to Eqs. (4.10) and (4.11), when an adult female finds an aquatic habitat to lay eggs, the potential number of eggs, $Eggs_{Potential}$, which it may preferentially lay is regulated by both the habitat capacity *HC* and the biomass already present in the habitat:

$$Eggs_{Potential}(gcn, w) = Eggs_{Max}(gcn) \times \left(1 - \frac{Biomass}{w * HC}\right)$$

where $Eggs_{Max}$ is the maximum number of eggs available to lay, *gcn* represents the gonotrophic cycle number, and *w* is the habitat sampling weight (i.e., 1, 2, or 3).

---

[6]Some of these terms were first introduced in Chapter 4, and are revisited here for easy reference.

[7]*IOD* is semantically equivalent to the *clustering coefficient* measure used in graph theory, which indicates the degree to which nodes in a graph tend to cluster together.

- *Resource Density*: Resource density of a particular resource type in a landscape is defined as the percentage of total area in the landscape occupied by objects of that resource type.[8] For example, a 5 × 10 landscape with 25 aquatic habitats have 50% density.
- *Vector Abundance (VA)*: At any specific point in simulated time, *VA* denotes the total number of adult female mosquito (vector) agents in the ABM; for each simulated time step, we keep track of *VA* by counting the aggregate total of adult female agents across every cell in the landscape.[9]

In Chapter 5, we presented simplified class diagrams for the agents and environments in the spatial ABM (see Figs. 5.2 and 5.3), in which the spatial attributes and methods were marked in gray. In the following, we describe some of those spatial attributes.

The *location* attributes of all habitats and agents are encoded as instances of the built-in Java *Point2D* class in the (x, y) coordinate space. It allows the ABM to implement the spatial properties of discrete locations for the *AquaticEnvironment*, *HumanEnvironment*, and *MosquitoAgent* classes.

As before, an instance of the *Simulation* class initiates and controls various aspects of a simulation run, which include creating other required class instances, running the simulation, keeping track of the global variables, assigning the initial mosquito agents to different spatial locations, and logging outputs to time-stamped output text files. It contains reference to a global environment, which is an instance of the *MosquitoEnvironment* class. The global environment in turn keeps track of all spatial environments, which are created as instances of either an *AquaticEnvironment* or a *HumanEnvironment* class. Each spatial environment instance has its spatial location and other attributes (e.g., habitat capacity for an aquatic habitat, number of persons living in a house). The mosquito agents are created as instances of the *MosquitoAgent* class with their initial spatial coordinates and are connected to their spatial environments by instances of the *AgentList* class. A simplified model architecture class diagram is also shown in Fig. 5.1.

6.2.2 Landscapes

As mentioned before, the spatial ABM implements its topology with a landscape-based approach, where each *landscape* comprises discrete and finite-sized cells (grids). A landscape is used to represent the coordinate space necessary for the spatial locations of the environments and the adult mosquito agents. Resources, in the forms of aquatic habitats and houses, are contained within a landscape. The density and spatial distribution of both types of resources inherently define the spatial heterogeneity of resources within a given landscape.

A *landscape* is denoted by its dimensions (*width* and *height*) and is defined as a collection of *height* numbers of horizontal rows and *width* numbers of vertical

---

[8]Two types of resources are considered in the current models: aquatic habitats and houses.
[9]*VA* is considered the primary output for all simulation results presented in this chapter.

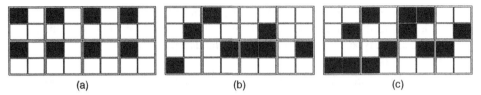

(a)   (b)   (c)

Figure 6.1   Examples of three types of landscapes: (a) regular, (b) random, and (c) hybrid. Gray and white rectangles represent spatial resources and empty cells in the mosquito environment, respectively. Updated from Arifin *et al.* [26]. Reprinted by permission of the publisher.

columns, having *width* × *height* numbers of cells. Each cell, with its spatial attributes, may represent a specific habitat environment (human or aquatic), or be part of the adult mosquito environment. Each landscape is modeled topologically as a 2-*D* torus space with a *nonabsorbing boundary*.[10] With a *nonabsorbing boundary*, when mosquitoes hit an edge, they reenter the landscape from the edge directly opposite of the exiting edge (and thus are not killed due to hitting the edge). For simplicity, we assume that each resource can occupy exactly one cell in a landscape.[11] Resource density of a landscape is regulated by its dimensions and the number of resources it contains. For example, placing 25 aquatic habitats in a 10 × 10 landscape produces 25% density; placing the same number of aquatic habitats in a 5 × 10 landscape produces 50% density. In this chapter, we use three types of landscapes, which are generated using our landscape generator software tools (described in Section 6.2.3):

- *Regular*: Resources are distributed according to a regular, well-defined pattern; every nonempty row contains the same number of resources; horizontal and vertical distances between any two neighboring resources always remain the same.
- *Random*: Resources are distributed randomly following a uniform random distribution.
- *Hybrid*: A blend of the previous two; every nonempty row contains the same number of resources; within a nonempty row, resources are placed randomly; this strategy allows to control both density and randomness.

Examples of the three types of landscapes are depicted in Fig. 6.1, in which each gray rectangle represents a resource (aquatic habitat or house), and each empty white rectangle represents a nonresource cell. Figure 6.1(a–c) depict examples of regular, random, and hybrid landscapes, respectively. Each landscape has a dimension of 8 × 4. Figure 6.1a and b have 25% resource density each; Figure 6.1c has 37.5% resource density.

6.2.3   Landscape Generator Tools

To facilitate the specification of parameters to the spatial ABM, we built landscape generator software tools as graphical user interfaces (GUIs). These tools help in generating

---

[10]See Chapter 9 for simulation results that are obtained using other types of boundaries.
[11]This assumption is relaxed in Chapter 10 by allowing a cell to contain multiple resources of different types.

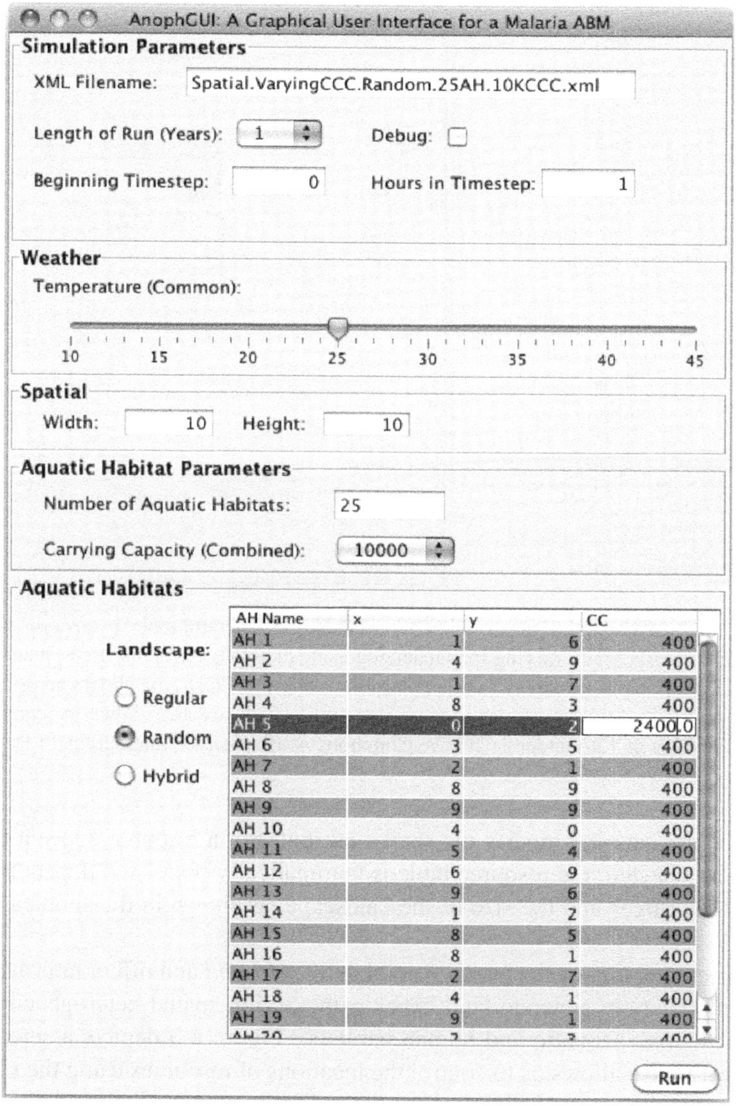

Figure 6.2   Screenshot of an early version of the landscape generator tool, *AnophGUI*. Updated from Arifin *et al.* [26]. Reprinted by permission of the publisher.

landscapes with varying spatial heterogeneity of both types of resources. The early version of the tools was named as *AnophGUI* and was first reported in [26]. Figure 6.2 depicts a screenshot of *AnophGUI*.

For a specific landscape composed of hundreds of resources, *AnophGUI* automates the task of generating spatial attributes (e.g., location, capacity) for these resources and allows the user to specify other simulation parameters (e.g., length of run), as well as relevant weather parameters (e.g., temperature). The user may also select

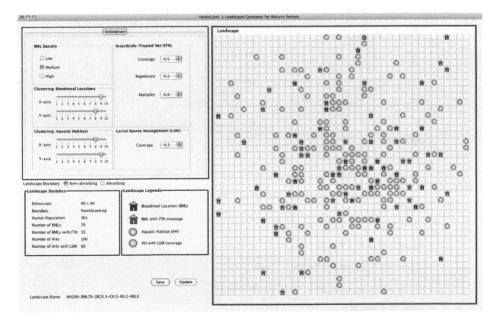

Figure 6.3   Screenshot of the latest version of the landscape generator tool, *VectorLand*. *VectorLand* can generate landscapes with varying spatial heterogeneity of both types of resources: aquatic habitats and houses. Locations of resources can be controlled using the *Clustering* sliders across both axes. Additional statistics about the generated landscape and legends are also shown in separate panels. Used from Arifin *et al.* [28] under a Creative Commons Attribution 4.0 International License.

different landscapes and modify the spatial attributes of a resource. Once a particular landscape is selected, the resource table is automatically populated depending on the number of resources and the size of the landscape, as shown in the southeast portion in Fig. 6.2.

The current version of the tool is named as *VectorLand* and offers improvement by allowing modelers to generate landscapes with varying spatial heterogeneity of both types of resources (aquatic and human habitats). Figure 6.3 depicts a screenshot of *VectorLand*. It also allows us to control the locations of resources using the *Clustering* sliders across both axes. Various vector control intervention parameters can be controlled using separate panels (currently, interventions LSM and ITNs are implemented, as described in Chapter 9). This screenshot depicts selecting medium house density, with 30% LSM coverage and 50% ITNs coverage. Additional statistics about the generated landscape and legends are also shown in separate panels. *VectorLand* is presented as a runnable program in the Book Companion Site.

We emphasize that *AnophGUI* and *VectorLand* are tools to generate landscapes, which are then used as spatial inputs to the ABM. These tools should not be treated as models in themselves.

6.3   RESOURCE CLUSTERING

The landscape generator software tools also allow us to generate landscapes in which the resources are clustered according to specific strategies (schemes). In this section, we discuss some examples using the following notation: the spatial location of a resource is denoted as a point $P(x, y)$ with coordinates $P.x$ and $P.y$. $N(\mu, \sigma)$ refers to a normal distribution (also known as *Gaussian* distribution) with mean μ and standard deviation σ. To control the distribution of point objects along both axes, we use bivariate normal distributions, denoted as $N_x(\mu_x, \sigma_x)$ and $N_y(\mu_y, \sigma_y)$ for x- and y-axis, respectively. For the two different resource types (A and B), we use $Type^A$ point objects and $Type^B$ point objects. *VectorLand* allows controlling the *IOD*s between resources of the same type as well as between different types.

We first calculate the *center* of the entire landscape grid, which is used as the mean for the subsequent bivariate normals. The *center* serves as a reference point for the set of point objects to be generated. After generating a new point (using any scheme), we ensure that it is nonoverlapping with the set of existing point objects and it resides within the edges of the landscape (since the landscape is modeled as a 2-D torus object, if a new point falls outside any edge, we wrap it around the edge). $Type^B$ point objects are generated after $Type^A$ point objects. Sample landscapes using different clustering schemes of resources are shown in Fig. 6.4.

The four schemes are described in the following:

Cluster around Center: In this scheme, all generated point objects are clustered around the center of the landscape. To control the distribution of point objects around the *center*, we use the bivariate normals $N_x(center_x, IOD_x^{A|B})$ and $N_y(center_y, IOD_y^{A|B})$.[12] Thus, the *IOD*s control the relative distance of new point objects from the *center*. Figure 6.4a depicts an example using this scheme.

Cluster around the First Object: In this scheme, all generated point objects *except the first* are clustered around the first point (which is denoted as *First-Point*). To generate *FirstPoint* itself with some controlled randomness from the *center*, we use a separate parameter *FirstPointSD* in the corresponding bivariate normals: $N_x(center_x, FirstPointSD)$ and $N_y(center_y, FirstPointSD)$. For both resource types, once the *FirstPoints* are generated, the remaining point objects are clustered around them using the bivariate normals $N_x(FirstPoint_x, IOD_x^{A|B})$ and $N_y(FirstPoint_y, IOD_y^{A|B})$. Thus, depending on the location of *FirstPoint*, the envelope of point objects can be arbitrarily *translated* within the landscape. Figure 6.4b depicts an example using this scheme.

Dynamic Clustering: This scheme is similar to *Cluster around the First Object* in generating the *FirstPoints*. However, for both resource types, the remaining

---

[12]The "|" symbol denotes "or".

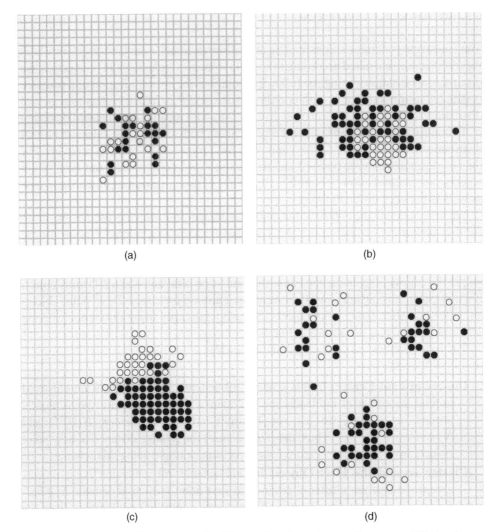

Figure 6.4 Examples of landscapes with different clustering schemes of resources. Filled and open circles denote different types of resources. (a) Cluster around center. (b) Cluster around the first object. (c) Dynamic clustering. (d) Multiple clusters ($n = 3$).

point objects are generated differently: for each new point, it randomly selects a point from the existing set, which is then used as a reference point (denoted as *Reference*). It then uses the bivariate normals $N_x(Reference_x, IOD_x^{A|B})$ and $N_y(Reference_y, IOD_y^{A|B})$. Thus, the envelope of point objects is *dynamically* expanded (hence the name *Dynamic Clustering*) depending on the most recently selected reference point *Reference*. Figure 6.4c shows an example using this scheme.

Multiple Clusters: In this scheme, the landscape is divided into n clusters (n can be specified in the *VectorLand* tool). If n is even, the landscape is equally divided into

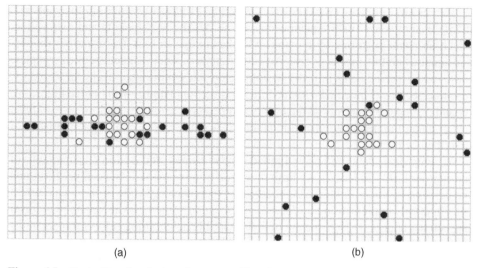

(a)   (b)

Figure 6.5   Controlling the clusters along a specific axis. Twenty resources of both types are used. (a) Along *x*-axis. (b) Along both axes.

n rectangular regions. If *n* is odd, the landscape is first equally divided assuming *n* + 1 clusters, and then the last two clusters are merged, forming a larger cluster. For each of the *n* clusters, the corresponding *centers* are calculated. Each cluster is assigned equal number of objects of both types (if the number of objects is not divisible by *n*, the remaining ones are arbitrarily assigned to the first cluster). Then, point objects within each cluster are generated using the *Cluster around Center* scheme. Figure 6.4d shows an example using *n* = 3 clusters.

VectorLand also allows us to control the relative stretch of resources along any axis. For example, as shown in Fig. 6.5, the filled circles of aquatic habitats (which represent one resource type) can be stretched along a single axis or along both axes.[13] In both cases, the open circles of houses (which represent the second resource type) are clustered around the center. Twenty resources of both types are used.

6.4   FLIGHT HEURISTICS FOR MOSQUITO AGENTS

In the spatial ABM, movement of adult female mosquito agents in a landscape is restricted: they move only when in *BMS* and *G* stages in order to seek for resources.[14] Since each landscape comprises discrete and finite-sized (50 m × 50 m) cells, our landscape-based modeling approach appeared to be especially suitable to capture the details of the resource-seeking process.

[13]In this example, we arbitrarily chose the *x*-axis; stretching along the *y*-axis has symmetric effects.
[14]These stages were marked in rectangle symbol in Fig. 4.1.

The resource-seeking (also known as *foraging*) process of the mosquito agents primarily encompasses two frequent events in the ABMs: host-seeking and oviposition, which an agent performs by moving in the landscape to seek for resources (houses and aquatic habitats, respectively). An adult female mosquito agent needs to complete these events periodically in order to complete each gonotrophic cycle. In summary, resource-seeking is modeled with random nondirectional flights with limited flight ability and perceptual ranges until the agents can perceive resources at close proximity, at which point, the flight becomes directional. It is guided by several flight heuristics as described below.

As empirical data indicates limited flight ranges and sensory perception of mosquitoes [200–203, 365], we limit the *speed* of movement to one cell per hour, and the *perception range* to be the eight adjacent (neighboring) cells of the focal/current cell (in effect, implementing a *Moore neighborhood*). Each gravid female may travel one cell per hour and reach one out of eight possible neighboring cells or remain in the current cell. The maximum distance that an agent may travel in a day is controlled by a *movement counter*, which is reset to 5 at the beginning of each day for a moving agent (thus, the counter controls the maximum daily range of movement, which translates to $250\sqrt[2]{2}m$).

To model the resource-seeking events in the spatial ABM, we replace the probability-based measures used in the nonspatial ABM by spatial, distance-based measures. For example, the 25% probability of finding a resource site (in the nonspatial model, see Chapter 5) is replaced by specifying the adult female mosquito's speed of movement as well as the density distributions of the resources in the corresponding landscape.

We pay special attention in modeling oviposition. As mentioned in Chapter 3, oviposition is one potential factor explaining heterogeneous biting and vector distribution in a landscape with a heterogeneous distribution of habitats; female mosquitoes tend to aggregate around places where they oviposit, thereby increasing the risk of malaria there, regardless of the suitability of the habitat for larval development [360]. Thus, even if an aquatic habitat is unsuitable for mosquito emergence, it can be a significant source for malaria.

The movement activities for both stages are depicted in the form of flowcharts in Fig. 6.6. In the *BMS* stage, the mosquito looks for human houses and the search continues until it successfully finds a house. In the *G* stage, the mosquito looks for an aquatic habitat, and once found, lays the eggs. The number of eggs it can lay is governed by the density-dependent oviposition rules (see Section 4.4 for details).

The flight heuristics are presented in a more detailed level in the form of flowcharts in Fig. 6.7 and are described below.[15] The host-seeking event starts when a female adult mosquito agent enters the *BMS* stage and searches for a human blood meal in a house. If the current cell contains a house, it immediately gets a blood meal and enters the *BMD* stage to digest the meal, rest, generate new eggs, and eventually enter the *G* stage to search for an aquatic habitat (if the current cell contains multiple houses, one is chosen

---

[15]Simulation results that are affected by the flight heuristics are presented in Chapter 9.

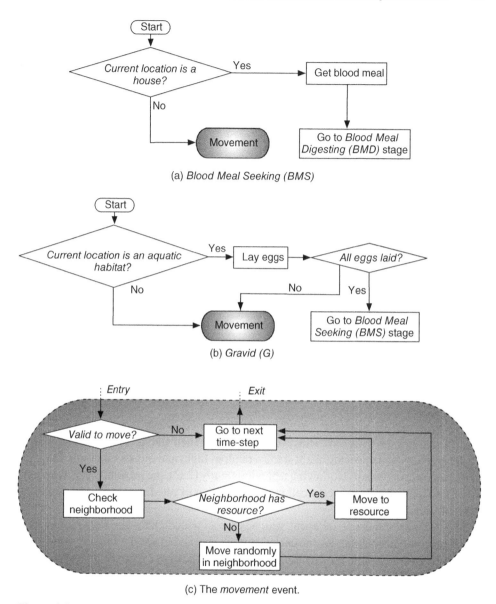

(a) *Blood Meal Seeking (BMS)*

(b) *Gravid (G)*

(c) The *movement* event.

Figure 6.6 Foraging event for mosquito agents. (a) Agent movement in *Blood Meal Seeking (BMS)* stage. (b) Agent movement in *Gravid (G)* stage. (c) The *movement* event. Updated from Arifin *et al.* [28] and used under a Creative Commons Attribution 4.0 International License.

at random). If the current cell does not contain any house, a new search event starts as follows. First, the agent's *movement counter* is checked. If the agent is permitted to move, its *Moore* neighborhood M is checked. If M contains multiple cells that have houses, a random cell C (from these cells) is selected, and the agent moves to cell C. If cell C contains multiple houses, a random house is selected, the agent gets a blood

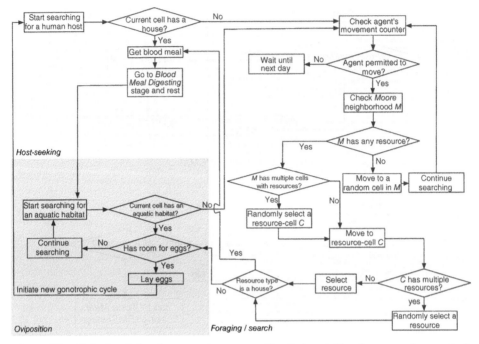

Figure 6.7 Flight heuristics for mosquito agents. Detailed activities by mosquito agents in host-seeking, oviposition, and foraging/search are shown. Updated from Arifin *et al.* [20] and used under a Creative Commons Attribution 4.0 International License.

meal, and continues as before. However, if the current cell and its *Moore* neighborhood do not contain any house, the agent starts a random flight and moves randomly into one of the adjacent eight cells (following a previous study [222], the probability of a random move into a diagonally adjacent cell is set as half that of moving into a horizontally or vertically adjacent cell).

In an oviposition event, an agent searches for an aquatic habitat. If the current cell contains an aquatic habitat, its current capacity is checked to see if it has any remaining capacity for new eggs, in which case, the agent lays the eggs (again, if the current cell contains multiple aquatic habitats, one is chosen at random). New agents, in the form of eggs, possess the same spatial locations as that of the aquatic habitat in which they are oviposited. Once all of the eggs are laid, it goes to the *BMS* stage, thus initiating a new gonotrophic cycle. Otherwise, it either remains in the same aquatic habitat or searches for another one to lay the remaining eggs, and this process continues until all eggs are laid. If the current cell does not contain any aquatic habitat, the search continues in the same manner as described above.

As evident from the above, in case of a directional flight, if multiple resources (houses or aquatic habitats) are found within a single cell, a random resource is selected. Note that this strategy can be easily extended/modified for future work to select a resource based on some preference criterion, for example, to select the house that has the fewest number of mosquitoes visited or to select the aquatic habitat that has the largest remaining capacity.

6.5 SIMULATION RESULTS

In this section, we present results of some initial simulation runs that use the spatial ABM and compare vector abundances as outputs.[16] We assume the following notation (for details about the terminology, see Section 6.2.1): AH denotes an aquatic habitat; HC denotes individual capacity of an aquatic habitat; CHC denotes the combined habitat capacity; VA denotes vector abundance; $density_{aquatic\_habitats}$ and $density_{houses}$ denote the densities of aquatic habitats and houses in a landscape, respectively. The x-axis denotes simulation time (in days), and the y-axis denotes VA. We refer to a specific graph in a figure by its corresponding legend entry (e.g., Spatial, 50%). Simulations are run for at least 1 year with 1000 initial adult mosquitoes and no initial eggs in any aquatic habitat.[17] In most cases, we present only relevant portions of the 1-year results.

In Section 6.5.1, we compare the results from the nonspatial and spatial ABMs by modeling one of the resource-seeking events (oviposition) in two different ways. In Section 6.5.2, using the spatial ABM, we compare vector abundance with two different landscapes. Sections 6.5.3 and 6.5.4 present results of varying the relative size and density of the aquatic habitats, respectively, with landscapes that all have the same combined habitat capacity (CHC). Lastly, Section 6.5.5 reports results of varying the overall capacity of the system by gradually increasing CHC.

6.5.1 Model Verification

In this section, we report the results of model verification by comparing outputs of the nonspatial model to the spatial model.[18] Model verification requires iterative evaluations of the corresponding ABMs. As we perform iterative refinements in several phases, the ABMs successively produce *more* similar outputs that are in increasing agreement among themselves. The close agreement in model verification results between the nonspatial and spatial ABMs as well as between different but comparable scenarios of the spatial ABM itself reflects successful model verification scenarios performed on the ABMs. This also rules out the effects of any potential inadvertent biases that may have been introduced by poor experimental or setup design in obtaining similar outputs from the ABMs.

As mentioned before, oviposition was modeled with 25% probability of success in each hour of searching in the nonspatial ABM (the value of 25% was chosen as

---

[16]Results of applying malaria control interventions are described in Chapter 9.

[17]All time units related to the simulation runs refer to *simulated time* as opposed to *physical time* or *wall clock time*; thus, a 1-*year* run indicates a virtual simulation run within the computer that represents an imitation of operations in the real world for the same time duration.

[18]For details about model verification by docking between several implementations of the nonspatial ABMs, see Chapter 8.

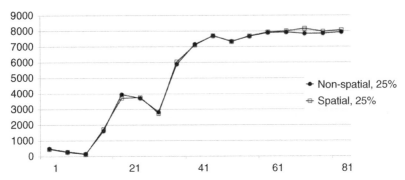

Figure 6.8   Model verification results. Both the nonspatial and the spatial ABMs yield consistent results with identical parameter settings. Each graph represents the average of 40 simulation runs and shows only relevant portions of the 1-year simulation results. Used from Arifin *et al.* [26]. Reprinted by permission of the publisher.

a baseline and should not be treated as absolute). The spatial ABM, on the other hand, replaces this by specifying the precise flight heuristics (see Section 6.4) and the speed of movement of the adult female mosquito agent, as well as the density distributions of the habitats in the corresponding landscape. Figure 6.8 shows the results of modeling oviposition in two different ways: *probability* based in the nonspatial model and *distance* based in the spatial model. Twenty-five percent $density_{aquatic\_habitats}$ is used in both cases. Each graph represents the average of 40 simulation runs and shows only relevant portions of the 1-year simulation results. With identical settings for other parameters, both ABMs yield consistent results.

6.5.2   Landscape Patterns

To explore the effects of using different landscape patterns, *regular* and *random* patterns are used for the spatial ABM. We use the same number (100) and density (25%) of aquatic habitats and the same *CHC* for both landscapes. As shown in Fig. 6.9, in these settings, different landscape patterns do not significantly affect the mean (stabilized) abundance (≈ 8000).

Note that this experiment uses relatively small landscapes (all of which have dimensions 20×20) and relatively high resource densities (25% densities of aquatic habitats). As a result, statistically similar results were obtained for both landscape patterns. With relatively larger landscapes having relatively lower resource densities, this may change due to the different, more *sparse* distributions of the resources. The spatial heterogeneity may in turn yield radically different abundances in those larger landscapes. For example, a 100×100 random landscape with only 5% $density_{aquatic\_habitats}$ will contain some isolated aquatic habitats having none or very few houses within their proximities. In this case, VA_{random} is expected to be much lower than $VA_{regular}$, since the agents originating from these isolated aquatic habitats will need to travel much further to find houses in the random landscape.

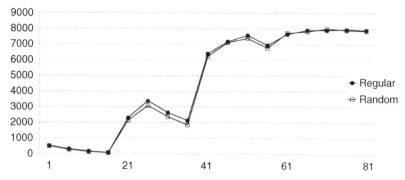

Figure 6.9 Results of using different landscape patterns. In the spatial ABM, the use of *regular* and *random* landscape patterns does not significantly alter the population levels. Each graph represents the average of 40 simulation runs and shows only relevant portions of the 1-year simulation results. Used from Arifin *et al.* [26]. Reprinted by permission of the publisher.

6.5.3 Relative Sizes of Resources

To explore the effects of relative sizes of resources, the relative sizes of the aquatic habitats in landscapes are varied in both the nonspatial and spatial ABMs. However, it is ensured that these landscapes have the same overall capacities (*CHC*). Recall that in the core model, the size of an aquatic habitat can be approximated by its capacity *HC* (see Section 4.4). For the spatial ABM, we use landscapes composed of one large aquatic habitat versus many smaller aquatic habitats. Different cases are constructed by increasing the numbers of aquatic habitats as squares of the first 10 integers (1−10) and using the same *density$_{aquatic\_habitats}$* for all cases in the nonspatial and the spatial ABMs. Figure 6.10 compares the results for 1 and 16 aquatic habitats, and Fig. 6.11 compares the results for 49 and 100 aquatic habitats (other results show similar trends).

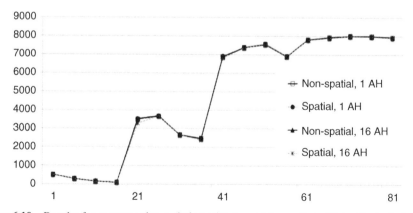

Figure 6.10 Results for resource size variation with 1 and 16 aquatic habitats. For both the non-spatial and the spatial models, the numbers of aquatic habitats are increased as squares of the first 10 integers. This figure shows *VA* with landscapes having 1 and 16 aquatic habitats. Used from Arifin *et al.* [26]. Reprinted by permission of the publisher.

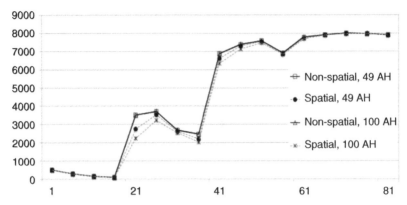

Figure 6.11 Results for resource size variation with 49 and 100 aquatic habitats. For both the non-spatial and the spatial models, the numbers of aquatic habitats are increased as squares of the first 10 integers. This figure shows *VA* with landscapes having 49 and 100 aquatic habitats. Used from Arifin *et al.* [26]. Reprinted by permission of the publisher.

As the average *VA* levels approach $\approx$8000, it becomes evident that once *CHC* is kept constant, *VA* does not change significantly if the numbers of aquatic habitats are varied. In addition, we find that a larger capacity aquatic habitat may produce and sustain *n* times adult population than the *per-AH* adult population produced by each of the *n* smaller aquatic habitats.

In Fig. 6.11, we also find that until the systems reach equilibrium (after the initial burn-in of the simulations), the nonspatial ABM ($VA_{Non-spatial,49AH}$ and $VA_{Non-spatial,100AH}$) always have equal or higher abundances than the spatial ABM ($VA_{Spatial,49AH}$ and $VA_{Spatial,100AH}$). This can be attributed to the travel time required by adult female mosquito agents. In the spatial ABM, the agents need to search for resource sites, incurring additional time delays to complete the host-seeking and oviposition events. Thus, the spatial ABM produces less abundances than the nonspatial ABM (in which agents do not require to travel in space to complete these events, as explained in Chapter 5). As the simulations continue after equilibrium, new aquatic agents (eggs, larvae, and pupae) cause the aquatic habitats to gradually become more full. As a result, the competition perceived by a gravid female agent to lay its eggs also increases, as governed by Eqs. (4.8), (4.9), and (4.11) of the core model (see Section 4.4). However, this does not impact the overall capacity of the system, which is already in equilibrium and hence has a steady, saturated flow of newly emerged adult agents from the aquatic habitats. Thus, after equilibrium, the models produce similar outputs.

6.5.4 Resource Density

To explore the effects of relative densities of resources, density of a single resource type (aquatic habitat) is varied in the spatial ABM. Using 10×10 hybrid landscapes with the same *CHC* of 100*K*, *VA* is compared with varying numbers of aquatic habitats.

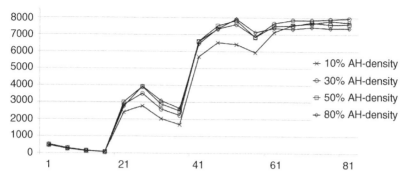

Figure 6.12   Results for resource density variation. This figure shows the effects of varying $density_{aquatic\_habitats}$ by increasing the number of *AHs* within the same 10×10 hybrid landscape. Each graph represents the average of 40 simulation runs and shows only relevant portions of the 1-year simulation results. Used from Arifin *et al.* [26]. Reprinted by permission of the publisher.

Note that in this setting, as the number of aquatic habitats increases in a landscape, its $density_{aquatic\_habitats}$ also increases. The numbers of aquatic habitats are increased from 10 to 80 in increments of 10. Figure 6.12 depicts selected results of varying resource density. For 10, 30, 50, and 80% cases, varying the $density_{aquatic\_habitats}$ does not significantly affect the average agent populations when the overall capacity *CHC* is unchanged (other results show similar trends).

We also note two interesting observations in Fig. 6.12:

- At around day 60 (until the populations reach equilibrium), $VA_{10\%}$ is less than $VA_{30\%}$, $VA_{50\%}$, and $VA_{80\%}$: In this case, due to lower $density_{aquatic\_habitats}$, average travel time *ATT* increases and becomes a limiting factor. For example, on the average, a gravid female agent may need to search many more cells in $VA_{10\%}$ to find a resource than in the other three higher density cases. Thus, less number of female agents may lay eggs in $VA_{10\%}$.

- After day 60 (after equilibrium), $VA_{30\%} > VA_{50\%} > VA_{80\%}$: As $density_{aquatic\_habitats}$ increases, both *HC* (per *AH*) and *ATT* decrease. However, even though a gravid female agent finds more frequent opportunities to visit aquatic habitats with increasing densities, it is also more restricted to lay eggs (see Eq. (4.11)). Thus, for an individual agent, *ATT* no longer remains a limiting factor in successfully finding a habitat and the smaller capacities of larger number of *AHs* dominate in restricting the abundances.

6.5.5   Combined Habitat Capacity (*CHC*)

Lastly, using 25% $density_{aquatic\_habitats}$, the overall capacity of a simulation is varied in 10×10 random landscapes in the spatial ABM. As shown in Fig. 6.13, the overall capacity *CHC* indeed drives abundance in all cases; as *CHCs* are gradually increased from $10K$ to $80K$, average *VAs* increase at a steady rate.

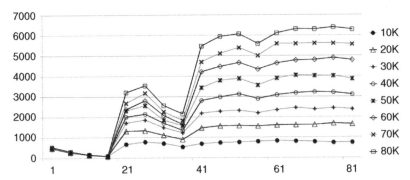

Figure 6.13 Results for system capacity variation. Using 10×10 hybrid landscapes, the system capacity *CHC* is gradually increased from $10K$ to $80K$. Each graph represents the average of 40 simulation runs and shows only relevant portions of the 1-year simulation results. Used from Arifin *et al.* [26]. Reprinted by permission of the publisher.

The first few dips in adult female agent populations in Figs. 6.8–6.13 can be attributed as artifacts of the *warm-up* periods of individual simulation runs.[19] As depicted in these figures, the first dip (at around days 10–15) is due to the deaths of the initial cohort of adult agents that entered the simulation system with the same initial age. The second dip (at around days 25–30) is due to the deaths of the first cohort of surviving adult agents (that emerged from the aquatic habitats in the *Immature Adult* stage, see Fig. 4.1), followed by a population-level rise caused by the next cohort. As the systems (represented by individual simulation runs) approach steady states, the subsequent dips diminish successively in magnitude and reflect the deaths and emergences of subsequent cohorts of adult agents.

6.6 SPATIAL HETEROGENEITY

In this section, we discuss some of the aspects of spatial heterogeneity, which encompasses the distributions and relative distances between various resources of both resource types (aquatic habitats and houses) sought by the adult female mosquito agents in a landscape. In some cases, spatial heterogeneity may directly influence the mosquito population levels, as shown by some of the results.

Spatial heterogeneity is controlled by two parameters: resource density and resource distribution of each resource type. To analyze how resource density affects abundance, we use landscapes with different resource densities and with varying *CHC*s. For this section, we denote each landscape by the tuple ($num_{habitats}$, num_{houses}, and *CHC*), where $num_{habitats}$ and num_{houses} denote the number of aquatic habitats and houses in the landscape, respectively.

In the spatial ABM, *VA* is eventually driven by two parameters: (1) *ATT* and (2) *CHC*. *ATT* is inversely proportional to densities of resources. Since female

[19] In M&S literature, the *warm-up* period is also known as the *burn-in* period.

mosquito agents must travel through the landscape in order to search for resources, *ATT* can increase or decrease with decreasing or increasing resource densities, respectively. For example, considering two hypothetical landscapes L_{sparse} and L_{dense} (having the same dimensions), where L_{dense} has more resource densities than L_{sparse}, agents in L_{sparse} would incur higher *ATT* than that incurred in L_{dense}. For an individual mosquito agent, this translates to the degree of ease with which the agent may find resources. As resource densities are increased in these landscapes, *ATT* gradually declines until resource densities reach critical thresholds, which are termed as the *critical resource densities*. Until a landscape possesses enough resources to reach this critical threshold, the abundance depends on both resource density and *CHC*. The less is the resource density, the higher is the *ATT*, and vice versa. When the resource density exceeds the critical threshold, *ATT* may no longer impact the agent's resource-seeking behavior. On the other hand, if a landscape possesses enough resources at or above the critical resource densities, abundance is driven primarily by *CHC* and does not change significantly until *CHC* is changed.

Although we did not empirically measure the average travel times or the critical resource densities for different landscapes, some preliminary simulation results confirm to the above insights, as described below. Starting with landscapes that all possess resource densities at or above the critical level, we found that as the resource densities of both resource types are increased (keeping the same landscape dimensions and the same *CHC*), abundance remains unchanged until the *CHC* is changed. For example, using 10×10 landscapes with $20K$ *CHC* each, $(10, 10, 20K)$, $(10, 20, 20K)$, $(20, 10, 20K)$, and $(20, 20, 20K)$ all yield the same *VAs* of ≈ 3000. Abundance, in these cases, is primarily controlled by *CHC*, and increasing the resource densities by increasing the number of resources (e.g., from 10 to 20 *AHs*) does not impact *VA* in these landscapes, which already had resource densities above the critical level. As *CHC* is increased to $40K$, abundance (≈ 6000) is still controlled by *CHC* and not by resource densities in landscapes $(20, 10, 40K)$ and $(20, 20, 40K)$.

Given these preliminary results with relatively smaller landscapes, we explored the effect of resource densities in a larger landscape (of dimension 30×30) with resource densities *below* and *above* the critical thresholds. The landscapes are shown in Fig. 6.14, in which each black circle represents an aquatic habitat and each gray rectangle represents a house. Figure 6.14a shows a landscape with 50 *AHs* and 20 houses with resource densities *below* the critical level, and Fig. 6.14b shows a landscape with 100 *AHs* and 100 houses with resource densities *above* the critical level. The landscapes are generated using the landscape generator software tool *AnophGUI*. Figures 6.15 and 6.16 depict the results that are produced using these landscapes.

In the case with resource densities *below* the critical level, as $density_{aquatic\_habitats}$ is increased (keeping $density_{houses}$ and *CHC* unchanged at 20 and $30K$, respectively), *VA* increases and eventually reaches ≈ 4500, as shown in Fig. 6.15. This supports the first part of our previous claim: as resource density is kept below the critical level, *ATT* gradually declines and *VA* successively increases. Two other observations are also made from Fig. 6.15: (1) with higher resource density cases, the rate of rise in *VA* is

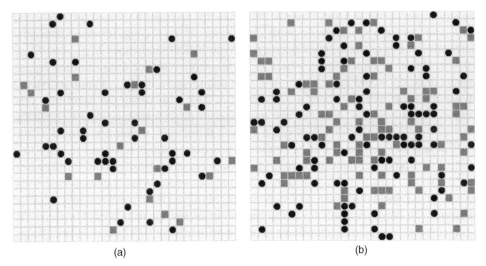

Figure 6.14 Sample 30 × 30 landscapes. (a) A landscape with resource densities *below* the critical level. (b) A landscape with resource densities *above* the critical level. Used from Arifin *et al.* [26]. Reprinted by permission of the publisher.

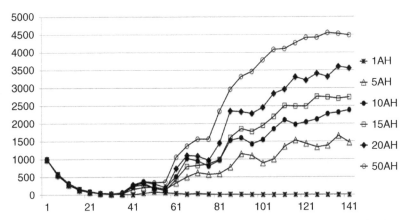

Figure 6.15 Results for resource density *below* the critical level. *VA* in a 30 × 30 landscape with 30*K CHC* and resource density *below* the critical level. Each graph represents the average of 40 simulation runs and shows only relevant portions of the 1-year simulation results. Used from Arifin *et al.* [26]. Reprinted by permission of the publisher.

always faster and (2) when a single aquatic habitat is present, the agent population dies out because it is too inadequate to sustain a population within the relatively larger dimensions of the landscape.

The case with resource densities *above* the critical level is explored next to investigate whether higher density of both resource types affects the upper limits of agent populations within the same landscape. As the results depict in Fig. 6.16, all cases with higher resource densities reach equilibrium with *VA* ≈4500. This supports the

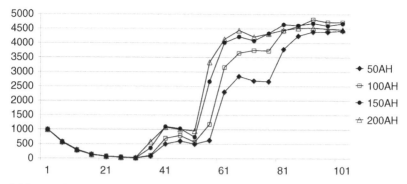

Figure 6.16   Results for resource density *above* the critical level. *VA* in a 30 × 30 landscape with 30*K CHC* and resource density *above* the critical level. Each graph represents the average of 40 simulation runs and shows only relevant portions of the 1-year simulation results. Updated and used from Arifin *et al.* [26]. Reprinted by permission of the publisher.

second part of our previous claim: as resource density is increased above the critical level (keeping the same dimensions and the same *CHC*), *VA* remains unchanged and is eventually limited by *CHC*. However, as shown in Fig. 6.16, since female mosquito agents are able to find resources more frequently in the higher resource density cases, the rate of rise in abundances after the second dips (between 45 and 76 days) is always faster.

6.7   SUMMARY

In this chapter, we presented a spatial extension of our previous nonspatial ABM. We described the spatial ABM in detail, including the mosquito agents, their spatial movement (regulated by flight heuristics), and the landscapes in which they move. Two versions of the landscape generator software tools were also presented and several resource clustering schemes were described with examples. We also discussed simulation results that examined preliminary model verification between the nonspatial and the spatial ABMs, the effects of varying the landscape patterns, the relative size and density of the aquatic habitats, and the overall capacity of the system. Lastly, we demonstrated the effects of spatial heterogeneity of the landscapes on agent populations. The spatial extension provided unique opportunities to investigate the effects of these spatial factors.

In the next chapter, we review and summarize some important contributions in verification, validation, and replication issues of ABMs, which in general deal with the measurement and assessment of accuracy of M&S research.

7

VERIFICATION, VALIDATION, REPLICATION, AND REPRODUCIBILITY

7.1 OVERVIEW

In modeling and simulation (M&S) research, verification and validation (V&V) processes are conducted during the development of a simulation model with the ultimate goal of producing an accurate and credible model [49, 481]. Quoting the popular aphorism in statistics, *"essentially, all models are wrong, but some are useful"*, which is generally attributed to the statistician George Box [78], the correctness of a model is crucially important for the developers, users, decision makers, and other individuals who are affected by decisions based on the model. Since simulation models are approximations of their real-world counterparts, they cannot exactly imitate the real-world system. Hence, a model's correctness should be confirmed to the degree needed for the model's intended purpose or application [474]. To this end, V&V, accreditation, quality assurance (QA), certification, replication and reproducibility (R&R), acceptability assessment, and uncertainty quantification are generally considered critical steps. If these steps are not properly conducted, there can be little trust in the insights and predictions generated by a simulation study. The importance and implications of these steps in M&S research have long been recognized [396–399, 403, 404, 406, 407].

Over the last decade, a multitude of techniques has been used to perform V&V as well as R&R of the agent-based models (ABMs), and reproducible M&S research has been identified as one of the M&S Grand Challenge activities [526]. While methods

Spatial Agent-Based Simulation Modeling in Public Health:
Design, Implementation, and Applications for Malaria Epidemiology, First Edition.
S. M. Niaz Arifin, Gregory R. Madey and Frank H. Collins.
© 2016 John Wiley & Sons, Inc. Published 2016 by John Wiley & Sons, Inc.

for V&V have been widely developed for discrete-event simulations, newer simulation approaches such as the agent-based, agent-directed, and multiagent simulation approaches introduced new V&V challenges.

In this chapter, we review and summarize some important contributions in V&V, QA, and R&R of simulation studies, with special focus on ABMs.[1] These essentially form the basis and act as a guide for our V&V and R&R results, which are described in the next two chapters (Chapters 8 and 9). Some commonly used methodologies and general techniques used for the assessment of accuracy of M&S research described in this and the next two chapters are alphabetically listed in Table 7.1.

The organization of this chapter is as follows. In Section 7.2, we review some of the earlier V&V works that involve advanced simulation methodologies, acceptability assessment of simulation studies, categorizations, taxonomies, and applications of M&S, and other areas of V&V and QA. Section 7.3 discusses some important R&R works, and Section 7.4 concludes.

7.2   VERIFICATION AND VALIDATION (V&V): A REVIEW

Many of the pioneering research in V&V were conducted by eminent M&S researchers such as Tuncer Ören, Osman Balci, and Levent Yilmaz. Some of the important works are discussed in the following sections.

7.2.1   Acceptability Assessment and Quality Assurance (QA)

Acceptability and credibility assessment, model reliability, and quality assurance (QA) are closely related to credibility of simulation studies, validation of models, and verification of simulation programs. Ören proposed a framework for assessing the acceptability of simulation studies which permitted the discussion of the concepts and criteria related to the acceptability of various components of a simulation study [396, 397]. The framework facilitated the analysis of simulation components such as simulation results, real-world and simulated data, parametric model, values of model parameters, experimentation specification, computer program representation and execution, modeling techniques, simulation techniques, and programming methodologies. The acceptability issues were described in detail in a highly cited paper by Ören with respect to the goal of simulation study, structure and data of the real system, parametric model, model parameter set, specification of the experimentation, norms of modeling methodology, experimentation technique, simulation methodology, software engineering and so on [397]. Ören discussed cognizant techniques such as perception, interpretation, goal-setting, and learning in simulative design, presented a glossary of QA terms [400]. Ören also described artificial intelligence (AI) concepts for M&S in different categories, including simulation environments, simulation models (models having time-varying structures, goal-directed models, models having perception

---

[1]Portions of the text in this chapter appeared in Arifin and Madey [21].

TABLE 7.1   Methodologies and Techniques Commonly Used for V&V in M&S Research

Methodology/ Technique	Definition/Interpretation/Goal	Synonymous Terms	References
Acceptability assessment	The official certification that a model, simulation, or federation of models and simulations is acceptable for use for a specific purpose	Accreditation, certification, credibility assessment	[39, 43, 45, 47, 397]
Calibration	The process of fitting a model to the observed data by adjusting the parameters; the investigation of potential changes and errors and their impacts on conclusions to be drawn from the model	Parameter estimation, parameter fitting, sensitivity analysis, uncertainty quantification	[63, 128, 224, 241, 277, 419, 541, 549]
Docking	A form of V&V that tries to align multiple models in order to investigate whether they yield similar results	Alignment, equivalence testing, model-to-model comparison	[22, 24, 35, 37, 89, 187]
Quality assurance	Ensuring that an M&S application possesses a desired set of characteristics to match a desired degree of quality	Quality assessment	[46, 399, 402, 448]
Replication	To allow independent researchers to address scientific hypotheses in a model and produce evidence for or against them in order to judge the scientific claims presented by the model	Alignment, cross-model validation, model-to-model comparison	[187, 263, 428, 530]
Reproducibility	The ability to independently verify, replicate, reproduce, and/or extend the prior findings reported by an established/published model		[184, 187, 472, 530]
Verification	The assessment of transformational accuracy of the model by addressing the question of "are we creating the model *right*?"		[40, 43, 45, 46, 47, 385, 473, 474]
Validation	The assessment of behavioral or representational accuracy of the model by addressing the question of "are we creating the *right* model?"		[40, 43, 45, 46, 47, 385, 473, 474]

The last column lists important references for each methodology.

abilities, and behaviorally anticipatory models), simulation query systems, machine learning in simulation, and simulation in computer-embedded machines [401, 402].

Ören listed a set of questions and meta-questions relevant to QA of system design for complex problems under six categories: (1) problem and problem solving paradigms, (2) goals, (3) performance measures, (4) decision and its components, (5) system, and (6) resources [398, 399]. He also presented a basis for the taxonomy of concepts related with QA in M&S, which included three major parts: (1) criteria for assessment, (2) types of assessments, and (3) a comprehensive categorized list of related terms [399].

In general, many applications in diverse research fields used the ideas related to acceptability assessment. For example, Ören *et al.* [404] offered M&S frameworks to clarify issues of model reliability and software QA for various types of errors that can be generated by simulations of nuclear fuel waste management programs, identifying potential problems with respect to reliability and quality concern such as decomposition, scope, fidelity, requirements, testing, correctness, and robustness, etc., and provided a list of the most common computerization errors [404]. Holmes discussed expert systems in AI and simulation for chemical process control, ocean surveillance, aircraft pilotage, scientific knowledge transfer, syntax programming, and real-time fault diagnosis [246]. Several simulation models which combined techniques from AI and M&S were discussed by Kim (ed.) [290]. Gupta *et al.* presented automatic calibration for hydrologic models, and compared those with multilevel expert calibration models [224]. Aarons *et al.* discussed QA issues in an early clinical drug development phase for pharmacokinetic (pharmacodynamic) M&S [1]. Refsgaard *et al.* classified QA guidelines for water management models, reviewed existing practices, and outlined new approaches [448].

Ören [403] discussed the professional *codes of ethics* in domains that are relevant to M&S, including science, engineering, business, computerization, software engineering, AI, software agents, the Internet, and defense industries. In order to promote the credibility and integrity of simulation as a field itself, he discussed a set of important philosophical questions related to simulation and ethics [403]. Defining the concept of *normative assessment* of simulation elements, Ören *et al.* proposed codes of ethics for simulation professionals, covering areas such as personal development and the profession, professional competence, trustworthiness, property rights and due credit, and compliance with the code [281, 405, 497]. Higdon *et al.* developed a statistical approach for characterizing uncertainty in predictions made by a simulation model [241].

7.2.2 Verification and Validation (V&V)

The general concepts of verification, validation, docking, testing, accreditation, and certification activities primarily deal with the measurement and assessment of accuracy of M&S [22–24, 43, 44, 385, 406, 474]. Verification involves transformational accuracy of the model artifacts in model development, in order to ensure that the implementation is a correct realization of the conceptual model [22, 23, 385]. Validation, on the other hand, involves substantiation that a model within its domain of applicability possesses a satisfactory range of accuracy consistent with its intended application [22, 23, 385]. In this section, we describe some of the previous works involving V&V, failure avoidance (FA), docking, alignment, and model-to-model comparison.

Balci presented a quality model for assessing the quality of large-scale complex M&S applications as integrated with V&V [46]. Balci *et al.* argued that certification of sufficient accuracy of M&S applications by conducting verification, validation, and accreditation (VV&A) requires multifaceted knowledge and experience that poses substantial technical and managerial challenges for researchers, practitioners, and managers, and proposed a simulation quality assurance (SQA) group for the success of a simulation study [40–44, 47]. Ören and Yilmaz [406] identified various sources of failures in order to take necessary precautions to minimize the risks associated with ABM and agent-directed simulation (ADS), and suggested new FA paradigms for V&V as well as QA.

Axtell *et al.* described the docking process of the Axelrod and Sugarscape models [35, 37]. After attaining docking of the two models, they used the richer set of mechanisms of the Sugarscape model to provide two experiments in sensitivity analysis for the cultural rule of Axelrod's model, and suggested that it could be beneficial if alignment and equivalence testing were more widely practiced among M&S modelers. Later, Galan and Izquierdo tried to replicate the simulation results reported by Axelrod on the evolution of social norms, eventually showing the importance of running stochastic simulations several times for longer time periods and exploring the parameter space adequately [187].

Sargent discussed different approaches and paradigms of V&V for the model development process using graphical data statistical references for operational validity [473]. Carley described the importance of docking in computational social and organizational science, and the relation of models to empirical data and characteristics of necessary infrastructure [91]. North and Macal implemented the Beer game using Mathematica, Repast, and Swarm, reproducing (i.e., docking) published results with the new implementations [384]. Burton argued that docking provides a guide in use of different computational laboratories to address organization questions [89]. Xu *et al.* discussed the results of docking a Repast simulation and a Java/Swarm simulation of social network models of the Open Source Software (OSS) community [573]. Edmonds and Hales replicated a published model involving cooperation between self-interested agents in two independent implementations to align the results and the conceptual design [164].

By using model-to-model comparison (docking), Xiang *et al.* demonstrated the V&V processes for a natural organic matter simulation model [251, 572]. Kennedy *et al.* presented V&V results involving two different case studies (a scientific model and an economic model), identifying general guidelines on the best approach to new simulation experiments and drawing conclusions on effective V&V techniques [278, 279]. Troitzsch discussed aspects of validating simulation models that are designed to describe, explain, and predict real-world phenomena [544]. Yilmaz described a process-centric perspective for the V&V of agent-based computational organization models, presenting a framework for the V&V of multiagent organizations and a set of formal validation metrics to substantiate the operational validity of emergent macro-level behavior [576].

7.3   REPLICATION AND REPRODUCIBILITY (R&R): A REVIEW

Replication and reproducibility (R&R) cover a wide spectrum of issues related to M&S. Like docking, R&R fall under the broader subject area of V&V. Many replication tasks may be viewed as a weaker form of docking, in which the goal of the modeler is to qualitatively (as opposed to quantitatively) replicate the results of previously published models. In the following, we describe some of the early and recent works involving R&R.

Replication is treated as the scientific gold standard to judge scientific claims. It allows independent researchers to address a scientific hypothesis and produce evidence for or against it [263, 428]. The importance, role, and potential for replication have been demonstrated in almost every branch of science, such as sociology and social sciences [123, 374], biology [312], epidemiology [239], economics [151, 227, 272], management [252], psychology [493], scientific discovery processes [444], scientific collaborations [110], information systems research [282], scientific study of religion [292], educational research [482], and many more. Replication exercises can also provide unique opportunities for V&V processes [585].

Reproducibility is another closely related issue that is confirmed by replication. It refers to the independent verification of prior findings and is at the core of the spirit of science [313, 471, 472]. As a fundamental principle of the scientific method, reproducibility refers to the ability to independently replicate, reproduce, and, if needed, extend computational artifacts associated with published work [184, 515]. Although computational science has led to exciting new developments, the nature of the work has also exposed shortcomings in the general ability of the research community to evaluate published findings [428, 515].

In M&S, goal-directed reproducible experimentation with simulation models is still a significant challenge [530]. As the use of computer simulation is becoming increasingly important, lack of proper documentation, validation, and distribution of models may hamper reproducibility, causing a credibility gap [577, 580]. Replicability of the *in silico* experiments and simulations performed by various published models bear special importance in order to minimize this credibility gap [28].[2]

Rand and Wilensky presented a case study that replicated the Axelrod-Hammond model; they showed that aligning the order of events lowered the variance of another model, causing the replicated model to be in statistical agreement with the original model; they also described the challenges in recreating the model and in determining whether the replication was successful [447, 562]. Pavón et al. proposed the use of agent-based graphical modeling languages to allow replication of simulations on

---

[2]See Chapter 9 for results of replicating published malaria models.

different platforms [424]. Rouchier et al. described advancements in model-to-model analysis [462]. Olaru *et al.* described the docking experience and validation stages performed when replicating a fuzzy logic model with an ABM [392]. Will and Hegselmann showed the importance of replication by reporting a failure to replicate the results presented on a published model [564].

Yilmaz emphasized that since science is a collective phenomenon, progress in simulation-based science requires the ability of scientists to create new knowledge, elaborate and combine prior computational artifacts, and establish analogy and metaphor across models [577]. Thus, models that are not designed and disseminated to be discovered, extended, or combined with other models may hinder scientific progress [577–579]. He suggested a set of guidelines for the authors, publishers, funding agencies, journals, and the broader scientific community, including (1) availability of links to data, source code, standard documentation, and experimental conditions, (2) open-source repositories and openly accessible simulations, (3) version control systems, (4) automated model documentation tools, and (5) annotation technologies and standard notation for metadata. Yilmaz also suggested other guidelines to promote reproducibility, such as (1) preference being given to highly qualified proposals with transparent and online scientific workflows, (2) incentives being provided to research groups for developing shared artifacts for reproducibility, and (3) maintaining and using a classification system of reproducibility categories (e.g., verifiable, verified, annotated, shared) [577].

Yilmaz identified issues, strategies, and implications for three dimensions (scholarly communication, methodology of scientific practice, and technical infrastructure dimensions for simulation model development) of simulation research, proposed a multidimensional software framework for establishing and maintaining open M&S platforms, and recommended systematic guidelines with regard to legitimization, dissemination, and access dimensions for authors and institutional environments [578, 579]. Yilmaz and Ören also introduced the *e-Portfolio* concept as an ensemble of integrated active documents that encompass published manuscript, computer code, data, and scientific workflow specification [578–580].

7.4 SUMMARY

This chapter presented a brief overview and literature review of some of the critical steps in the M&S research, including V&V, accreditation, quality assurance (QA), certification, replication and reproducibility (R&R), acceptability assessment, and uncertainty quantification. Our contributions on some of these steps (especially V&V and R&R) are described in the next two chapters (Chapters 8 and 9) with respect to the biological core model of *An. gambiae* and the ABMs that were described in Chapters 4–6.

8

VERIFICATION AND VALIDATION (V&V) OF ABMs

8.1 OVERVIEW

In Chapter 7, we presented an overview of some of the critical steps in the modeling and simulation (M&S) research, including verification and validation (V&V) and replication and reproducibility (R&R).[1] In this chapter, we discuss our V&V experiences from a series of simulations performed during the development phases of the ABMs described in Chapters 5 and 6.[2]

This chapter is organized as follows. Section 8.2 introduces our V&V experiences with ABMs by categorizing these into two parts, based on the *phase-wise docking* and the *compartmental docking* paradigms. Details of these paradigms, including the V&V results, are presented in Sections 8.3 and 8.4. Section 8.5 concludes with a summary.

8.2 VERIFICATION AND VALIDATION (V&V) OF ABMS

Assessing the credibility of complex simulation models can be challenging. In M&S research, V&V techniques are used to determine whether the model is an accurate

---

[1]R&R, which fall under the broader subject area of V&V, are discussed in Chapter 9 along with the results of replicating other published malaria models.
[2]Portions of this chapter appeared in Arifin *et al.* [23, 22].

Spatial Agent-Based Simulation Modeling in Public Health:
Design, Implementation, and Applications for Malaria Epidemiology, First Edition.
S. M. Niaz Arifin, Gregory R. Madey and Frank H. Collins.
© 2016 John Wiley & Sons, Inc. Published 2016 by John Wiley & Sons, Inc.

representation of the real system. *Verification* involves transformational accuracy of the model artifacts in model development and can be performed using a variety of testing techniques. The goal of verification is to ensure that the implementation is a correct realization of the conceptual model. The primary goal of verification is to compare multiple models with each other in order to ensure that the implementations are correct. *Validation*, on the other hand, involves substantiation that a model within its domain of applicability possesses a satisfactory range of accuracy consistent with its intended application. Validation ensures that the model is semantically right and is indeed modeling the phenomena of the real system being simulated. A model is considered valid for a set of experimental conditions if its accuracy is within an acceptable range. In order to improve the model, V&V processes are iteratively performed by comparing the model to actual system behavior until model accuracy is judged to be acceptable.

As mentioned in Chapter 1, several language-specific implementations of the same conceptual core model (described in Chapter 4) have been developed by individual researchers within our research group over the recent years.[3] These implementations naturally led to the development of multiple versions of the ABMs, which were programmed by independent modelers in two programming languages (Java and C++). The primary reasons of developing these multiple versions were (1) to compare programming language-specific dependencies as well as other V&V features and (2) to explore a variety of malaria-related research problems.[4] The notion of the conceptual core model played a central role in the long development process of these versions. As our experiences showed, the mental images of the conceptual model, which initially resided amorphously only in the modelers' brains, vastly differed among individual modelers due to countless ambiguities. Thus, its transformation from an abstract notion of a conceptual model into a computational and verifiable entity (an ABM) created many unique V&V challenges. Our V&V experiences focused on examining potential mismatches between these implementations and versions.

Table 8.1 lists the V&V techniques we used for the ABMs. Some of these techniques were listed in a taxonomy of V&V techniques for conventional simulation models proposed by Balci [44]. In addition, we also used the new dynamic techniques of *phase-wise docking* and *compartmental docking*, which are marked with *. All techniques are classified under the three primary categories of informal, static, and dynamic (as proposed by Balci [44]). The more frequently used techniques are marked in bold. Among these, face validation was by far the most frequently used.

As mentioned in Table 7.1, *docking* is a form of V&V that tries to align multiple models in order to investigate whether they yield similar results. Docking is also known as alignment or model-to-model comparison [22, 24, 37]. It is useful to confirm whether the claimed results of a given simulation are reliable and can be reproduced by someone starting from the scratch. As noted by Axelrod [34], without this confirmation, some published results may be simply mistaken due to programming errors, misrepresentation of what was actually simulated, or errors in analyzing or reporting the results.

---

[3]See Chapters 5 and 6 for the implementation details of the ABMs.

[4]For example, two different versions explored the efficacy of vector control interventions [28] and the sterile insect technique to control the population of *Anopheles gambiae* [196].

TABLE 8.1   V&V Techniques Used for the ABMs

Category	V&V Technique
Informal	Calibration, documentation checking, **face validation**, inspections, reviews, walkthroughs
Static	Cause–effect graphing, control flow analysis, **data dependency analysis, data flow analysis, failure analysis**, semantic analysis, **state transition analysis**
Dynamic	Acceptance testing, bottom-up testing, comparison testing, data interface testing, **debugging, docking (compartmental, phase-wise)***, execution testing, functional (black-box) testing, **graphical comparisons, partition testing**, performance testing, predictive validation, **sensitivity analysis**, special input testing, statistical techniques, structural (branch, condition, loop, path) testing, submodel testing, top-down testing, **visualization**

Docking can also be useful for testing the robustness of inferences from models and to determine if one model can subsume another.

Other than face validation, we used *docking* as the primary method of V&V of the ABMs. In the next two sections, we present the workflows and results of *phase-wise docking* and *compartmental docking*.

8.3   PHASE-WISE DOCKING

As the name suggests, phase-wise docking is performed in different phases. We denote the ABMs used for docking according to the programming language-specific implementations Java and C++, where the former had three different versions developed in different phases. These language-specific implementations and versions of the ABMs are henceforth referred to as *J1, J2, J3*, and *CPP*.[5] All of these ABMs followed the specifications of the core model (see Chapter 4).[6]

8.3.1   Assumptions for the ABMs

Some of the important assumptions of the core model and the ABMs used for phase-wise docking are described as follows. The stage transition times for mosquito agents, which are somewhat different (simplified) than those described in Chapter 4, are described in Table 8.2. For some of the adult stages, duration in each stage is determined by separate probability distributions for each possible pair of stages, which closely match published data for *An. gambiae*. For egg laying (oviposition) in the *Gravid* stage, the maximum number of eggs a female may oviposit ($Eggs_{Max}$) is drawn from a normal distribution with mean $\mu = 80$ and standard deviation $\sigma = 20$.

---

[5]'J' and 'CPP' stand for programming languages Java and C++, respectively. Different versions of the ABMs developed in Java and C++ are denoted by, for example, *J1* and *CPP*.

[6]However, since the core model was continually evolving at the time while docking was performed, we used one fixed version of it for the purpose of docking.

TABLE 8.2   Simplified Stage Transition Times for Phase-Wise Docking

Stage Transition	Duration
Egg → Larva	In egg stage for 24 hours
Larva → Pupa	Temperature dependent; see Eqs. (4.2–4.4)
Pupa → ImmatureAdult	In pupa stage for 24 hours
Immature Adult → Mate Seeking	1, 2, or 3 days [$p(1) = 0.1; p(2) = 0.8; p(3) = 0.1$]
Mate Seeking → Mate Seeking	0 (immediate transition; males only)
Mate Seeking → Blood Meal Seeking	0 (immediate transition; females only)
Blood Meal Seeking → Blood Meal Digesting	2 or 3 days [$p(2) = 0.7; p(3) = 0.3$]
Blood Meal Digesting → Gravid	0 (immediate transition)
Gravid → Blood Meal Seeking	0 (immediate transition when no eggs remaining)

Age-specific mortality rates are used for the *Larva* stage and for all the adult stages (see Section 4.6). For some transitions, $p(i)$ denotes the probability of transition on day i.

Figure 8.1 shows the workflow of phase-wise docking, illustrating different phases of the separate implementations. The programming language-specific implementations

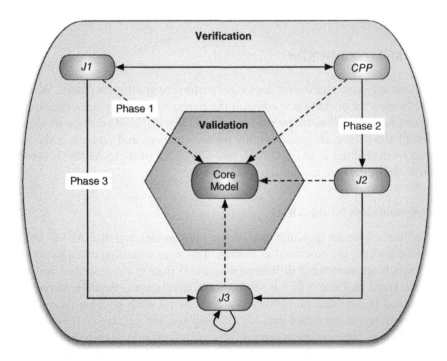

Figure 8.1   The phase-wise docking workflow. The programming language-specific implementations and versions of the ABMs developed in Java and C++ are denoted as *J1*, *J2*, *J3*, and *CPP*. Unidirectional solid arrows indicate immediate successorship between the implementations. Bidirectional solid arrow indicates *verification* relationships between *J1* & *CPP*. Dashed arrows indicate *validation* relationships with the core model. Used from Arifin *et al.* [23].

and versions of the ABMs developed in Java and C++, are denoted as *J1*, *J2*, *J3*, and *CPP*. Since Java and C++ were developed by separate programmers (with C++ built first), it was necessary to develop Java in phases to achieve incremental docking, as discussed below:

Phase 1: The first Java implementation *J1* is built from the core model independently of *CPP*. Verification starts with comparing the outputs of *J1* against *CPP*. Results show substantial differences, highlighting different conceptual images (of the core model) among the developers, and thus necessitating further investigation.

Phase 2: Before delving too deep in analyzing the differences, we develop *J2* as a simple clone of *CPP*. When compared, results show close agreement between the two models. This phase, though seems trivial, eliminates the source of any potential language-specific discrepancies and programming errors, as well as reduces the gaps in developers' conceptual images of the model.

Phase 3: The goal of the final phase *J3* is to *dock* with *CPP* and to validate these against the core model. Being the most time-consuming, *J3* is iterative in nature, since the set of existing minor discrepancies requires numerous fine-grained iterations for docking.

At this point, we address some minor issues. First, we verify that initial parameter settings and constants used are identical for all models. Next, we log all randomly generated numbers with the specified distribution parameters used and observe that the appropriate distributions are being generated, ruling out any potential difference due to the random number generator libraries.[7] Naturally, the models involve a mix of decimals and integers that require floating-point arithmetic. Calculation nuances created by these mixed architectures may cause unintended differences between model outputs. For example, integer division may result in type-coercion and rounding, causing cascaded loss of precision through the models leading to divergent results. To avoid these issues, we explicitly typecast all arithmetic involving a mix of decimals and integers to decimals.

8.3.2 Phase-Wise Docking Results

Figure 8.2 shows the phase-wise docking results for *Phase 1*. The following three major differences are identified when the mosquito abundance graphs from different implementations (*CPP* with *J1* and *J3*) are compared:

Difference 1: Both the adult and the aquatic mosquito populations differ dramatically.

---

[7]To generate random numbers in the simulations, we use GSL (the GNU Scientific Library) [189] for C++ and Repast [452] for all Java versions. Both implementations use the Mersenne Twister pseudorandom number generator (PRNG) [345], which is by far the most widely used PRNG and provides fast generation of high-quality pseudorandom numbers.

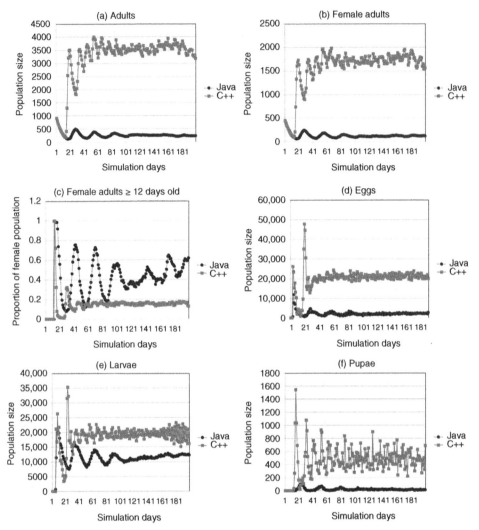

Figure 8.2   Phase-wise docking results for Phase 1. Mosquito abundance graphs from *J1* & *CPP* outputs are plotted for different populations. The *x*-axis denotes simulation time (in days) and the *y*-axis denotes abundances. Used from Arifin *et al.* [23].

Difference 2: The proportion of *older* female adult mosquito agents (with age ≥ 12) is significantly higher in *J1* than *CPP* (see Fig. 8.2c).

Difference 3: Aquatic population sizes are consistently lower in *J1* than *CPP* (see Fig. 8.2d–f)

To address the first difference, we verify the age-specific mortality functions for the adults. Comparisons of the specific routines calculating $ASMR_{age(adult)}$ reveal that once calculated, *CPP* places an artificial bound to kill only 80% when it is to eliminate all

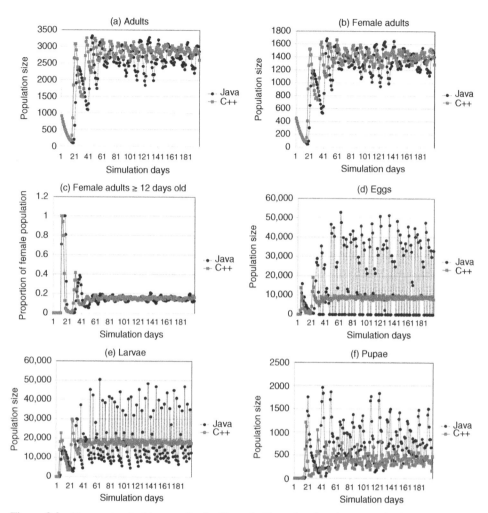

Figure 8.3 Phase-wise docking results for Phase 3. Mosquito abundance graphs from *J3* & *CPP* outputs are plotted for different populations. The *x*-axis denotes simulation time (in days) and the *y*-axis denotes abundances. Used from Arifin *et al.* [23].

members of a given age group. However, this modification, applied to *J3*, seems to have little significant impact on the results.

This step reveals another critical error. In *J1*, an agent enters the simulation with an age of 0, and the age is increased by one each day. This continues without any resetting of age when the agent enters the *Immature Adult* stage (see Fig. 4.1). However, in *CPP*, the age is reset to 0 once this transition occurs. This partially explains the second difference, that is, why the proportion of *older* female adult mosquito agents (with age ≥12) is significantly higher in *J1* than *CPP* (see Fig. 8.2c). While resetting the age reduces the oscillation in the proportion of older female agents, it does not significantly raise the mean number of adult mosquitoes close to *CPP*.

To address the third difference, we note that the number of eggs in *J1* is consistently less than *CPP*, causing *J1* to inject less agents into the system. This, in conjunction with the second difference, suggests that younger mosquito agents are killed more rapidly than the older ones, a counterintuitive indication given the death rate equations, which are designed to kill the older mosquito agents at a higher rate. To eliminate this, we verify the age-specific mortality rates for the aquatic stages. This reveals that *J1* and *CPP* calculate the age-adjusted *1-day-old equivalent larval population* N_e (see Section 4.6.1) differently. *CPP* computes N_e once at the start of each day using the previous day's aquatic populations. *J1*, on the other hand, recomputes N_e for every oviposition event, creating a selection bias for female mosquitoes trying to lay eggs ahead of others *within* the same simulation day, and thus causing more repulsive force to the female agents trying later. This, when implemented, has some impact to increase the amount of eggs being laid in *J3*. It also reveals a transition logic variance in *CPP* for egg development time: eggs take 2 days instead of 1 (see Table 8.2). When implemented, this reduces the difference in number of adults by approximately 500.

At this point, *J3* & *CPP* are not completely docked, especially in terms of the aquatic mosquito populations, as evident from Fig. 8.3. To achieve a complete dock, we use the compartmental docking technique, which is described in the next section.

8.4   COMPARTMENTAL DOCKING

In a complex ABM, synergies arising from seemingly insignificant differences in separate implementations may lead to significant mismatch in overall model output. Hence, it is crucial, and sometimes necessary, to *compartmentalize* the artificial simulation world, that is, to separate it into isolated compartments so that errors in one specific compartment are not propagated and thus cannot influence the discovery (and correction) of errors in other compartments.

In this section, we present the results of *compartmental docking* obtained by following the *divide and conquer* paradigm. To manage increased complexities that arise from different population compartments in our complex ABMs, we compartmentalized the simulation world with respect to the adult and aquatic mosquito populations in order to prohibit the propagation of errors between the compartments. We ensured that the pieces were working as intended, and then combined these to perform more complex simulations. Using four separate implementations (that sprung from the same core model), we describe a series of docking experiments, analyze the results, and show how they lead to a successful dock between all four implementations, and hence achieve a complete fourfold docking of the models. The complete fourfold docking encompassed *verification* between the four ABMs, as well as *validation* against the core model with respect to these implementations.

This section particularly addresses the following V&V issues:

- How the results from the four agent-based implementations compare to each other and to the corresponding results from theoretical models

- How to verify the age structure of mosquito populations and the age-specific mortality rates (for both adult and aquatic mosquito agent populations)
- How to verify the oviposition mechanism and the calculation of *1-day-old equivalent larval population N_e* at each step of the simulation (see Section 4.6.1) by temporarily removing all sources of randomness

8.4.1   Implementations of the ABMs

The compartmental docking workflow is depicted in Fig. 8.4. As before, the programming language-specific implementations and versions of the ABMs, developed in Java and C++, are henceforth referred to as *J1, J2, CPP1,* and *CPP2,* all of which followed the specifications of the core model (see Chapter 4).[8]

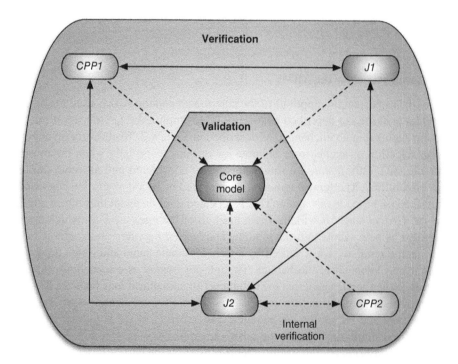

Figure 8.4   The compartmental docking workflow. The programming language-specific implementations and versions of the ABMs developed in Java and C++ are denoted as *J1, J2, CPP1,* and *CPP2.* Bidirectional arrows indicate *verification* relationships between the four implementations. The dashed arrow, between the re-factored implementations *J2* and *CPP2,* indicates *internal verification,* since these two are docked with respect to each other. Unidirectional dashed arrows indicate *validation* relationships between the core model and the four implementations. source© 2010 IEEE. Reprinted, with permission, from Arifin *et al.* [22].

---

[8]As mentioned before, 'J' and 'CPP' stand for programming languages Java and C++, respectively. Different versions of the ABMs developed in Java and C++ are denoted by, for example, *J1* and *CPP1.*

CPP1 was the earliest implementation of the core model [586]. It was developed in the C++ programming language utilizing the GSL [189]. This implementation was portable and could be compiled to run on any platform for which an ANSI compliant C++ compiler is available. A drawback of this implementation was the lack of built-in visualization tools. The first Java implementation *J1* was built over multiple phases using Java [23]. It provided some key advantages such as built-in graphical visualization tools that allowed the agents to be readily inspected (aiding in the debugging process), high efficiency, and less error-prone code.

The re-factored implementations, *CPP2* and *J2*, reflected a unified architecture and encoded a mosquito's life cycle and behavior in a structure called a *strategy* [195]. The strategy was flexible and could adapt to characterize new genus, species or variation within one species. The architecture was well suited for parallelization across many cores or computers. For compartmental docking, *CPP2* and *J2* were verified with respect to each other (internal verification), and a single output was compared with those of *CPP1* and *J1*.

8.4.2 Assumptions for the ABMs

Some of the important assumptions of the core model and the ABMs used for the compartmental docking are described as follows. The simplified stage transition times for mosquito agents remain unchanged as described in Table 8.2. To allow for an unbiased, uniform selection of agents from separate age-groups (especially when the mosquito agents die out), only *female* mosquito agents are considered and all male mosquito agents are omitted. The female mosquito agents feed on blood meals, lay eggs, and go back to feed on blood meals again. This is repeated until an agent dies. Once a female enters the *Gravid* stage, it remains there until all of her eggs are laid, which are then instantiated as new agents into the system. The *habitat capacity* of an aquatic habitat represents the repulsive force sensed by a *Gravid* female agent and limits the number of eggs it may oviposit in the habitat. Though not treated as a hard limit, this is an indication to the female agent that the habitat is full, and thus it may be more beneficial to lay eggs elsewhere. As before, age-specific mortality (see Section 4.6) is used for the larva stage and for all the adult stages. The ordering of the key processing steps performed in a single time-step in the ABMs remains the same (see Fig. 5.6).

A simplified life cycle of mosquito agents is used for the purposes of compartmental docking, as shown in Fig. 8.5. Two slightly different versions were used: one with a single aquatic habitat (Fig. 8.5a), and the other with multiple aquatic habitats (Fig. 8.5b). In the simplified life cycle, the *aquatic* phase is unchanged and consists of the following three aquatic stages: *Egg*, *Larva*, and *Pupa*. The *adult* phase, however, consists of four adult stages as follows: *Immature Adult*, *Blood Meal Seeking*, *Blood Meal Digesting*, and *Gravid*. Male agents are omitted. Adult female agents cycle through obtaining blood meals (in *Blood Meal Seeking* stage), developing eggs (in *Blood Meal Digesting* stage), and ovipositing the eggs (in *Gravid* stage) until they die. One important, though biologically unrealistic, assumption is the stage duration for the *Gravid* stage: a female mosquito agent is forced to remain in the *Gravid* stage for a duration

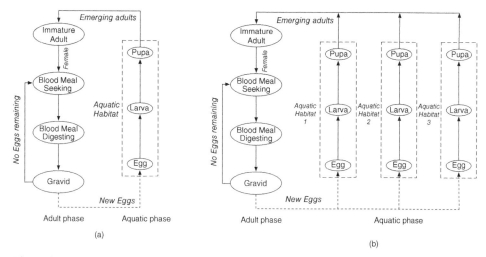

Figure 8.5 Simplified life cycle of mosquitoes for compartmental docking. Two slightly different versions were used as follows: (a) A model with a single aquatic habitat and (b) A model with multiple aquatic habitats. The *aquatic* phase is unchanged, consisting of three aquatic stages: *Egg*, *Larva*, and *Pupa*. The *adult* phase, however, consists of four adult stages: *Immature Adult*, *Blood Meal Seeking*, *Blood Meal Digesting*, and *Gravid*. Each oval represents a stage in the model. Male agents are omitted. Adult female agents cycle through obtaining blood meals, developing eggs, and ovipositing the eggs until they die. © 2010 IEEE. Reprinted, with permission, from Arifin *et al.* [22].

(in days) that equals the number of oviposition attempts taken to successfully lay all its remaining eggs.

For the compartmental docking experiments, the mosquito populations were first compartmentalized into adult and aquatic populations by following the *divide and conquer* paradigm, and then recombined at the end. These were performed in multiple phases (as before). After the completion of each phase, we compared the fourfold outputs from the ABMs, analyzed and fixed potential misinterpretations, and proceeded to the next phase. For all experiments, a fixed habitat capacity (*HC*) of 3000 was used for all aquatic habitats.

For the adult mosquito population compartment, we used 2, 2, and 0 days as the stage durations for *Immature Adult*, *Blood Meal Seeking*, and *Blood Meal Digesting*, respectively. Female mosquito agents stayed in the *Gravid* stage until all eggs are laid and transitioned back to *Blood Meal Seeking* the following day (see Fig. 8.5). Starting with a small sample of 100 female adult agents, this compartment ensured that the age structure and age-specific mortality rates for the adult stages match the corresponding theoretical values (obtained by separate calculations). It also verified the simplified oviposition mechanism.

The aquatic mosquito population compartment started with 1000 female egg agents that initially resided in a single aquatic habitat (with 3000 habitat capacity). It ensured that the age structure of all aquatic states, the age-specific mortality rates of larvae, and the base mortality rates of eggs and pupae populations match the corresponding theoretical values (obtained by separate calculations). It also verified the temperature-dependent larval development rate (see Eqs. 4.2–4.4).

At the end, we recombined the adult and aquatic mosquito population compartments. Starting with 100 female adult agents and 1000 female egg agents (initially residing in a single aquatic habitat with 3000 habitat capacity), it verified the transitions from the aquatic to the adult phase (i.e., from *Pupa* stage to *Immature Adult* stage). It also checked the simplified oviposition mechanism, the actual number of eggs laid in the aquatic habitat, and other stage durations as described in Table 8.2.

8.4.3 Compartmental Docking Results

The compartmental docking issues that are discovered and updated in the three different phases are listed in Tables 8.3 and 8.4. The first column in Table 8.4 denotes the phase.

Figure 8.6 shows the compartmental docking results for *Phase 1*. In this phase, four V&V issues were identified that caused differences in the outputs of the ABMs, including differences in the adult mosquito populations, the oviposition

TABLE 8.3   Compartmental Docking Issues in Phase 1

Compartmental Docking (V&V) Issue	Resolution
The adult agent populations were slightly less in magnitude in *CPP1* and *J1* than those in *J2* and *CPP2*. The aquatic agent populations in *CPP1* and *J1* were killed at higher rates than suggested by the mortality rate equations and constants	These were resolved after all implementations used the same habitat capacities for the single aquatic habitat
In *CPP1* and *J1*, gravid female mosquito agents laid all eggs on the first oviposition attempt. This created an egg-laying pattern where bursts of eggs were laid on the same day, followed by a hiatus (few days when no eggs were laid), then another burst, and so on. In *J2* and *CPP2*, however, the eggs were laid over a period of successive days (no hiatus)	This issue suggested a mismatch in the egg-laying code. It was partially resolved after all implementations ensured to use the same equations and constants for calculating how many eggs a female could lay in different egg-laying attempts
In *CPP1* and *J1*, female mosquito agents laid eggs 1 day sooner (during the first oviposition attempt) than in *J2* and *CPP2*	It was revealed that in *CPP1* and *J1*, female mosquito agents laid eggs at the end of the *Blood Meal Digesting* stage, rather than waiting until the first day of being *Gravid* (see Fig. 8.5). *CPP1* and *J1* were updated to ensure that eggs were laid while in the *Gravid* stage
In *J1*, after all female mosquito agents laid all eggs in the *Gravid* stage, they did not transition back to the *Blood Meal Seeking* stage on the same day	*J1* was updated to ensure that the female agents transitioned back to the *Blood Meal Seeking* stage from the *Gravid* stage on the same day once all eggs were laid

TABLE 8.4   Compartmental Docking Issues in Phases 2–3

Phase	Compartmental Docking (V&V) Issue	Resolution
2	In *CPP1* and *J1*, female mosquito agents were allowed to lay all eggs on the very first egg-laying attempts at the beginning of simulations (around days 5–6). However, as suggested by Eq. (4.11), laying all eggs in a single egg-laying attempt was possible only if the aquatic habitat was empty	We found that in *CPP1* and *J1*, egg laying was indeed complete after three attempts, and made a simple adjustment in the delay before female mosquito agents could leave the *Gravid* stage
2	In *CPP2* and *J2*, an upper bound of 80% was placed on the larval mortality rate	We ensured that *CPP1* and *J1* use the same upper bound
2	In egg laying, *CPP2* and *J2* inadvertently used $Eggs_{Remaining}$ (the number of eggs remaining to lay) instead of $Eggs_{Max}$ (the maximum number of eggs) in calculations of Eq. (4.11)	We ensured that *CPP2* and *J2* use $Eggs_{Max}$
2	In *J1*, *Gravid* female agents incorrectly laid all eggs and the biomass of the aquatic habitat did not reflect the number of eggs actually laid	In the calculation of $Eggs_{Laid}$ (the number of eggs allowed to lay), some *double*-precision variable values were coerced to *integer*-precision variable values, causing the expressions evaluating to 0 for these instances. This, in turn, affected the related variables ($Eggs_{Potential}$, $Eggs_{Laid}$, and $Eggs_{Remaining}$). We updated *J1* using explicit typecasting to *double*-precision variable values
3	In *CPP1* and *J1*, different numbers of adult mosquito agents were killed	We found that in *J1*, an extra constant was inadvertently used in the age-specific mortality rate function for adult mosquito agents (see Section 4.6.2); we omitted the constant in *J1* to match the correct form of the corresponding equation

mechanism (concerning the pattern and the exact timing of egg laying), and stage transitions. At the end of *Phase 1*, these issues were resolved, as described in Table 8.3.

The compartmental docking results for *Phase 2* are shown in Fig. 8.7. In this phase, another four V&V issues were identified that caused differences in the outputs of the ABMs, including a delay before female mosquito agents could leave the *Gravid* stage, an upper bound on the larval mortality rate, use of an inappropriate variable (a bug in the code), and explicit typecasting to double-precision variable values. At the end of *Phase 2*, these issues were resolved, as described in Table 8.4.

In *Phase 3*, a single V&V issue was identified that involved killing different numbers of adult mosquito agents after the simulations ran for some initial time

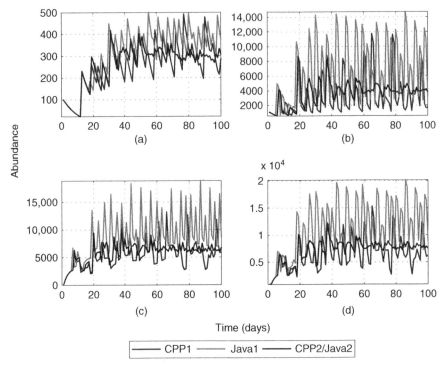

Figure 8.6   Compartmental docking results for *Phase 1*. Each subfigure depicts the fourfold outputs from the four ABMs: *CPP1*, *J1*, and *CPP2/Java2* (since *CPP2* and *J2* were verified with respect to each other, their outputs were merged as a single graph). Different mosquito populations are shown: (a) adult agents, (b) all agents (adults and aquatic), (c) the 1-day-old equivalent larval population N_e (see Eq. 4.9), and (d) biomass (see Eq. 4.8). The legend at the bottom shows the corresponding ABMs. Within each subfigure, each color-coded plot represents outputs from a specific ABM, with color keys presented in the legend. The *x*-axis denotes simulation time (days) and the *y*-axis denotes abundance. The first 100 days of the simulations are shown. © 2010 IEEE. Updated, with permission, from Arifin *et al.* [22].

(see Table 8.4). After close re-examinations of the code, we found that one version erroneously included an extra constant for the adult age-specific mortality rate function. Once it was resolved, the fourfold outputs of the four ABMs produced a *complete* fourfold dock, as shown in Fig. 8.8.

8.5   SUMMARY

This chapter described the V&V challenges from a series of simulation experiments involving several ABMs, all of which originated from the same conceptual model. Using the *phase-wise docking* technique, we showed how to obtain a partial dock of several independently developed models in two programming language-specific implementations (Java and C++). *Phase-wise docking* helped in *verification* of the ABMs

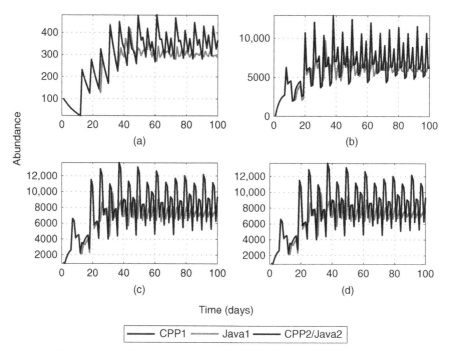

Figure 8.7 Compartmental docking results for *Phase 2*. Each subfigure depicts the fourfold outputs from the four ABMs: *CPP1*, *J1*, and *CPP2/Java2*. Different mosquito populations are shown: (a) adult agents, (b) all agents (adults and aquatic), (c) the 1-day-old equivalent larval population N_e (see Eq. 4.9), and (d) biomass (see Eq. 4.8). The legend at the bottom shows the corresponding ABMs. Within each subfigure, each color-coded plot represents outputs from a specific ABM, with color keys presented in the legend. The x-axis denotes simulation time (days) and the y-axis denotes abundance. The first 100 days of the simulations are shown. © 2010 IEEE. Updated, with permission, from Arifin *et al.* [22].

and in *validation* of the ABMs against the core model. It revealed incorrect assumptions and errors, which, being unnoticed, initially led to erroneous results. We also described how the major findings helped to clarify concepts and eliminate ambiguities by identifying differences in model specification, interpretation, implementation and enhancement phases, and revealing semantic errors. The importance of rigorous docking was illustrated by the discovery of some incorrect assumptions and programming errors, which, being unnoticed, led to erroneous results. Results showed that synergies arising from seemingly insignificant differences in separate implementations may lead to significant mismatch in overall model output, suggesting that docking should be iterative, and should involve well-planned feedback from earlier implementations.

The fourfold *compartmental docking* technique obtained by following the *divide and conquer* paradigm encompassed verification between the four ABMs, as well as validation against the core model with respect to these implementations. Isolating the agent world into the adult and the aquatic mosquito populations allowed us to design specific experiments that suit each compartment. The major findings, as described in

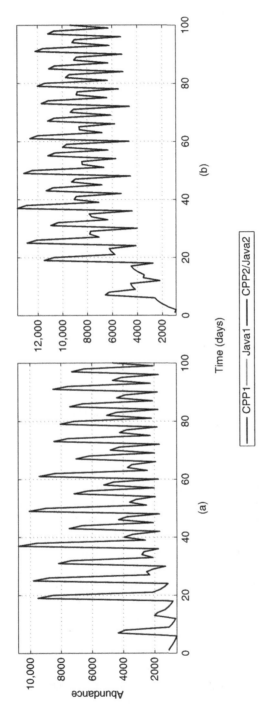

Figure 8.8 Compartmental docking results for *Phase 3*. Each subfigure depicts the fourfold outputs from the four ABMs: *CPP1*, *J1*, and *CPP2/Java2*. Different mosquito populations are shown: (a) all agents (adults and aquatic) and (b) biomass (see Eq. (4.8)). The legend at the bottom shows the corresponding ABMs. The *x*-axis denotes simulation time (days) and the *y*-axis denotes abundance. The first 100 days of the simulations are shown. © 2010 IEEE. Updated, with permission, from Arifin *et al.* [22].

Tables 8.3 and 8.4, helped to clarify model concepts and to eliminate ambiguities. This exercise also served as a case study to illustrate the importance of docking complex simulation models, since even the best simulation programs may imply dubious assumptions, leading to erroneous results. Rigorous docking can detect such problems, uncovering these incorrect assumptions [563]. The compartmental docking process served the dual purpose of increasing confidence to the core model and revealing conceptual errors in model implementations. It produced incremental agreements in model outputs as well as served the dual purpose of increasing confidence to the core model and revealing conceptual errors in model implementations.

Both techniques of phase-wise docking and compartmental docking should collectively serve as a case study of docking public health simulation models, similar to the works done in other fields [37, 384, 392, 572, 573]. The novelty of our approach, however, lies in demonstrating the importance of docking by showing that it can increase confidence to the core model, reveal conceptual and/or programming errors and eliminate dubious assumptions, thus reinforcing the findings in [91, 164, 447, 563, 564].

In Chapter 9, we present the R&R results that are obtained by replicating other published malaria models.

9

REPLICATION AND REPRODUCIBILITY (R&R) OF ABMs

9.1 OVERVIEW

As we mentioned in Chapter 7, replication and reproducibility (R&R) cover a wide spectrum of issues related to modeling and simulation (M&S) research and fall under the broader subject area of verification and validation (V&V). Replicability of the *in silico* experiments and simulations performed by various malaria models bear special importance. Although computational science has led to exciting new developments, the nature of the work has also exposed shortcomings in the general ability of the research community to evaluate published findings [428]. Replication, which is treated as the scientific gold standard to judge scientific claims, allows independent researchers to address a scientific hypothesis and produce evidence *for* or *against* it [263, 428].[1] Replication confirms reproducibility, which refers to the independent verification of prior findings, and is at the core of the spirit of science [471, 472]. In M&S, replication is also known as model-to-model comparison, alignment, or cross-model validation. One of its goals is to try to align multiple models in order to investigate whether they produce similar results [278, 572]. When the original models (e.g., the source codes)

---

[1]For this chapter, replication refers to running multiple simulations with the same configuration (i.e., using the same set of values for all parameters and the same starting conditions) repeatedly with different random seeds.

Spatial Agent-Based Simulation Modeling in Public Health:
Design, Implementation, and Applications for Malaria Epidemiology, First Edition.
S. M. Niaz Arifin, Gregory R. Madey and Frank H. Collins.
© 2016 John Wiley & Sons, Inc. Published 2016 by John Wiley & Sons, Inc.

are available, the stricter form of model verification known as *docking* may also be performed.[2]

In this chapter, we present simulation results of replicating another published malaria ABM by improving/extending some of its dubious assumptions.[3] The published ABM explored the impact of applying two stand-alone vector control interventions [221, 222]. For brevity, we hereafter refer to the two studies as GN-LSM and GN-ITNs, and their ABM used as GN-ABM, where GN refer to the initials of last names of the authors.[4] Critical examination of these studies reveals that although they provide reasonably plausible results, some unrealistic assumptions may be extended to include two major modeling improvements concerning simulation stochasticity and boundary conditions, which are described next. In the process of replicating other published ABMs, we also present the details of modeling the two vector control interventions – LSM and ITNs – with our spatial ABM.[5]

This chapter is organized as follows. In the remainder of this section, we discuss the two important issues of simulation stochasticity and boundary conditions (most of the simulation results presented in this chapter focus on these issues). Section 9.2 introduces the malaria control interventions and describes the modeling details of LSM and ITNs. It also discusses the population profiles and the coverage schemes used with ITNs and the settings for examining the impact of applying LSM and ITNs in isolation and in combination. Section 9.3 presents the simulation results. Section 9.4 discusses some R&R challenges of the ABMs and offers recommended guidelines for future ABM modelers. Section 9.5 discusses some key insights and Section 9.6 concludes.

9.1.1 Simulation Stochasticity

As highlighted by recent simulation research, most simulation models (including ours) that involve substantial stochasticity should conduct sufficient number of replicated runs, and some form of aggregate measures of these replicated runs should be reported as results (as opposed to reporting results from a single run). For example, Thiele *et al.* discussed the importance of varying parameter values and starting conditions for parameter fitting and replication [541].[6] They argued that to learn about the relative importance of the various mechanisms represented in a model and to test its robustness against the output to parameter uncertainty, modelers should explore the sensitivity of model output to changes in parameters. Sufficient number of replications is required to ensure that, given the same input, the aggregate response can be treated as a deterministic number and not as random variation of the results. This allows modelers to obtain a *more complete* statistical description of the model variables.

---

[2] See Chapter 8 for our V&V experiences, results, and lessons learnt by *docking* from a series of simulation experiments with the ABMs.

[3] Portions of the text and figures presented in this chapter appeared in Arifin *et al.* [28, 29].

[4] LSM and ITNs stand for the two malaria control interventions: larval source management and insecticide-treated nets, respectively.

[5] The spatial ABM was presented in Chapter 6.

[6] Parameter fitting is closely related to sensitivity analysis.

The same principle also applies to a set of stochastic (Monte Carlo) simulation models in other domains (e.g., traffic flow, financial problems, risk analysis, and supply chain forecasting), where, in most cases, the standard practice is to report the averages and standard deviations of the measures of interest (known as the *Measures of Effectiveness* or MOEs) [98, 111].

Since our spatial ABM involves substantial stochasticity in the forms of probability-based distributions and equations, performing sufficient number of replicated runs is important for selecting the optimal experimental sample size and also for validation of the results. In the ABM, mosquito agents' decisions are often simulated using random draws from certain distributions. These sources of randomness are used to represent the diversity of model characteristics and the behavior uncertainty of the agents' actions, states, and so on. For example, when a host-seeking mosquito agent searches for a blood meal in an ITN-covered house, a 20% ITNs coverage would mean that it may find a blood meal with a probability of 0.2, which can be simulated using random draws from a uniform distribution. As another example, the number of eggs in each egg batch of a *Gravid* mosquito is simulated using random draws from a *normal* distribution with *mean/average* = 170 and *standard deviation* = 30. The randomness has significant impact on the results of the simulation and different simulation runs can therefore produce significantly different results (due to a different sequence of pseudorandom numbers drawn from the distributions).

9.1.2   Boundary Types

The second issue involves the use of a specific boundary type, which may greatly impact the outcomes resulting from the simulated movement of agents' in the artificial landscape of the ABM. Boundary conditions, along with initial conditions, constitute one of the most important aspects of modeling [186, 237]. Since the boundary conditions directly define the set of rules followed by agents when they hit an edge, this is especially important for spatial models. An improper choice of the boundary conditions can sometimes produce undesired artifacts, leading to an unrealistic simulated system size [237].

In general, three different boundary types are commonly used in ABMs:

1. Nonabsorbing: With a *nonabsorbing* (also known as *periodic*) boundary, when agents hit an edge, they reenter the landscape from the edge directly opposite of the exiting edge (and thus are not killed due to hitting the edge). Thus, agents can leave the domain through one end and automatically reappear on the other end; this periodic boundary condition implies that the number of agents in the system is conserved; periodic boundaries are widely used because of their simplicity and because they effectively shape an infinite domain [186].

2. Absorbing: With an *absorbing* boundary, agents are permanently removed (effectively killed) when they hit an edge of the landscape's boundary.

3. Reflecting: With a *reflecting* boundary, agents are reflected when they hit an edge of the landscape's boundary.

For our malaria ABM, unless the underlying landscape reflects a completely isolated geographic location (e.g., an island far away from the mainlands), the *nonabsorbing* boundary seems to be the most logical choice, since it captures the mosquito population dynamics more realistically. This is especially true when the resource densities are high and the resources are more evenly distributed across the landscape.[7]

The published malaria ABM studies – GN-LSM [222] and GN-ITNs [221] – use absorbing boundaries for all landscapes. On the other hand, our spatial ABM uses non-absorbing boundaries and models all landscapes topologically as 2-D torus spaces.[8] However, to compare with GN-LSM, we first report results that are obtained using absorbing boundaries. Simulation results depicting the effects of using absorbing and nonabsorbing boundaries are presented in Section 9.3.2.

9.2 VECTOR CONTROL INTERVENTIONS

In this section, we present the modeling details of applying the two vector control interventions – LSM and ITNs. These frontline vector control tools, along with others such as long-lasting impregnated nets (LLINs) and indoor residual spraying (IRS), have gained unprecedented increases in their coverages in the last decade (2000–2010) of worldwide malaria control efforts [181]. Impact of these interventions, often applied in isolation and in combination, have been investigated by numerous early and recent studies [28, 115, 160, 218, 221, 222, 228, 289, 299, 391, 558, 574]. In addition to the time-tested, established tools such as ITNs, IRS, and LSM, new and novel intervention tactics and strategies, in the forms of new drugs, vaccines, insecticides, improved surveillance methods, and so on, are also being investigated [216]. Some of the promising approaches include genetically engineered mosquitoes through sterile-insect technique (SIT) or release of insects containing a dominant lethal (RIDL) [297, 434], fungal biopesticides that increase the rate of adult mosquito mortality [229], the development of genetically modified mosquitoes (GMMs) or transgenic mosquitoes manipulated for resistance to malaria parasites [340], transmission blocking vaccines (TBVs) against malaria that are intended to induce immunity against the stages of the malaria parasites [96], and so on.

As mentioned in Chapter 2, chloroquine and DDT inspired a global malaria eradication campaign over half a century ago. The campaign achieved substantial progress in many areas, especially outside Africa. However, with diminished political and financial commitments, and with the emergence and spread of chloroquine-resistant *Plasmodium* parasites and DDT-resistant *Anopheles* mosquitoes, a global resurgence of malaria followed, including in areas where it had been largely eliminated [216]. In recent malaria research, the international community has continued to face difficult decisions

---

[7]Recall that houses and aquatic habitats are considered as ecological resources for the mosquito agents in a landscape.

[8]A *2-D torus* object represents a geometrical surface of revolution generated by revolving a circle in a 2-D space about an axis coplanar with the circle; in ABM, a toroidal space resembles a donut topology, allowing an agent to reenter the space from the opposite edge when it moves off one edge.

in balancing efforts in discovery, development, and implementation of new tools. The emergence of artemisinin resistance and the lack of sufficient knowledge, tools, and multinational cooperation to effectively prevent the spread of resistant parasites still prevails [216].

There is now a consensus that malaria elimination with current tools is far more likely if the best available tools are used in combinations [335], and the most effective control programs usually apply a combination of such tools [115, 160, 216, 391, 574]. The potential of applying current vector control interventions in various transmission settings in an integrated vector management (IVM) approach is promoted by the World Health Organization (WHO) and demonstrated by recent studies [181, 182]. Because of its improved efficacy, cost-effectiveness, ecological soundness, and sustainability, IVM is increasingly being recommended as an option for sustainable malaria control [377]. However, in many cases, the costs of universally implementing the existing interventions (e.g., ITNs and IRS) may exceed the available resources, necessitating an urgent need to develop new interventions and improved intervention strategies that, given these limited resources, may provide maximal benefit by reducing transmission levels below a critical threshold to eliminate malaria. Since the existing interventions are insufficient to meet the global eradication goal and the efficacy of current interventions will be lost to a changing parasite or mosquito species in the near future, new concepts, tools, and interventions are required.

As we described in Chapter 6, the resource-seeking (foraging) process of the female mosquito agents primarily encompasses two frequent events in the ABMs: oviposition and host-seeking, which occur in aquatic habitats and houses, respectively. An agent performs these events by moving in the spatial landscape to seek for these resources.[9] The two vector control interventions, LSM and ITNs, target the aquatic habitats and houses, respectively. In the remainder of this section, we briefly describe LSM and ITNs and their modeling details within our spatial ABM. We also discuss the population profiles and the different coverage schemes used with ITNs and the simulation settings for examining the impact of applying LSM and ITNs in isolation and in combination.

9.2.1   Larval Source Management (LSM)

LSM, also known as source reduction, is one of the oldest tools in the fight against malaria. Large-scale LSM proved to be a highly effective malaria control method in the first half of the twentieth century [181]. It refers to the management of aquatic habitats in order to restrict the completion of immature stages of mosquito development. Recent studies suggest that LSM can be successfully used for malaria control in African transmission settings by highlighting its historical and recent successes and can be integrated in an IVM approach working toward malaria elimination [181, 182]. In areas with moderate and focal malaria transmission, where larval habitats are accessible and well defined, LSM is also cost-effective when compared to other frontline vector

---

[9]See Figs. 6.6 and 6.7 for the flight heuristics and movement activities for mosquito agents, which describe the movement rules (in the form of flowcharts) *without* any intervention being applied.

control tools such as IRS and LLINs [570]. LSM can be further classified into (1) habitat modification, (2) habitat manipulation, (3) biological control, and (4) larviciding [181]. It provides the dual benefits of not only reducing numbers of house-entering mosquitoes but also those that bite outdoors.

For the spatial ABM, LSM refers to the permanent elimination of targeted aquatic habitats, which in practice may be achieved by various methods that include landscaping, drainage of surface water, land reclamation and filling, coverage of large water storage containers, wells and other potential breeding sites, and so on.

9.2.2   Insecticide-Treated Nets (ITNs)

ITNs, particularly the long-lasting insecticidal nets (LLINs), are considered among the most effective vector control strategies currently in use [77, 231, 335, 574]. Scale-up applications of ITNs can offer direct personal protection to users as well as indirect, community protection to nonusers (through insecticidal and/or repellent effects), and hence are advocated to combat against the major malaria vectors (including *Anopheles gambiae*) in Africa [221, 231]. However, in Africa, due to a wide array of variations in entomological and epidemiological conditions, results of randomized community trials show varying effects of ITNs on the major vector populations [116, 221, 336, 409].

Primarily due to mathematical convenience, earlier models that studied the impact of ITNs on malaria transmission assumed a uniform contact structure between mosquitoes and hosts across the landscape [289, 314]. However, empirical data indicating limited flight ranges and sensory perception of mosquitoes suggest that proximity between the mosquitoes and their hosts can play a crucial role in the mosquito biting behavior [200–203, 365]. Hence, spatially explicit models are needed to analyze the local host-seeking process of the mosquitoes and to study the responses of mosquitoes to ITNs. Such models can also provide evidence for the need of entomological surveillance for evaluation of scale-up ITNs programs [221].

Response of host-seeking mosquito agents to ITNs is modeled as a series of three ITNs parameters: coverage C, repellence R, and mortality M.[10] When a host-seeking female mosquito agent (being in the *BMS* state) finds a house, coverage is checked first to ensure whether the house is ITNs-covered. If it is covered, repellence comes into action; the mosquito may be repelled by ITNs and thus forced to search for another house. If it can avoid repellence, a random host is picked in the house. If the host sleeps under a bed net, mortality comes into action; it may be killed due to the insecticidal effect of the bed net. If it survives the mortality, depending on the ITNs coverage scheme (see below), it either picks another random host in the same house or must search for another house. If, on the other hand, the host does not sleep under a bed net, feeding is assumed to be always successful.

---

[10]Note that for ITNs, we use the term *mortality* to refer to the *insecticidal effect* of the bed nets, that is, the additional mortality concurred by ITNs.

TABLE 9.1   Population Profiles for Varying Levels of ITNs Coverage

ITNs Coverage	Partial Coverage Scheme				Complete Coverage Scheme			
	Household Coverage (%)	Population Coverage (%)	Bed Net Users	Nonusers	Household Coverage (%)	Population Coverage (%)	Bed Net Users	Nonusers
0.4	40	21.62	40	145	40	41.08	76	109
0.6	60	32.43	60	125	60	59.46	110	75
0.8	80	43.24	80	105	80	82.70	153	32
1.0	100	54.05	100	85	100	100	185	0

9.2.3   Population Profiles for ITNs

Population profiles for ITNs are created by modeling humans as *static* agents residing in the houses with an average occupancy.[11] Table 9.1 shows the population profiles for varying levels of ITNs coverages with a total human population of 185. The table also shows the differences in household- and population-level coverage, as well as the variation in number of bed net users and nonusers, for varying levels of ITNs coverage with multiple coverage schemes (see Fig. 9.1). The human population is distributed over 50 houses. Each house has an average (mean) occupancy of 3.7 (with standard deviation of 1.2) having at least two residents.

9.2.4   Coverage Schemes for ITNs

In malaria literature, multiple definitions of the term *ITNs coverage* can be found. The Roll Back Malaria (RBM) Partnership uses ITNs coverage as the proportion of households owning a bed net or sleeping under a bed net [421] (this definition is also used by Gu and Novak [221]). On the other hand, the WHO reports ITNs coverage as the number of bed nets distributed per person at risk [567]. In some studies, ITNs coverage is also defined as the proportion of populations sleeping under treated bed nets [289], and is used more widely in recent malaria models [115, 160, 289, 574]. However, this distinction in multiple definitions of ITNs coverage, primarily concerning coverage levels of households and individuals, has not been addressed (within a single study) by most recent models. Although different studies used different schemes [115, 160, 221, 289, 574], none (including ABMs and mathematical models of malaria) actually compared their relative impacts side by side. Without a precise definition of the scheme used in a particular model, the task of replication becomes much harder. Hence, we argue that the comparison of results from using the three schemes may guide future modelers to select the appropriate scheme to use in their models.

The WHO emphasizes the importance of scale-up ITNs coverage beyond vulnerable population (children under 5 years of age and pregnant women) as a priority for

---

[11] In the context of our spatial ABM, a *static* agent does not move in space.

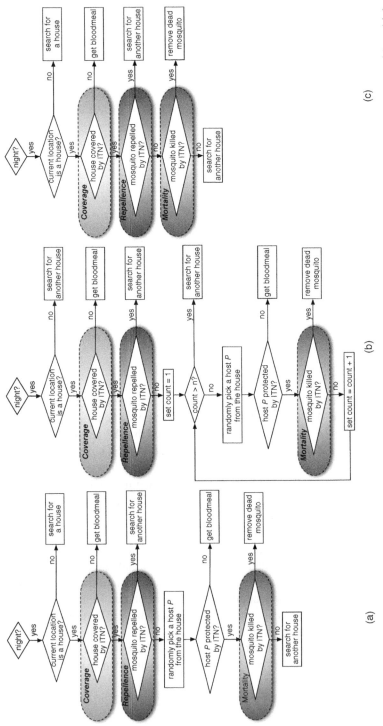

Figure 9.1 Coverage schemes for ITNs. (a) Household-level partial coverage with single chance. (b) Household-level partial coverage with multiple chances. (c) Household-level complete coverage. Used from Arifin *et al.* [28] under a Creative Commons Attribution 4.0 International License.

128

combating malaria in tropical Africa [566]. Also, several studies have shown that the patterns of coverage and effective coverage are important determinants of ITNs/LLINs success [218]. Simplistic ITNs/LLINs models in which the coverage scheme is not carefully designed can lead to overly optimistic results [288, 314, 500]. Based on these, we argue that simulating different definitions of ITNs coverage and assessing their relative impacts are important, especially when replicating and validating results of an earlier model that used either of these definitions (e.g., [221]). We simulate and compare three different definitions/schemes of ITNs coverage that differ by the number of persons actually covered by bed nets in an ITNs-covered house: (1) household-level *partial* coverage with *single chance* for host-seeking, (2) household-level *partial* coverage with *multiple chances* for host-seeking, and (3) household-level *complete* coverage. These three schemes are depicted as logical flowcharts in Fig. 9.1.

We define household-level coverage as

$$Household\ level\ coverage\ (\%) = \frac{Number\ of\ houses\ with\ coverage}{Total\ number\ of\ houses} \times 100 \qquad (9.1)$$

and population-level coverage as

$$Population\ level\ coverage\ (\%) = \frac{Number\ of\ bed\ net\ users}{Total\ human\ population} \times 100 \qquad (9.2)$$

The same household-level coverage in different schemes may yield different population-level coverage. The distinction between *partial* (with single or multiple chances) and *complete* schemes becomes apparent when we compare the respective numbers for varying levels of ITNs coverage in Table 9.1: for any coverage level (column 1), with the same household-level coverages (compare columns 2 and 6), the complete coverage scheme has almost twice the population-level coverages than that in the partial coverage schemes (compare columns 3 and 7). The same applies to the corresponding number of bed net users (compare columns 4 and 8).

In household-level *partial* coverage with *single chance* for host-seeking, each house with ITNs coverage is assigned a single bed net, and two randomly selected persons in the house are protected by the bed net (irrespective of the total number of persons in the house). Once a host-seeking mosquito enters an ITNs-covered house and is not deterred by the repellence, it gets a single chance of obtaining a blood meal by picking a random host in the house. Since at most two persons can sleep under the bed net, the probability of a random host sleeping under the bed net is $2/n$, where n is the number of persons in the house. Thus, the probability to obtain a blood meal from a nonprotected host in the house is $1 - 2/n$. If the host is protected (sleeps under the bed net), the mosquito cannot get a blood meal but still runs the risk of being killed by the ITNs mortality (insecticidal effect of the bed nets). If it can survive, it must start searching for another house. Otherwise (i.e., if the host is unprotected), the mosquito gets a blood meal.

The second scheme, household-level *partial* coverage with *multiple chances* for host-seeking, works similarly as the first one, except for the fact that a host-seeking mosquito gets n chances in the same house (where n is the number of persons in the house). If it cannot get a blood meal within n chances and still survives the ITNs mortality, it must start searching for another house. Note that with this scheme, even though the mosquito gets multiple chances for host-seeking, it also encounters the risk of being exposed to the ITNs mortality each time (if the randomly selected host sleeps under bed net). With both these schemes, even when all houses are ITNs-covered (i.e., 100% household-level coverage), a portion of the population may still remain unprotected, and thus, vector population may not be completely suppressed.

With the last scheme, household-level *complete* coverage, if a house is ITNs-covered, all persons in the house are protected by bed nets (and hence we use the term *complete*). This can simulate, for example, an ITNs study over a region where there are enough bed nets to protect every person in an ITNs-covered house. In this scheme, when a host-seeking mosquito enters an ITNs-covered house and is not deterred by the repellence, it cannot get a blood meal (because all persons are covered) and must search for another house. Thus, it incurs additional delays and risks for the mosquito to be eventually successful in obtaining a blood meal.

9.2.5 Applying LSM in Isolation

To explore the impact of LSM in isolation (i.e., without any other intervention) and to replicate the results of GN-LSM, we discretize and digitize the 40×40 grid-based landscapes used in GN-LSM [222]. In the digitization process, the original tiny landscapes from GN-LSM are enlarged and gridlines are added to aid in measuring the objects' coordinates. The coordinates are then measured by inspection. To locate the center of each object (an aquatic habitat or a house), we use distances (in both x- and y-axes) from the nearest gridlines. Whenever multiple objects overlap and appear to be rendered on top of one another, we use the best guess to infer the center coordinates. The landscapes are then generated using our landscape generator tool *VectorLand*.[12] Each of the 18 landscapes, as depicted in Fig. 9.2, contains 70 aquatic habitats (circles) and three different arrangements of 20 houses (house icons): diagonal, horizontal, and vertical.

For each arrangement, different LSM scenarios (targeted and nontargeted) are also constructed, as was done by Gu and Novak [222]. The three targeted interventions T1, T2, and T3 refer to the removal of aquatic habitats within 100, 200, and 300 m of surrounding houses, accounting for 4, 17, and 28 of 70 habitats, respectively. C1, C2, and C3 refer to nontargeted, random removal of the same numbers of aquatic habitats as the corresponding targeted interventions. Removal of an aquatic habitat makes it completely inaccessible to gravid mosquitoes and no eggs can be laid in it during oviposition. In practice, this is usually done by habitat modification (a category of LSM), which results in permanent change of land and water and is performed by means that include landscaping, drainage of surface water, land reclamation and filling, coverage of large water storage containers, wells and other potential breeding sites, and so on [181]. Increasing LSM coverage, although affecting the larval population (by killing the biomass in the corresponding aquatic habitats), does not increase the mortality of

---

[12]The landscape generator tool, *VectorLand*, was presented in Section 6.2.3.

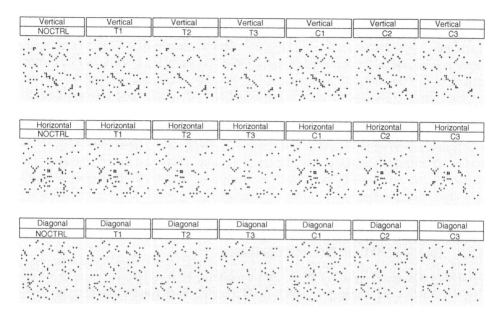

Figure 9.2 Landscapes for Applying LSM in Isolation. The 40 × 40 grid-based landscapes are digitized and reproduced from the GN-LSM study [222]. Each landscape contains 70 aquatic habitats (circles) and 20 houses (house icons). Within each landscape, the houses are arranged either diagonally, horizontally, or vertically. For each arrangement, seven scenarios of LSM are shown; from left to right: NOCTRL means no LSM; T1, T2, and T3 refer to targeted removal of aquatic habitats within 100, 200, and 300 m of surrounding houses, accounting for 4, 17, and 28 of 70 habitats, respectively. C1, C2, and C3 refer to nontargeted, random removal of the same numbers of aquatic habitats as the corresponding targeted interventions. Used from Arifin *et al.* [28] under a Creative Commons Attribution 4.0 International License.

adult mosquitoes; it just decreases the probability of successfully finding an aquatic habitat (and hence delaying the process) by adult females trying to oviposit. Note that the digitization of these landscapes from GN-LSM [222] (and later from GN-ITNs [221]) is conducted primarily for validation, comparison, and replication purposes. It is much easier and less time-consuming to generate new landscapes with any desired spatial distribution and parameter combinations using *VectorLand* (as we did for applying LSM and ITNs in combination, see Section 9.2.7). However, to be able to directly compare our results with GN-LSM and to adhere to the requirements of a standard replication process, the digitization of the original landscapes was necessary.

To compare the impact of LSM using the above landscapes, we use a fixed daily mortality rate (DMR) of 0.2 for the absorbing boundary in order to match the DMR of the GN-LSM study [222]. However, the core model [29], as described in Chapter 4, uses age-specific mortality rates for all the adult stages and the larva stage. Hence, in simulations that use nonabsorbing boundaries (in this chapter), we use age-specific mortality rates for these stages. For each of the 21 landscapes, we run 50 replicated simulations and report the average results. Thus, a total of 1050 (21 × 50) simulations are reported.

9.2.6   Applying ITNs in Isolation

To examine the impacts of applying ITNs in isolation, a single 40×40 grid-based land-scape is digitized and reproduced from the GN-ITNs study [221] using our landscape generator tool *VectorLand*, as shown in Fig. 9.3. The landscape contains 90 aquatic habitats (circles) that are randomly distributed and 50 houses (house icons) that are arranged diagonally.

We use representative sample values for the three ITNs parameters of coverage, repellence, and mortality, as shown in Table 9.2. These values provide 60 ($4 \times 3 \times 5$) distinct parameter combinations. Using the three ITNs coverage schemes (see Section 9.2.4) and these 60 combinations, we run 50 replicated simulations for each and report the average results. Thus, a total of 9000 ($3 \times 60 \times 50$) simulations are reported. Nonabsorbing boundaries are used in all simulations.

9.2.7   Applying LSM and ITNs in Combination

To apply LSM and ITNs in combination, we use three 40×40 landscapes, as shown in Fig. 9.4. Each of the landscapes contains 200 aquatic habitats and different densities of houses: Low (20), Medium (70), and High (200), with corresponding human population densities of 100, 350, and 1000, respectively. Aquatic habitats and houses are shown

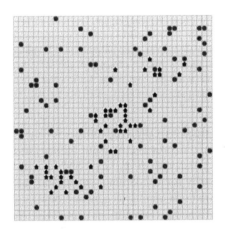

Figure 9.3   Landscape for Applying ITNs in Isolation. The 40×40 landscape is digitized and repro-duced from the GN-ITNs study [221]. It contains 90 aquatic habitats (circles) that are randomly distributed and 50 houses (house icons) that are arranged diagonally. Used from Arifin *et al.* [28] under a Creative Commons Attribution 4.0 International License.

TABLE 9.2   Parameter Space for ITNs

Parameter	Values
Coverage (C)	0.4, 0.6, 0.8, 1.0
Repellence (R)	0.2, 0.5, 0.9
Mortality (M)	0.0, 0.25, 0.5, 0.75, 1.0

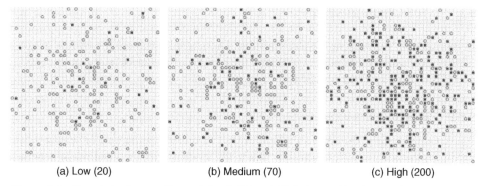

| (a) Low (20) | (b) Medium (70) | (c) High (200) |

Figure 9.4   Sample landscapes for applying LSM and ITNs in combination. Each 40×40 landscape contains 200 aquatic habitats and different densities of houses ($density_{houses}$). (a) $density_{houses} = Low(20)$ with human population of 100. (b) $density_{houses} = Medium$ (70) with human population of 350. (c) $density_{houses} = High(200)$ with human population of 1000. Aquatic habitats and houses are shown as circles and house-shaped icons, respectively. For 240 distinct parameter combinations (see Table 9.3), similar landscapes are generated and 50 replicated simulations are run for each. Used from Arifin *et al.* [28] under a Creative Commons Attribution 4.0 International License.

TABLE 9.3   Parameter Space for LSM and ITNs

Parameter	Values
$density_{houses}$	Low (20), Medium (70), High (200)
Population density	Low (100), Medium (350), High (1000)
LSM coverage	0.0, 0.1, 0.3, 0.6, 0.9
ITNs coverage	0.0, 0.25, 0.5, 1.0
ITNs mortality	0.0, 0.3, 0.7, 1.0

as circles and house-shaped icons, respectively. All landscapes are generated using the landscape generator tool *VectorLand*.

Parameter values used to run simulations with LSM and ITNs in combination are shown in Table 9.3. The four parameters $density_{houses}$, LSM coverage, ITNs coverage, and ITNs mortality provide 240 ($3 \times 5 \times 4 \times 4$) distinct combinations.[13] For each combination, we generate similar landscapes (using *VectorLand*), run 50 replicated simulations, and report the average results. Thus, a total of 12,000 (240×50) simulations are reported. For all cases, the household-level complete coverage scheme is used for ITNs (see Section 9.2.4) and ITNs repellence (R) is ignored (i.e., R is set to 0.0). Initially, aquatic habitat density is fixed at $50 \, \mathrm{km}^{-2}$ (in 40×40 landscapes, since each cell represents $50 \, \mathrm{m} \times 50 \, \mathrm{m}$, the 200 aquatic habitats are distributed across an area of $4,000,000 \, \mathrm{m}^2$ or $4 \, \mathrm{km}^2$) and later reduced as LSM coverage is increased. Nonabsorbing boundaries are used in all simulations.

---

[13]Values of the second parameter, *population density*, are matched with the corresponding values of the first parameter, $density_{houses}$, as listed in Table 9.3. For example, we use *low (100)* population density with $density_{houses} = 20$.

9.3 SIMULATION RESULTS

In this section, we present the R&R results. These results explore the effects of simulation stochasticity, boundary types, and the two malaria control interventions (LSM and ITNs) using our spatial ABM.

9.3.1 Simulation Stochasticity

As explained before, different simulation runs (with identical parameter settings) can produce significantly different results due to the stochasticity involved while generating random draws from the probability distributions. The effects of smoothing out the simulation stochasticity by performing sufficient number of replicated simulation runs are shown in Fig. 9.5. It depicts the importance of multiple simulation runs, instead of a single run, where we derive the *maximum*, *minimum*, and *average* abundance values obtained in each time step across 50 replicated runs. Four LSM scenarios are shown (see Fig. 9.2): Fig. 9.5(a) and (b) refer to scenarios C1 and C2, respectively, and use absorbing boundaries with nontargeted, random removal of aquatic habitats. Figure 9.5(c) and (d) refer to the same scenarios and use nonabsorbing boundaries. Within each scenario, the three time-series plots represent the maximum, the minimum, and the average mosquito abundances, respectively, obtained across all 50 replicated runs in each time step. Note that the scales along *y*-axis of different scenarios are purposefully modified (zoomed in) to highlight the actual differences between the three cases.

As evident from each of the four scenarios in Fig. 9.5, the *average* plot lies within a band (envelope) defined by the *maximum* and *minimum* plots. If replication was not performed by averaging multiple simulation runs, the results could have potentially taken any trajectory bounded within the band and thus would have been less reliable. Also note that for all scenarios, the *average* plot is much smoother than the *maximum* and *minimum* plots. This suggests much less abrupt changes in the *average* plots (which, in the *maximum* and *minimum* plots, were possibly caused by the random events across the simulation runs). All simulation results reported in this chapter represent the same replication policy of multiple runs.

9.3.2 LSM in Isolation

Figures 9.6 and 9.7 show the impact of applying LSM in isolation with absorbing boundaries and nonabsorbing boundaries, respectively (the reproduced landscapes used for LSM application were shown in Fig. 9.2). To compare our results with the GN-LSM study [222], we calculate the percent reduction (PR) values in abundance, which are shown in Table 9.4.

Although the two models (i.e., the GN-ABM [222] and our ABM) differ in several assumptions, in most cases, we observe general agreement in changes in PRs (i.e., an increase or decrease) as we move from one landscape to another, as shown in Figs. 9.6 and 9.7 and Table 9.4. For all three landscape types (*Diagonal*, *Horizontal*, and *Vertical*), in our model, the absorbing boundary almost always (in 17 out of 18 scenarios, i.e., 94% cases) yields larger PR than that of the nonabsorbing case for the same

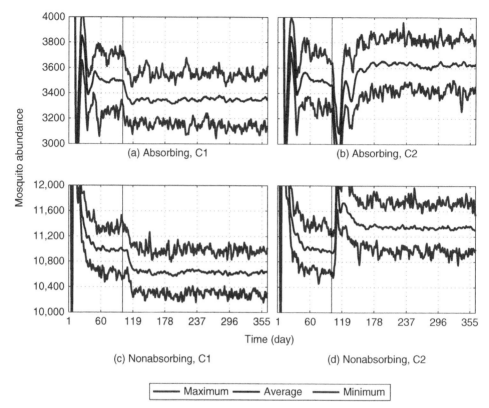

Figure 9.5 Sufficient number of replicated simulation runs can smooth out the simulation stochasticity effects. The importance of performing multiple simulation runs (instead of a single run) can be seen by comparing abundances for *maximum*, *minimum*, and *average* cases. Four LSM scenarios are shown (see Fig. 9.2): (a) and (b) refer to scenarios C1 and C2, respectively, and use absorbing boundaries with nontargeted, random removal of aquatic habitats. (c) and (d) refer to the same scenarios and use nonabsorbing boundaries. Within each scenario, the three time-series plots represent the maximum, the minimum, and the average mosquito abundances, respectively, obtained across all 50 replicated runs in each time step. Used from Arifin *et al.* [28] under a Creative Commons Attribution 4.0 International License.

scenario. While this trend is generally expected due to the additional (but unrealistic) killing effect of the absorbing boundary, this indicates the validity of results obtained from comparing the models using different boundary types.

It is interesting to observe that in Figs. 9.6 and 9.7, except for scenario T1, abundances in all other scenarios for the *Horizontal* landscape are greater than those for the *Diagonal* and *Vertical* landscapes. This is because the average distance between aquatic habitats and blood meal locations (when both of these resource types are ranked according to distances from one another) for the *Horizontal* landscape is less than those for the *Diagonal* and *Vertical* landscapes. As a result, female mosquito agents need to travel shorter average distances in the *Horizontal* case in order to find resources and thus completing their gonotrophic cycles. For scenario T1 (which is obtained by removing four

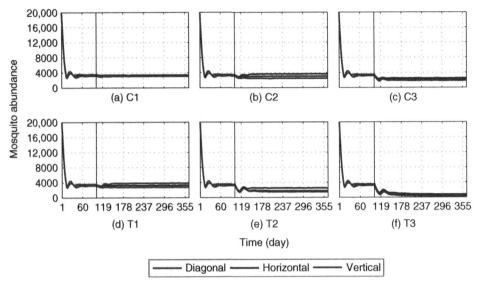

Figure 9.6   The figure depicts the full 1-year results of applying LSM in isolation with absorbing boundaries as we replicate the results of GN-LSM [222]. Each subfigure represents a specific LSM scenario. The *x*-axis denotes simulation time (days) and the *y*-axis denotes mosquito abundance. The three targeted interventions T1, T2, and T3 refer to the removal of aquatic habitats within 100, 200, and 300 m of surrounding houses, accounting for 4, 17, and 28 of 70 habitats, respectively. C1, C2, and C3 refer to nontargeted, random removal of the same numbers of aquatic habitats as the corresponding targeted interventions. Within each subfigure, the *Diagonal*, *Horizontal*, and *Vertical* plots represent abundances (for the specified LSM scenario) for three different arrangements of houses in the landscapes (see Fig. 9.2 for the landscapes). With an *absorbing boundary*, mosquitoes are killed when they hit an edge of the landscape's boundary. Each simulation is run 50 times and the average results are reported. This figure represents averages of a total of 900 (18 × 50) simulations. Used from Arifin *et al.* [28] under a Creative Commons Attribution 4.0 International License.

aquatic habitats from the baseline landscapes), however, abundance for the *Diagonal* landscape is greater than that for the *Horizontal* landscape. To explore why, we measure the *effective shortest distance* (*ESD*) between each of the four removed aquatic habitats and to their seven nearest blood meal locations. *ESD* measures the shortest distance, in units of number of cells, between the source and the destination cells (recall that each cell in the landscape is 50 m × 50 m; thus, *x ESD* means $x \times 50$ m) and includes diagonal paths wherever necessary, since mosquitoes are allowed to move diagonally in the ABM. It turns out that $ESD_{Diagonal} = 143$ and $ESD_{Horizontal} = 197$, that is, $ESD_{Diagonal} < ESD_{Horizontal}$ (see Fig. 9.2 for the specific landscapes). This suggests that removal of these four aquatic habitats in scenario T1 has less impact for the *Diagonal* landscape than for the *Horizontal* landscape – female mosquito agents can find blood meals more easily by traveling less distances in the former (*Diagonal*) case, resulting greater abundance.

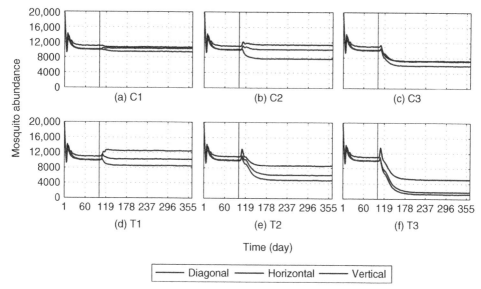

Figure 9.7   The figure depicts the full 1-year results of applying LSM in isolation with nonabsorbing boundaries as we replicate the results of GN-LSM [222]. Each subfigure represents a specific LSM scenario. The *x*-axis denotes simulation time (days) and the *y*-axis denotes mosquito abundance. The three targeted interventions T1, T2, and T3 refer to the removal of aquatic habitats within 100, 200, and 300 m of surrounding houses, accounting for 4, 17, and 28 of 70 habitats, respectively. C1, C2, and C3 refer to nontargeted, random removal of the same numbers of aquatic habitats as the corresponding targeted interventions. Within each subfigure, the *Diagonal*, *Horizontal*, and *Vertical* plots represent abundances (for the specified LSM scenario) for three different arrangements of houses in the landscapes (see Fig. 9.2 for the landscapes). With a *nonabsorbing boundary*, when mosquitoes hit an edge of the landscape's boundary, they enter the landscape from the edge directly opposite of the exiting edge and thus are not killed due to hitting the edge. Each simulation is run 50 times and the average results are reported. This figure represents averages of a total of 900 (18 × 50) simulations. Used from Arifin *et al.* [28] under a Creative Commons Attribution 4.0 International License.

9.3.3   Impact of Boundary Types

As stated above, use of absorbing boundaries yields less abundances than those with nonabsorbing boundaries. For all three landscape types (*Diagonal, Horizontal,* and *Vertical*), the absorbing boundary almost always (17 out of 18 scenarios, i.e., in 94% cases) yields larger PRs in abundances than the corresponding nonabsorbing boundary case with the same scenario. In addition, we found that even before applying LSM (i.e., before day 100), abundances are too low with absorbing boundaries when compared to those with nonabsorbing boundaries (see Figs. 9.6 and 9.7). Since at the beginning of all simulations, female mosquito agents start their activities from randomly selected houses, a good portion of them aggregate around these clumped houses. We verified that in most cases, these clumped houses have comparatively

TABLE 9.4   Percent Reductions in Abundance with LSM

		C1	T1	C2	T2	C3	T3	Ref.
Diagonal	GN-LSM (Absorbing)	4.2	38.4	8	100	69.6	100	[222]
	Absorbing	2.08	−21.63	3.56	43.82	31.74	85.32	[28]
	Nonabsorbing	−1.82	−23.24	0.22	39.55	29.72	82.65	[28]
Horizontal	GN-LSM (Absorbing)	8.9	−5.7	44	100	34.3	100	[222]
	Absorbing	4.35	7.37	−3.96	29.03	29.3	78.82	[28]
	Nonabsorbing	3.25	6.71	−3.27	22.29	34.16	54.01	[28]
Vertical	GN-LSM (Absorbing)	2.8	30.6	16.67	100	33.14	100	[222]
	Absorbing	5.21	15.45	24.17	55.54	43.21	91.79	[28]
	Nonabsorbing	5.32	14.32	23	52.13	40.45	88.20	[28]

far smaller average distances to their nearest edges in the landscape (see Fig. 9.2 for the landscapes). As a result, female mosquito agents that start moving around from these houses find an edge much quicker (and thus being killed) than those that start from the other houses. Thus, more mosquitoes die out due to the additional unrealistic killing effects imposed by the absorbing edges, suggesting the importance of using nonabsorbing boundaries in the ABM to avoid the potential bias created by absorbing boundaries.

9.3.4   ITNs in Isolation

Impact of ITNs in isolation on mosquito abundance is shown in Figs. 9.8–9.10, using household-level *partial* coverage with single chance for host-seeking, *partial* coverage with multiple chances for host-seeking, and *complete* coverage, respectively.[14] The reproduced landscape from GN-ITNs [221] used for ITNs application was shown in Fig. 9.3.

As shown in Figs. 9.8 and 9.9, the two partial coverage schemes with *single* or *multiple* chances (see Section 9.2.4) produce little differences when compared. Searching for a host within the same house for *n* times does not give much leverage to the mosquito agent, because each time, if the randomly picked host is protected by a bed net, the risk of being exposed to the insecticidal effect of ITNs (and thus getting killed) still exists. Since we replicate GN-ITNs [221] that is based on *partial* coverage, we compare their abundance results in Fig. 9.9, which shows household-level *partial* coverage with multiple chances for host-seeking. As coverage *C* increases, abundance is eventually reduced from 4000 to ≈2000, as shown in Fig. 9.9(d–l). This seems more plausible as opposed to achieving a 100% reduction in abundance as was shown by GN-ITNs [221], because with the partial coverage scheme, since only 54% of the human population are protected by bed nets, a portion of the mosquitoes can still find enough blood meals, and hence a complete suppression of the mosquito population cannot be expected.

As shown in Fig. 9.10, with the household-level complete coverage scheme, abundance is reduced from 4000 to ≈1000 when coverage is in the range $60\% < C \leq 80\%$

---

[14]See Section 9.2.4 and Fig. 9.1 for the ITNs coverage schemes.

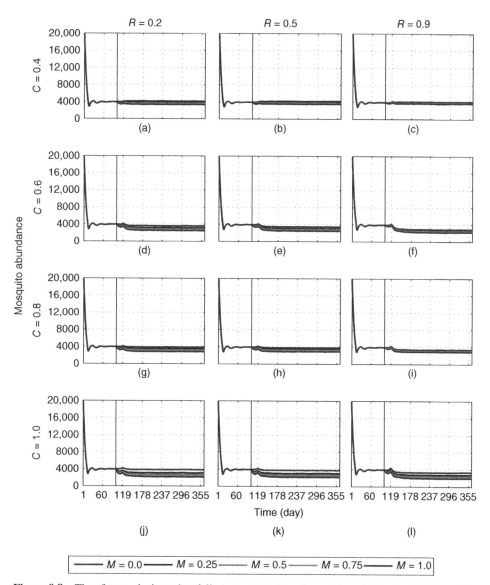

Figure 9.8 The figure depicts the full 1-year results of applying ITNs in isolation with household-level partial coverage and single chance for host-seeking as we replicate the results of GN-ITNs [221]. Each subfigure represents a specific combination for the three ITNs parameters of coverage, repellence, and mortality. The x-axis denotes simulation time (days) and the y-axis denotes mosquito abundance. Each row represents a specific coverage (C) for ITNs (e.g., $C = 0.8$). Each column represents a specific repellence (R) for ITNs (e.g., $R = 0.5$). Within each subfigure, each color-coded plot represents a specific mortality (M) value for ITNs (e.g., $M = 0.25$), with mortality (M) color keys at the bottom of the figure. The figure represents averages of a total of 3000 ($4 \times 3 \times 5 \times 50$) simulations. Nonabsorbing boundaries are used. For the partial coverage schemes, see Section 9.2.4. Used from Arifin *et al.* [28] under a Creative Commons Attribution 4.0 International License.

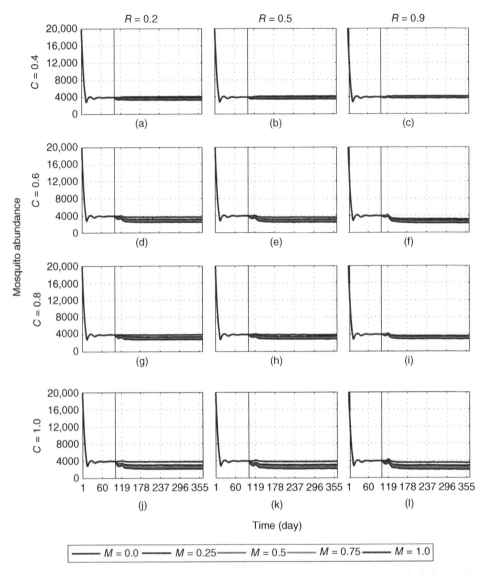

Figure 9.9 The figure depicts the full 1-year results of applying ITNs in isolation with household-level partial coverage and multiple chances for host-seeking as we replicate the results of GN-ITNs [221]. Each subfigure represents a specific combination for the three ITNs parameters of coverage, repellence, and mortality. The x-axis denotes simulation time (days) and the y-axis denotes mosquito abundance. Each row represents a specific coverage (C) for ITNs (e.g., $C = 0.8$). Each column represents a specific repellence (R) for ITNs (e.g., $R = 0.5$). Within each subfigure, each color-coded plot represents a specific mortality (M) value for ITNs (e.g., $M = 0.25$), with mortality (M) color keys at the bottom of the figure. The figure represents averages of a total of 3000 ($4 \times 3 \times 5 \times 50$) simulations. Nonabsorbing boundaries are used. For the partial coverage schemes, see Section 9.2.4. Used from Arifin *et al.* [28] under a Creative Commons Attribution 4.0 International License.

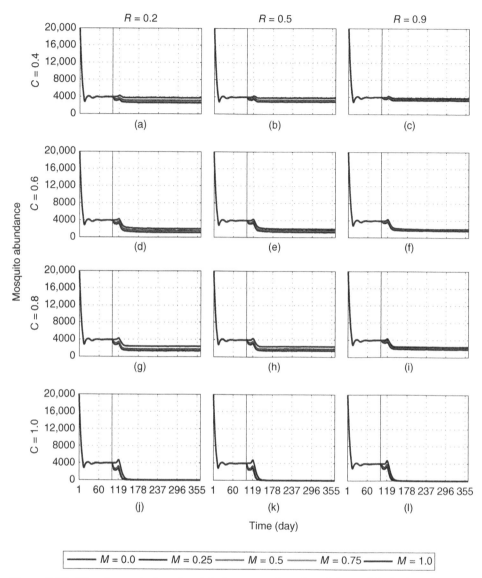

Figure 9.10 The figure depicts the full 1-year results of applying ITNs in isolation with household-level complete coverage as we replicate the results of GN-ITNs [221]. Each subfigure represents a specific combination for the three ITNs parameters of coverage, repellence, and mortality. The x-axis denotes simulation time (days) and the y-axis denotes mosquito abundance. Each row represents a specific coverage (C) for ITNs (e.g., $C = 0.8$). Each column represents a specific repellence (R) for ITNs (e.g., $R = 0.5$). Within each subfigure, each color-coded plot represents a specific mortality (M) value for ITNs (e.g., $M = 0.25$), with mortality (M) color keys at the bottom of the figure. The figure represents averages of a total of 3000 ($4 \times 3 \times 5 \times 50$) simulations. Nonabsorbing boundaries are used. For the complete coverage scheme, see Section 9.2.4. Used from Arifin *et al.* [28] under a Creative Commons Attribution 4.0 International License.

and repellence R is not too high (see Fig. 9.10(d, e, g, and h)). As C approaches 100% (i.e., all humans are protected by bed nets), irrespective of repellence, abundance can be completely suppressed, as seen in Fig. 9.10(j)–(k). However, too high repellence (e.g., $0.5\% \leq R \leq 0.9$), though unlikely to be present in commonly used insecticides in real-world scenarios, can have a detrimental effect on vector control (by increasing abundance) with the same levels of coverage and mortality, but the degree of this negative impact is reduced as coverage increases (see Figs. 9.9(b, c, e, f, h, and i) and 9.10(b, c, e, f, h and i).

Figures 9.11 and 9.12 show the PR values in mosquito abundance for selected and all parameters, respectively. These results are obtained by applying ITNs with household-level partial coverage (with multiple chances) and complete coverage for host-seeking. As seen in Fig. 9.12(e–g), when $R \leq 0.5$, around 60% PR can be

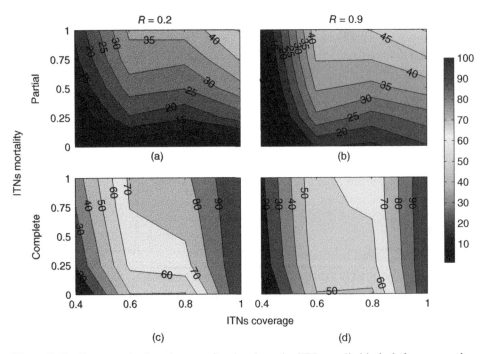

Figure 9.11   Percent reductions in mosquito abundance by ITNs, applied in isolation, comparing household-level partial coverage (with multiple chances for host-seeking) and complete coverage. Each subfigure represents a specific combination of coverage scheme (partial or complete) and repellence (R) for ITNs: (a) and (b) show the partial scheme with $R = 0.2$ and $R = 0.9$, respectively. (c) and (d) show the complete scheme with $R = 0.2$ and $R = 0.9$, respectively. The x-axis denotes ITNs coverage and the y-axis denotes ITNs mortality. The upper row represents household-level partial coverage and the lower row represents household-level complete coverage, as marked on the left. Each column represents a specific repellence (R) value, as marked on the top. ITNs are applied at day 100 in the 40 × 40 grid-based landscape with 50 houses having a total human population of 185. The percent reduction (PR) values are represented as filled contour plots in each subfigure. The color bar on the right quantifies the PR isolines. Results for the entire parameter space are depicted in Fig. 9.12. Used from Arifin *et al.* [28] under a Creative Commons Attribution 4.0 International License.

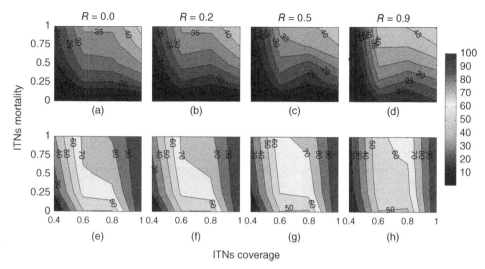

Figure 9.12   Percent reductions in mosquito abundance by ITNs, applied in isolation, comparing household-level partial coverage (with multiple chances for host-seeking) and complete coverage. This figure shows results for the entire parameter space. For other details, see Fig. 9.11. Used from Arifin *et al.* [28] under a Creative Commons Attribution 4.0 International License.

achieved with coverage and mortality being as low as ≈60% and ≈30%, respectively. However, when $0.5 < R \leq 0.9$, to achieve the same PR, the coverage needs to be as high as ≈85%. Also, $R = 0.9$ means 90% of the host-seeking mosquitoes are driven away from the house before the ITNs mortality can play any role (see the complete coverage scheme in Section 9.2.4). This is why mortality seems to have less impact in Fig. 9.11d than in Fig. 9.11c.

Interestingly, with the complete coverage scheme, even with no ITNs mortality, very high PR (around 80%) can be achieved with high coverage (≈90%), irrespective of repellence (see Fig. 9.11c and d). With 90% coverage, around 90% of the population sleep under bed nets. Since the ABM assumes complete usage of bed nets and the *An. gambiae* mosquitoes are almost exclusively anthropophilic and highly endophagic, no blood meal can be obtained from sources other than humans, or during daytime. Thus, though no mosquitoes are killed due to ITNs mortality, they cannot complete their gonotrophic cycles (because ≈90% of the host-seeking attempts fail), and eventually, the mosquito population dies out.

9.3.5   LSM and ITNs in Combination

In this section, we present the simulation results of applying LSM and ITNs in combination. Figures 9.13 and 9.14 show the PR values in mosquito abundance as a function of LSM coverage and ITNs coverage. Each subfigure represents a filled contour plot where the isolines are labeled with specific PRs, whose magnitudes are shown in the color bar on the right. Each row represents a specific mortality (M) value for ITNs

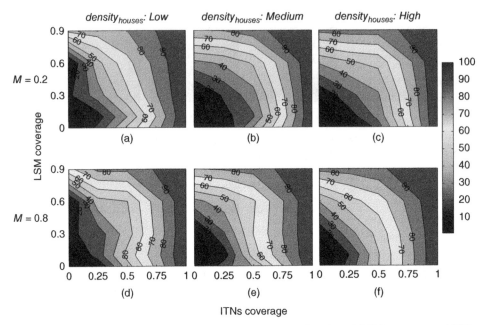

Figure 9.13 Percent reductions in mosquito abundance as a function of LSM coverage and ITNs coverage when LSM and ITNs are applied in combination. The *x*-axis denotes ITNs coverage and the *y*-axis denotes LSM coverage. Each subfigure represents a filled contour plot where the isolines are labeled with specific percent reduction (PR) values, with specific combination of density of houses (*density_houses*) and mortality (*M*) for ITNs: subfigures (a)–(c) represent *M* = 0.2 with *density_houses* of *Low, Medium*, and *High*, respectively; subfigures (d)–(f) represent *M* = 0.8 with *density_houses* of *Low, Medium*, and *High*, respectively. ITNs repellence (*R*) is fixed at 0.5. Each simulation is run for 1 year; both LSM and ITNs applied at day 100 and continued up to the end of the simulation. The color bar on the right quantifies the PR isolines. The figure represents average percent reduction values of a total of 6000 (3 × 5 × 4 × 2 × 50) simulations. For ITNs, household-level complete coverage scheme is used (see Fig. 9.1c). Nonabsorbing boundaries are used. Sample landscapes with the three *density_houses* levels are shown in Fig. 9.4. The figure depicts selected results that involve a subset of the parameters from Table 9.3. Used from Arifin *et al.* [28] under a Creative Commons Attribution 4.0 International License.

(e.g., *M* = 0.2), as marked on the left. Each column represents a specific *density_houses*, as marked on the top.

Figures 9.13 and 9.14 indicate some interesting observations. First, impact of ITNs mortality (*M*) becomes increasingly important as the *density_houses* increases. Comparing the subfigures columnwise, increasing ITNs mortality (*M*) has less impact on the landscape with *Low density_houses* than with *Medium* or *High* cases. With *Low density_houses*, number of available human hosts are also low, making the number of host-seeking events much lower than the other two cases. Less host-seeking events in turn mean reduced probability of a mosquito being in contact with ITNs. As a result, increasing ITNs mortality (*M*) cannot affect PR values as greatly as it can with the other two cases. In general, as ITNs mortality and *density_houses* increase, more successes with the

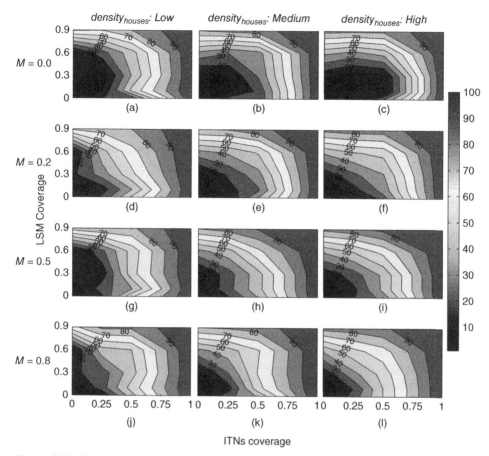

Figure 9.14   The figure depicts percent reductions results that involve the entire parameter space from Table 9.3 as a function of LSM coverage and ITNs coverage when LSM and ITNs are applied in combination. This figure shows results for the entire parameter space. For other details, see Fig. 9.13. Used from Arifin *et al.* [28] under a Creative Commons Attribution 4.0 International License.

combined interventions are observed, indicating the importance of at least some ITNs mortality being there when ITNs are applied.

Increase in ITNs mortality (M) also influences the general shape of the PR isolines. With *High density$_{houses}$* (column 3), as M increases, the combined interventions become more effective, as seen by the increases of higher PR values: for $PR > 40\%$, the corresponding area increases from 70.83% (for $M = 0.2$) to 83.33% (for $M = 0.8$). This trend is also seen for *Low* and *Medium* densities (columns 1 and 2), with the *Low* density column having the least impact.

Next, considering the impact of each intervention in isolation (i.e., looking exactly at both the x- and y-axes PR values with $y = 0$ and $x = 0$, respectively), on a per-row or per-column basis, the rate of changes in PR is similar across all subfigures. For example, with *Low density$_{houses}$* at Fig. 9.13a and c (i.e., column 1), looking at the y-axis (i.e., at $x = 0$, meaning when ITNs are ignored, and LSM coverage is gradually increased), the isolines of PR values intersect the y-axis at approximately similar intervals (e.g., PR_{10} with LSM coverage ≈ 0.18, PR_{20} with LSM coverage ≈ 0.63). Similar trends are observed across the x-axis, and also for columns 2 and 3. This ensures that without the presence of the other intervention, both LSM and ITNs, with their respective parameters varied, yield significant impact on abundance and reinforces the importance of ensuring the individual efficacy of each intervention.

Next, when ITNs mortality (M) is nonzero (i.e., the bed nets are at least partially lethal to mosquitoes), increasing ITNs coverage is more effective in reducing mosquito abundance (i.e., increasing PR) than increasing LSM coverage, which is observed by the more pronounced increase in PR across the x-axis than up the y-axis. This observation is in agreement with similar results obtained in reducing the basic reproductive number of malaria (R_0) by Yakob and Yan [574]. However, with nonlethal ITNs ($M = 0$), the efficacy of both interventions approach more equivalency as the $density_{houses}$ approaches from *Low* to *High*. Also, comparing the subfigures column-wise, integrating both interventions yield more synergistic effect as the $density_{houses}$ approaches from *Low* to *High*. Again, this trend agrees with similar results obtained in reducing R_0 in [574].

Not surprisingly, the increase in PR values indicate more synergistic patterns when all parameters are in effect (i.e., have some nonzero values). For example, looking at Fig. 9.14(b, c, e, and f), where the $density_{houses}$ is *Medium* to *High*, and M is in the range 0.2–0.8, increasing coverages of both interventions yield more synergistic benefits, as indicated by the more convexity of the PR isolines in general. In these cases, with sufficient number of host-seeking events, and ITNs in action with some mortality (insecticidal effect), both interventions play important roles in reducing abundance and thus increasing PRs.

Other synergistic effects are also observed in the results. As shown in Figs. 9.13 and 9.14, the combined impact is additive (and not multiplicative) and is more effective with high $density_{houses}$, confirming similar findings by a previous study [574]. For example, with higher $density_{houses}$, impact of ITNs mortality (M) becomes increasingly important. As shown in Fig. 9.13, increasing ITNs mortality affects the shape of the low-to-medium range (10–40%) PR isolines. With no insecticidal effect of ITNs (i.e., $M = 0.0$), looking at Fig. 9.14(a–c), as $density_{houses}$ increases, more host-seeking events occur, causing more mosquitoes to seek for aquatic habitats in order to lay eggs. But with increasing LSM coverage, they are denied more opportunities to lay eggs (as more aquatic habitats are eliminated), causing the lower range (10–40%) PR isolines to reduce vertically (down the y-axis). However, as both $density_{houses}$ and ITNs coverage increase (but mortality still remains zero), more host-seeking events actually encounter ITNs, but with no mortality in effect, ITNs cannot have significant impact, thus extending the lower range (10–40%) PR isolines horizontally (across the x-axis). As ITNs mortality increases (see Fig. 9.14d–1), this extension effect is gradually reduced and more impact is seen with higher $density_{houses}$.

9.4 REPLICATION AND REPRODUCIBILITY (R&R) GUIDELINES

In this section, we present some R&R guidelines for future modelers from our experiences. Replicating earlier ABMs that examined the impact of LSM and ITNs in isolation posed some unique challenges. For example, the unavailability of source codes of the original models inhibits from performing direct model-to-model comparison (docking). In addition, the structural characteristics of ABMs, which are fundamentally different from other types (e.g., mathematical) of models, also rule out the possibility of systematic verification of model features.

The overall exercise drew important R&R issues from which model differences may arise, and/or the process of replication may become more time-consuming and challenging. In the following, we discuss some of them:

Conceptual Image of the Model: As we mentioned before, at least during the initial stages of an M&S project, mental/conceptual images of the model often reside amorphously only in the modelers' brains and may vastly differ among individual modelers due to countless ambiguities. Its transformation into a computational/verifiable entity (the ABM) can be a challenging process itself. In other words, the intended logical view of the ABM may be perceived differently by different modelers, thus creating different conceptual, mental images of the logical view.

Choice of Tools: The appropriate selection of computer programming languages and tools from the myriad options offered these days warrants special attention. Issues such as the availability and limitations of a particular programming language, the use of specific data structures and other language constructs, and even the coding style of individual modelers, can compound the differences that may arise from using a specific language (e.g., C++ vs Java). For specific purposes, choice of proprietary versus open-access computing tools (e.g., Matlab vs Python for simulation output data analysis) can be important too.

Availability of Additional Resources: In some cases, additional resources used by the model, if not defined or made explicitly available by the original authors, may pose subtle challenges. For landscape-based ABMs, examples of these resources include artificial maps, object listings in landscapes, GIS data layers, and so on. Although the importance of these resources may seem somewhat arbitrary in the broader context, goals, and outputs of the original models, their precise specification still remains important for the purposes of replication. For example, as described in Section 9.2.5, the absence of spatial coordinates listings of the objects (which may be provided as supplementary materials) not only forces future modelers to spend considerable amount of time in reproducing the landscapes, it also increases the possibility of judgment errors being introduced in this phase. Due to the lack of additional information, some part of the process often needs to rely on best guesses.

Clear, detailed description of the parameter space for all model parameters used by the ABM, including their initial and other time-varying conditions, may substantially help in minimizing the conceptual image gaps. However, as the past experience shows [22, 23, 25], merely stating model parameters, logical flowcharts, initial conditions, and so on cannot entirely solve the above problems, primarily because (1) the possibility of different logical workflow paths in the programmed code still remains open and (2) many implementation details still cannot be covered. Based on this modeling exercise, we recommend the following guidelines for future ABM modelers:

Code and Data Sharing: The source code and executable programs of the ABMs should be shared with the research community. As argued by Peng, enough information about methods and code should be available for independent researchers in computational sciences to reach consistent conclusions in order to ensure a minimum standard of reproducibility [428]. Many reputed journals across multiple disciplines have also implemented different code-sharing policies. For example, the journal *Biostatistics* [66] has implemented a policy to encourage authors of accepted papers to make their work reproducible by others. In this journal, based on three different criteria termed as "code," "data," and "reproducible," the associate editor for reproducibility (AER) classifies the accepted papers as *C*, *D*, and/or *R*, respectively, on their title pages [427, 428]. As reproducibility is critical to tracking down the bugs of computational science, code sharing may be specially important for ABMs. Having multiple research groups examining the same model and generating new data or output may lead to robust conclusions [472]. Some recent malaria models have partially followed this path by providing controlled access to their models. For example, the *OpenMalaria* epidemiology model [394] provides a general open-access platform for comparing, fitting, and evaluating different model structures. The advanced individual-based model *EMOD* from Intellectual Ventures Lab [169] is available within controlled execution environments.[15] However, for certain reasons (e.g., during preliminary design and development phases, exploratory feature testing phases), it may not always be feasible to share the source code. In these cases, we recommend that at least the associated executable programs and/or other tools (with detailed instructions on how to run the programs) be made available as supplementary materials for ABM-based studies that are accepted for publication.

Open Access (OA) Research: To facilitate code and data sharing, the recent trends of Open Access research, which have become increasingly important and popular in recent years, can be followed. *Open Access (OA)* provides unrestricted online access to peer-reviewed scholarly research and is primarily intended for scholarly journals, theses, book chapters, and monographs. The impact of OA on research and scholarship on every phase of the scientific research process has been recognized by high-level research funders, policy makers, university administrators,

---

[15]Note that in Chapter 11, *EMOD* is presented along with two important epidemiological scenarios in Africa.

librarians, publishers, and scholars [268]. Over the past decade, OA has become central to advancing the interests of researchers, scholars, students, librarians, businesses, and the public, and has been identified as an integral part of the infrastructure supporting scholarly research, as a key driver of scientific productivity, and as an accelerator for innovation and commercialization [268, 519]. OA solves the *pricing crisis* by preventing libraries from buying access to the required literature and the *permission crisis* by preventing libraries and their patrons from making full and legitimate use of the materials [519]. As shown by recent studies, articles available through OA have greater research impacts across multiple disciplines with high citation advantages, and scholars in diverse disciplines are increasingly adopting OA practices [14, 69, 176]. The additional usage rights associated with OA are often granted through the use of various *Creative Commons (CC)* licenses [131]. CC is a nonprofit organization that enables the sharing and use of creativity and knowledge through free legal tools; it develops, supports, and stewards legal and technical infrastructure that maximizes digital creativity, sharing, and innovation. Although not an alternative to copyright, a CC license is one of several public copyright licenses that enable the free distribution of an otherwise copyrighted work. Thus, modelers can use CC to provide free, easy-to-use copyright licenses in a simple, standardized way to give others the right to share, use, and build upon their models, data, results, and other works.

Relevant Documentation: Documentation is an important part of software engineering. Well-written documentation should be provided by modelers who share the source code and/or executable programs of their ABMs. Many peer-reviewed reputed journals (e.g., the *PLOS Computational Biology* [437]) emphasize that the source code must be accompanied with documentation on building and installing the software from the source, including instructions on how to use and test the software on supplied test data [438]. An ABM documentation may include statements describing the attributes, features and characteristics of its agents and environments, the overall architecture or design principles of the code, algorithms and application programming interfaces (APIs), manuals for end users, interpretation of additional materials (e.g., object-based landscapes), and so on. To this end, free and commercial software tools are available that can help automating the process of code annotation, code analysis, and software documentation [275, 330, 338, 485].

Standardized Models: For a given ABM, its general workflow should include and follow standardized components such as formal input/output requirements and program logic. The need for standardization becomes more important when the broader utility of the model is considered within an integrated modeling platform. For example, both *OpenMalaria* [394] and *EMOD* [169] are currently being integrated within the open-access execution environment of the Vector-Borne Disease Network (VecNet) [548]. The proposed VecNet cyberinfrastructure (VecNet CI), within a shared execution environment, establishes three modes of access sharing for model developers: (1) shared data: model developers run their models on their own compute resources and upload the output data to the

VecNet CI for public consumption; (2) shared execution: model developers share their software with VecNet CI developers only, allowing the CI and its operators to incorporate their model into the CI execution environment; and (3) shared software: model developers share their software at large with the public. Once integrated, these models can utilize other components of the VecNet CI, including the VecNet Digital Library, web-based user interface (UI), tools for visualization, job management, and query and search, in order to, for example, import and use model-specific data to run specific scenarios or campaigns of interest and display their output using the visualization and/or the UI tools of the VecNet CI. It is envisaged that most ABMs in the future will be accommodated within the integrated modeling frameworks of similar cyberinfrastructure platforms. To expedite the future integration process, ABMs should plan and follow a well-defined integration path from the early phases of model development.

9.5 DISCUSSION

Some of the key insights obtained by exploring the individual and combined efficacies of LSM and ITNs are discussed in this section.

In general, with LSM applied in isolation, our replicated results agree with the major findings by GN-LSM [222] that LSM coverage of 300 m surrounding all houses can lead to significant reductions in abundance, and, while targeting aquatic habitats to apply LSM, distance to the nearest houses can be an important measure. However, as shown by our model, some of the underlying assumptions in the earlier models could have seriously affected the predicted outcomes. To be specific, reporting results from a single simulation run and the use of absorbing boundaries could lead to substantially different results, invalidating the findings and thereby diminishing the predictive power of the models. Also, without a more sophisticated spatial metric that can capture the interrelations of different resources in different landscapes, simplistic features such as the general arrangement pattern of houses (e.g., diagonal, horizontal, or vertical) is insufficient to capture a landscape's potential to transmit the disease. For example, comparing the most restrictive cases of LSM application, the reduction in abundance is more prominent with a nonabsorbing boundary (from ≈10,000 to ≈1800, as shown in Fig. 9.7f), than with absorbing boundaries (from ≈3000 to ≈500, as shown in Fig. 9.6f). Due to the random distributions of houses and aquatic habitats in the three selected landscape patterns, the reduction effects remain unpredictable, depending on factors such as the proximity of the resources to the boundaries of the landscapes. Thus, when applied to different (e.g., more general or specific) conditions, these assumptions may produce misleading results. The modified assumptions, as implemented in this study, provide new insights and potentially more accurate results under certain conditions.

It is implausible to expect 100% reductions in abundance even with the most restrictive application of LSM (see T3 in Table 9.4). This is because even with absorbing boundaries, some mosquitoes would always survive by roaming around in different parts of the landscape, instead of hitting the edges of the boundary (and hence dying out). This is observed in the results – the highest PR value obtained is 91.79% with scenario T3 using an absorbing boundary, as opposed to 100% that was observed in several cases in the GN-LSM study [222].

In few cases, negative PR values are obtained (see Table 9.4), counterintuitively suggesting that the abundances actually increase after applying LSM. A closer look at the landscapes (see Fig. 9.2) reveals that these cases are associated with the removal of a small fraction of all aquatic habitats (4 out of 90 for C1 and T1) by LSM. Recall that in the ABM, abundance is primarily governed by the capacity of aquatic habitats and the density-dependent oviposition mechanism (see Chapter 4). Removal of only a few nearby habitats may actually save a mosquito from wasting its time trying to search, locate, and compete in laying eggs in the already crowded habitats, and instead be more productive by finding comparatively less-crowded habitats that are within close vicinity.

This points to an important insight: if the mosquito population in the environment is not unrestricted (i.e., it is restricted to be within the limit of the environment's overall capacity, as in the ABM), and some stages of the mosquito biology are governed by special mechanisms (e.g., density-dependent oviposition), then removal of only an insufficient number of aquatic habitats may, in some cases, increase the abundance. Thus, before actually applying LSM, it may be crucial to estimate its impact (to achieve the desired level of success) by simulating varying levels of coverage.

The choice of using fixed- versus age-dependent mortality rates can have significant impact on the results, which can be compounded by the choice of boundary type as well. As stated before, we use fixed mortality rates of 0.2 for the absorbing boundary and age-dependent mortality rates (for all adult stages and the larva stage) for the non-absorbing boundary. We get unbounded abundance using mortality rates < 0.2 with the absorbing boundary and using any fixed mortality rates (other than the age-dependent mortality rates) with the nonabsorbing boundary (these results are not shown).

With ITNs applied in isolation, different definitions of ITNs coverage can lead to significantly different results. The household-level partial coverage schemes can provide only $\approx 50\%$ reduction in abundance with 100% coverage and 100% mortality. This means that even when each house is equipped with one bed net (which, overall, covers only $\approx 54\%$ of the human population), this scheme cannot perform even anywhere close to suppress abundance. On the other hand, the household-level complete coverage scheme can provide as much as 70% reductions in abundance with $\geq 85\%$ coverage and mortality as low as 25%. With this scheme, when the coverage is 100%, abundance can be completely suppressed even when no mortality is in action (i.e., $M = 0.0$), as shown in Fig. 9.10(j–l). This is expected, since every person in every house is protected by bed nets, the host-seeking mosquitoes cannot find unprotected hosts to obtain blood meals. While modeling the impact of ITNs, these distinctions should be clearly marked and the choice of the ITNs coverage scheme should be made carefully.

In general, repellence, which drives the host-seeking mosquito away from a house, can have a detrimental effect on vector control when the risk (additional delay in search and so on) of finding an unprotected host in another house is less than that in the same house. With the complete coverage scheme, since every person in the house (with ITNs coverage) is protected by bed net, the above turns out to be true. However, as coverage increases, more houses fall within the range of coverage, and the probability of finding an unprotected host (in another house) during the next search decreases. Thus, with increasing coverage, the negative impact incurred by too high repellence gets reduced, as evident in Fig. 9.10(a–i).

On the other hand, with household-level partial coverage schemes (both with single or multiple chances), this effect is almost absent (see Figs. 9.8 and 9.9). Recall that with the partial coverage schemes, every person in the same house (with ITNs coverage) may not be protected by a bed net. Thus, the mosquito may find an unprotected host in the same house. If it is repelled too often (due to high repellence), it is being deprived of its current positional advantage and the risk of finding an unprotected host in another house may not be well justified.

Interestingly, the use of a specific boundary type does not have significant impact for the particular landscape (see Fig. 9.3). We simulated and compared the three schemes of ITNs coverage using absorbing and nonabsorbing boundary and found no significant differences as long as the age-dependent mortality rates are used with both boundary types.

With the combined application of LSM and ITNs, the results indicated that varying human population densities can affect the degree of synergistic benefits that may be obtained from such efforts, as was previously shown by a mathematical model [574]. To the best of our knowledge, this is the first ABM-based study to explore this particular combination of LSM and ITNs (acknowledging that some other combinations were explored by other ABMs, e.g., [160]).

9.6 SUMMARY

In this chapter, we presented the results of replicating another published malaria ABM by improving/extending some of its dubious assumptions. In the process of replication, we also presented the details of modeling two vector control interventions – LSM and ITNs – with our spatial ABM. As we explored the individual and combined efficacies of LSM and ITNs, we systematically compared our results with those of other published malaria models. By improving and/or extending some of the original assumptions such as reporting results from single simulation runs and use of absorbing boundaries, we showed that these assumptions may lead to less reliable results. Some challenges faced while replicating earlier models are also discussed and several guidelines (code and data sharing, relevant documentation, and standardized models) obtained from this exercise are recommended for future ABM modelers.

As the results indicated, replicability of the experiments and simulations performed by models published earlier bear special importance. Due to several factors that include new tools and technologies, massive amounts of data, interdisciplinary research, and so on, the task of replication may become even more complicated. Future modelers may avoid these unforeseen complications to a considerable extent by following the R&R guidelines that we proposed from our experiences.

Modeling the malaria control interventions and exploring their efficacies with our spatial ABM can be treated as one of its ideal example applications. In Chapter 10, we present another useful application that integrates a GIS with the spatial ABM and thereby takes the virtual world of mosquito agents one step closer to the real world of mosquitoes.

10

A LANDSCAPE EPIDEMIOLOGY MODELING FRAMEWORK

10.1 OVERVIEW

This chapter presents a landscape epidemiology modeling framework that integrates a geographic information system (GIS) with our spatial agent-based model (ABM) of malaria.[1] The field of *landscape epidemiology* emerged from the theory that most vector-borne diseases (VBDs) are commonly tied to the landscape as environmental determinants control their distribution and abundance [423]. It draws some of its roots from the field of *landscape ecology*, which is concerned with analyzing patterns and processes in different ecosystems [295].

Landscape epidemiology studies the patterns, processes, and risk factors of diseases across time and space, and describes how the temporal dynamics of host, vector, and pathogen populations interact spatially within a permissive environment to enable disease transmission [166, 295, 450]. The spatially defined *focus*, or *nidus*, of disease transmission may be characterized by several factors such as vegetation, climate, latitude, elevation, and geology. The ecological complexity, dimensions, and temporal stability of the nidus are determined largely by pathogen natural history and vector bionomics [450].[2]

---

[1] The spatial ABM was presented in Chapter 6.

[2] See, for example, the review by Reisen [450], which describes the evolution of landscape epidemiology as a science and exemplifies selected aspects by contrasting the ecology of two different disease outbreaks in North America caused by (1) the mosquito-borne West Nile virus (WNV) and (2) a zoonotic VBD called the Lyme disease transmitted by ticks and the bacterial species *Borrelia burgdorferi*.

Spatial Agent-Based Simulation Modeling in Public Health:
Design, Implementation, and Applications for Malaria Epidemiology, First Edition.
S. M. Niaz Arifin, Gregory R. Madey and Frank H. Collins.
© 2016 John Wiley & Sons, Inc. Published 2016 by John Wiley & Sons, Inc.

Spatial epidemiology, medical geography, geographical epidemiology, and *health geomatics* are all effectively synonymous terms for landscape epidemiology. These disciplines generally focus on the study of geographical distribution of disease spread or population at risk [68, 76, 165, 432].[3] The emergence and spread of infectious diseases in a changing environment require the development of new methodologies and tools. As such, disease dynamics models on geographic scales ranging from village to continental levels are increasingly needed for quantitative prediction of epidemic outcomes and design of practicable strategies for control [296, 358].

The close relationships between place, space, disease, and human health are well known for many decades [303]. Disease ecology and epidemiology consider population, society, and both the physical and biological environments to be in dynamic equilibrium. Significant stress on this equilibrium can produce cascading effects on any of these components [349]. For example, major changes in land use, migration, population pressure, or other factors can show significant abnormality in human-environment relationship, causing the appearance or diffusion of existing and new diseases [160, 349].

One of the first applications of spatial analysis in epidemiology is the 1832 work that represented the 48 districts of the city of Paris by halftone color gradient according to the number of deaths by cholera per 1000 inhabitants [141]. Perhaps more famous is John Snow's 1854 pioneering work and classic discovery of the association between cholera and the originating Broad Street station water pump in London, providing strong evidence in support of his theory that cholera was a water-borne disease. The *John Snow map* depicted a cholera outbreak in London using points to represent the locations of some individual cases, and was unique in using cartographic methods not only to depict but also to analyze clusters of geographically dependent phenomena [211, 249, 359]. Understanding the complex spatiotemporal relationships between environmental factors and disease outbreaks and identifying exposures to environmental hazards in high-risk populations are essential elements of an effective public health management program [542]. To this regard, GIS can provide cost-effective tools for evaluating interventions and policies, potentially affecting health outcomes. As shown by recent research, GIS and related spatial statistical methods are regarded as important tools in epidemiology to identify areas with increased risk of diseases and to determine spatial association between disease and risk factors [367, 466].

Understanding a landscape epidemiology system requires more than an understanding of the different types of populations (host, vector, and pathogen) that comprise the system. For example, it also requires understanding how the individuals interact with each other and how the results can be more than the sum of the parts. As we described in Chapter 3, an ABM often exhibits emergent properties arising from the interactions of the agents that cannot be deduced simply by aggregating the properties of the agents.

---

[3]See, for example, Jones *et al.* [267] and Kearns and Moon [274] for introductions to medical geography.

Thus, an ABM can be a very practical method of analysis of the dynamic consequences of agents within a landscape epidemiology model.[4]

A GIS is a system designed to capture, store, manipulate, analyze, manage, and present all types of geographical data. The idea of integrating GIS with ABMs is not new. Several studies, ranging across multiple domains, have shown such integration. For example, Brown *et al.* addressed the coupling of GIS-based data models with agent-based process models and analyzed different requirements for integrating ABM and GIS functionality [82]. They illustrated the integration approach with four ABMs: urban land use change, military mobile communications, dynamic landscape analysis and modeling system, and infrastructure simulations.

However, with the exception of the individual-based model named *EMOD* (epidemiological modeling, see Chapter 11), no ABM of malaria has yet shown how to effectively integrate simulation outputs from an ABM with a GIS and other geospatial features, and thereby harness the full power of GIS. There is also a vacuum of knowledge in building robust integration frameworks that can guide the use of ecological, geospatial, environmental, and other types of features (related to malaria transmission) as model inputs, as opposed to simply use these features as cartographic outputs from the models (as done by most previous studies). In recent years, despite the proliferation of spatial models that acknowledge the importance of spatially explicit processes in determining disease risk, the use of spatial information beyond recording spatial location and mapping disease risk is rare [260]. Although numerous recent tools have been developed using GIS, global positioning systems (GPSs), remote sensing, and spatial statistics, there is still a lack of and hence a serious need to develop efficient and useful tools for research, surveillance, and control programs of VBDs.

In this chapter, we present a landscape epidemiology modeling framework by integrating our spatial ABM of malaria with a GIS.[5] To account for three output indices and five scenarios (that represent two coverage levels of the two malaria control interventions being modeled), we run a total of 750 simulations for 2 years and report their average results. Using spatial statistics tools, we perform hot spot analysis for all scenarios in order to determine the statistical significance of the simulation results. In addition, we apply ordinary kriging with circular semivariograms on the output indices.

Besides being useful for simulation modelers in different branches of science and engineering, this work can provide important insights from the epidemiological perspective and thus would be valuable for epidemiologists, disease control managers, and public health officials for research as well as in practical fields. In particular, we believe that the insights gained through this study can assist these stakeholders in refining further research questions and surveillance needs, and in guiding control efforts and field studies. Although the landscape epidemiology modeling framework described in this chapter utilizes an ABM of malaria-transmitting mosquitoes, it is applicable to a

---

[4]See Section 3.4 for a brief discussion about the power of ABMs to model *emergence* and *aggregation*.

[5]Portions of the text and figures presented in this chapter appeared in Arifin *et al.* [20, 27].

wider range of other infectious VBDs (e.g., dengue, yellow fever), and hence may find its use in a much wider scenario.

The model described in this chapter has been designed specifically around the mosquito *Anopheles gambiae*. As mentioned before, the *An. gambiae* complex is a closely related group of eight named mosquito species found primarily in Africa and includes the three nominal species *An. gambiae*, *Anopheles coluzzii*, and *Anopheles arabiensis*, which are among the most efficient malaria vectors known. While the respective ecologies and involvement in malaria transmission among other members of the *An. gambiae* complex differ in important ways, this model could effectively apply to all three and even to many of the several dozen other major malaria vectors in the world.

Results presented in this chapter use the following features:

- Use of improved models: The core model and the corresponding ABM reflect the most recent updates with enriched features, which allows us to model the population dynamics of *An. gambiae* mosquito agents in a more comprehensive way.[6] Since the most recent ABM is tested using the rigorous verification, validation, and replication techniques, the results entail much higher confidence from both the epidemiological and the simulation perspectives.[7]
- Malaria control interventions: This chapter extends the modeling of malaria control interventions and exploring their efficacies on a real geographical region.[8]
- Reporting aggregate measures by replication: The importance of replication was discussed in detail in Chapter 9. Following the same replication policy, 50 replicated runs for all simulations are performed and their averages are reported in this study.

As mentioned in Chapter 4, the core model describes the complete *An. gambiae* mosquito life cycle, which consists of aquatic and adult phases (see Fig. 4.1). It also presented several important features of the *An. gambiae* life cycle, including the development and mortality rates in different stages, the aquatic habitats, and oviposition. Another important feature, vector senescence, was adopted to account for the age-dependent aspects of the mosquito biology, and implemented using density- and age-dependent larval and adult mortality rates.

In Chapters 6 and 9, we used various artificial landscapes for our spatial ABM. The landscapes were topologically modeled as 2-D torus spaces with nonabsorbing boundaries and contained the houses and aquatic habitats that served as important ecological resources for the mosquito agents to obtain human blood meals (in houses) and to lay eggs (in aquatic habitats).[9] The same landscape-based modeling approach is extended here by including real-world landscapes from a specific study area (see Section 10.3).

---

[6]The core model and the spatial ABM were presented in Chapters 4 and 6, respectively.

[7]The processes and results of verification, validation, and replication of the ABMs were presented in Chapters 8 and 9.

[8]See Chapter 9 for results that explored the efficacies of malaria control interventions on artificial landscapes.

[9]See Chapter 9 for a comparison of results involving absorbing and nonabsorbing boundaries.

This chapter is organized as follows. Section 10.2 discusses several studies that use GIS and other spatial techniques in public health and epidemiology, with special focus on malaria. Section 10.3 describes the study area and briefly mentions some features of the spatial ABM (which are used in this chapter). Section 10.4 presents the GIS by describing the processing steps of the GIS data layers, the GIS feature counts, and the GIS-ABM workflow. Section 10.5 describes the simulation setup, the hypothetical scenarios based on malaria control interventions, and the output indices. It also introduces the two spatial analyses techniques of hot spot analysis and kriging analysis. Section 10.6 describes the spatial results. Section 10.7 offers some relevant discussion and Section 10.8 concludes.

10.2   GIS IN PUBLIC HEALTH

In this section, we discuss several studies that use GIS, GPS, geostatistics, spatial statistical methods, and/or other geospatial features in the fields of public health and epidemiology, with a special focus on malaria.

In general, GIS and related technologies have been extensively used in public health and epidemiology studies. For example, Brownstein *et al.* applied GIS and remote sensing to determine the distribution of human risk for WNV by spatial analysis of the initial case distribution for the New York City area [83]. De Lepper *et al.* summarized several interesting applications of GIS in public and environmental health [143]. Clarke *et al.* and Croner *et al.* presented general reviews of epidemiology, human health, and GIS, discussing the expanding opportunities of GIS for public health and epidemiology [119, 132]. Bullen *et al.* used GIS to identify a nested hierarchy of localities for the management of primary health care in West Sussex, England [88]. Kistemann *et al.* presented a review of recent developments using GIS within the domains of environmental health sciences, disease ecology, and public health [293]. Dangendorf *et al.* applied GIS in the field of drinking water epidemiology research and found GIS extremely useful to perform area-based correlation studies and to analyze the exposure of populations in drinking water epidemiology [134]. Theseira discussed the use of Internet GIS technology for sharing health and health-related data based on the issues that arose during the formative period of the Multi-agency internet geographic information service (MAIGIS) project [540]. Ward and Brown presented a framework for incorporating the prevention of Lyme disease transmission into the landscape planning and design process [551]. Schröder presented applications of GIS, geostatistics, metadata banking, and classification and regression trees (CARTs) by environmental monitoring [484]. Kandwal *et al.* explored various GIS-based functionalities for health studies and their scope in analyzing and controlling epidemiological diseases with emphasis on HIV/AIDS [271]. Khormi and Kumar presented a review of mosquito-borne diseases, with examples of the use of spatial information technologies to visualize and analyze mosquito vector and epidemiological data [283]. Ozdenerol *et al.* presented a review of the recent literature to explore spatiotemporal patterns of WNV using GIS and other geospatial technologies [411].

In particular, for malaria as a disease, GIS has been used for measuring the distribution of mosquito species, their habitats, the control and management of the disease, and so on. For example, Gimnig *et al.* discussed the application of GIS to the study of mosquito ecology and mosquito-borne diseases (including malaria) [204]. Hightower *et al.* applied spatial analysis and examined spatial hypotheses for a malaria field study in Western Kenya to produce maps with highly accurate locational information for all of the geographic features of interest [242]. Mbogo *et al.* studied the seasonal dynamics and spatial distributions of *Anopheles* mosquitoes and *Plasmodium falciparum* parasites along the coast of Kenya [350]. Using handheld GPS, they recorded latitude and longitude data at each site and produced the spatial distribution maps for three *Anopheles* species. Li *et al.* presented a spatially distributed mosquito habitat modeling approach, integrating a Bayesian modeling method with Ecological niche factor analysis (ENFA) using GIS [316]. They used data for seven environmental variables to represent the environmental conditions of larval habitats in the Kenya highlands. The Malaria Atlas Project (MAP) developed the science of malaria cartography by modeling the global spatial distribution of *P. falciparum* malaria endemicity [236]. Focusing on the spatial heterogeneity of malaria transmission intensity, they effectively produced and used maps as essential tools for malaria control [232].

Zhou *et al.* used GIS layers of larval habitats, land use type, human population distribution, house structure, and hydrologic schemes, overlaid with adult mosquito abundance, to investigate the impact of environmental heterogeneity and larval habitats on the spatial distribution of adult *Anopheles* mosquitoes in western Kenya [588]. Mmbando *et al.* studied the spatial variation and socioeconomic determinants of *P. falciparum* infection in northeastern Tanzania using handheld GPS units [367]. Their results showed a significant spatial variation of *P. falciparum* infection in the region, identifying altitude, socioeconomic status, high bed net coverage, and urbanization as important factors associated with the spatial variability in malaria. Ndenga *et al.* used GPS units to classify aquatic habitats within highland sites in western Kenya [380]. They recorded the latitude, longitude, and altitude of the habitats, classified them as natural swamp, cultivated swamp, river fringe, puddle, open drain or burrow pit, and showed that the productivity of malaria vectors from different habitat types are highly heterogeneous.

10.3   THE STUDY AREA AND THE ABM

The study area selected for this study is located within a subsection of the Siaya and Bondo Districts (Rarieda Division, Nyanza Province) in western Kenya. It comprises a village that is selected from a set of 15 villages with an area of approximately $70\,km^2$. The greater area is locally known as *Asembo*, which covers an area of $200\,km^2$ with a population of approximately 60,000 persons [433]. It lies on Lake Victoria and experiences intense, perennial (year-round) malaria transmission [378]. The primary reason for selecting Asembo is the availability of relevant data from the Asembo Bay Cohort Project [352] and the Asembo ITNs project [433]. In a series of 23 articles, these studies

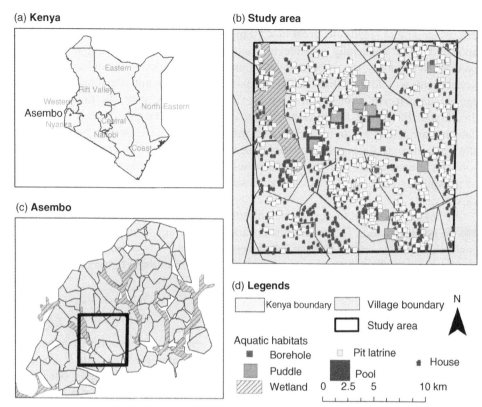

Figure 10.1   The study area. (a) Kenya boundary and administrative units (provinces). (b) Study area with selected data layers; the outlined polygon represents a subset of villages selected for the simulation runs in this study. (c) Village cluster in Asembo. (d) Legends. Used from Arifin *et al.* [20] under a Creative Commons Attribution 4.0 International License.

reported important public health findings from a successful trial of ITNs in western Kenya [273].

The study area is shown in Fig. 10.1; Fig. 10.1a shows the boundary and administrative units for Kenya, Fig. 10.1b shows the selected data layers within the village cluster (see Section 10.4), and Fig. 10.1c shows the selected village cluster in Asembo, Kenya.

Our spatial ABM can handle a landscape with finite maximum dimensions (without explicit parallelization or multiple runs). Hence, a subset of villages with 95×96 cell dimensions is selected for all simulation runs in this study, as outlined by the polygons in Fig. 10.1b and c. Other features of the spatial ABM, which are used in this chapter, are briefly mentioned as follows.

10.3.1   Features of the Spatial ABM

As mentioned in Chapter 6, in the spatial ABM, movement of an adult female mosquito agent in its resource-seeking process is guided by several flight heuristics (see Section 6.4 and Fig. 6.7). Since each landscape (used in this chapter) comprises discrete and finite-sized cells of 50 m × 50 m, the landscape-based modeling approach appeared to be especially suitable to capture the details of the resource-seeking process. In summary, the resource-seeking process is modeled with random nondirectional flights with limited flight ability and perceptual ranges until the female mosquito agents can perceive resources at close proximity, at which point, the flight becomes directional. In case of a directional flight, if multiple resources (houses or aquatic habitats) are found within a single cell, a random resource is selected. Note that this strategy can be easily extended/modified for future work to select a resource based on some preference criterion, for example, to select the house that has the fewest number of mosquitoes visited and to select the aquatic habitat that has the largest remaining capacity.

As before, a mosquito agent's neighborhood is modeled as an eight-directional *Moore* neighborhood. The maximum distance that an agent may travel in a day is controlled by a *movement counter*, which is reset to 5 at the beginning of each day for a moving agent. Thus, the counter controls the maximum daily range of movement, which translates to $250\sqrt[2]{2}$ m.

10.3.2   Vector Control Intervention Scenarios

The combined impacts of two vector control interventions-larval source management (LSM) and insecticide-treated nets (ITNs)—are evaluated for this study.[10] For this study, LSM refers to the permanent elimination of targeted aquatic habitats. For ITNs, the *household-level complete coverage* scheme is used, which ensures that if a house is covered, all persons in the house are protected by bed nets (see Section 9.2.4 and Fig. 9.1); the two other relevant parameters, killing effectiveness and repellence, are both fixed at 50%.[11]

Four different scenarios are constructed using two representative coverage (C) levels of *low* (20%) and *high* (80%). For a specific coverage, aquatic habitats and houses that will be covered by the corresponding intervention are selected randomly. The actual number of objects covered approximate the desired coverage levels. A baseline scenario (with no intervention) is also added for comparison. The scenarios are summarized in Table 10.1, in which 975 aquatic habitats and 941 houses are used to calculate the desired coverage (C) levels of *low* (20%) and *high* (80%) (see Section 10.4.3). The first column denotes the scenario and lists the interventions applied. The last two columns list the coverage (C) levels for aquatic habitats and houses, respectively, which are covered by the corresponding intervention in the landscape.

---

[10] See Chapter 9 for the modeling details of LSM and ITNs.

[11] *Killing effectiveness* refers to an increased mortality, toxicity, or killing efficiency due to the insecticidal killing effects of the ITNs; the insecticide kills the mosquitoes that come into contact with the ITNs. *Repellence* refers to the insecticidal excito-repellent properties of the ITNs, which repel the blood meal-seeking mosquitoes; it adds a chemical barrier to the physical one, further reducing human-mosquito contact and increasing the protective efficacy of the ITNs.

TABLE 10.1 Vector Control Intervention Scenarios

Scenario	Coverage (C) $(\%)$	
	% Aquatic Habitats Covered by LSM	% Houses Covered by ITNs
Baseline	0	0
$LSM_{Low} - ITNs_{Low}$	$208/975 = 0.21$	$204/941 = 0.22$
$LSM_{Low} - ITNs_{High}$	$215/975 = 0.22$	$751/941 = 0.8$
$LSM_{High} - ITNs_{Low}$	$774/975 = 0.79$	$195/941 = 0.21$
$LSM_{High} - ITNs_{High}$	$781/975 = 0.8$	$736/941 = 0.78$

10.4 THE GEOGRAPHIC INFORMATION SYSTEM (GIS)

The GIS-processed data layers are synthesized in the spatial ABM with the landscape-based approach mentioned above. In this approach, each *landscape* comprises discrete and finite-sized cells (grids) and is used to represent the coordinate space necessary for the spatial locations of the environments and the adult mosquito agents. Resources, in the forms of aquatic habitats and houses, are contained within a landscape. Each cell, with its spatial attributes, may represent a specific habitat environment (human or aquatic), or be part of the terrestrial mosquito environment. Landscapes are topologically modeled as 2-D torus spaces with a *nonabsorbing (periodic) boundary*.[12]

10.4.1 The GIS-ABM Workflow

The ArcGIS software [16] is used to produce, process, and analyze the relevant data layers, and to convert the layers into plain-text ASCII format.[13] A customized Java program called the *Input Formatter* converts the ASCII files into the XML format and feed these as inputs to the spatial ABM.[14] Note that the XML input files may also contain information about vector control interventions. The spatial ABM then runs simulations with the supplied input files. Once the simulations are completed, the outputs are analyzed using a custom-built Perl module called the *Output Analyzer*. Plots and other figures are produced from the analyzed outputs. To perform spatial analyses (hot spot analysis and ordinary kriging), another set of ASCII files are produced from the analyzed outputs and fed into the GIS. The spatial maps are then

[12]Recall from Section 9.1.2 that with a *nonabsorbing (periodic) boundary*, when mosquitoes hit an edge of a landscape, they reenter it from the edge directly opposite of the exiting edge, and thus are not killed due to hitting the edge.

[13]ASCII stands for *American Standard Code for Information Interchange*; it is a character-encoding scheme used to represent text in computers.

[14]XML stands for *Extensible Markup Language*; it is a free, open standard, markup language that defines a set of rules for encoding documents in a format that is both human-readable and machine-readable.

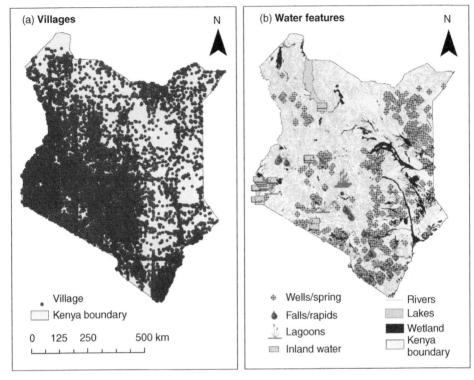

Figure 10.2   Selected sets of GIS features for Kenya. (a) Villages. (b) Water sources.

produced by the GIS by portraying simulation outputs (e.g., mosquito abundances) on top of the relevant data layers.

10.4.2   GIS Processing of Data Layers

ArcGIS Desktop 10 [17] is used to produce, process, and analyze the relevant data layers. Different types of water features and villages (including houses) are identified, extracted, and projected to the *Arc 1950 UTM Zone 36S* projection system for all over Kenya, as shown in Fig. 10.2: Fig. 10.2a and b show the villages and selected water sources, respectively. The selected water features include rivers, lakes, wetlands, wells/springs, falls/rapids, lagoons, and so on. Each water feature type is assigned a unique ID.

The selected features are scaled down to a village cluster around Asembo. Water features for different types of aquatic sites are included. Since the spatial ABM deals with spatial features at the habitat levels, the study area is further scaled down to village and household levels, and then to subsets of villages levels. Some of the water features are ranked by precedence by subgrouping the water source data layers based on their attributes. Similar types of water features in the same data layer are combined.

The selected data layers are then converted into the raster format with a cell resolution of 50 m × 50 m. All point shapefiles for aquatic habitats and houses are converted

TABLE 10.2   GIS Feature Types and Counts for the ABM

Type	Count	Assigned Capacity
Pool	4	2000
Puddle	13	1000
Pit latrine	395	500
Borehole	4	300
Wetland	559	10
House	941	5

using the *Point to Raster* tool.[15] Since pit latrines are usually found inside the household boundaries, the shapefile for pit latrines is created from the shapefile for houses. It is possible to have more than one feature type within a single cell. In these cases, to calculate the number of features of each type in each cell, the summation of value fields of the corresponding data features is used. Finally, the raster files are converted into the ASCII format and are ready to be used as inputs to the spatial ABM.

10.4.3   Feature Counts

A total of 975 aquatic habitats, categorized into five different types, are identified in the selected area as follows: (1) pools (large), (2) puddles (small), (3) pit latrines, (4) boreholes, and (5) wetland. Boreholes, also known as borrow pits, have significant potential as breeding sites in the area. They represent human-made holes or pits in the ground when local people use clay or soil for building houses, making pots, and so on, thereby leaving depressions in the ground that easily get filled with rain water. Pit latrines are very common to the households in the area. The wetland represents a stretch of marsh lying to the northwest corner of the area, which is dominated by herbaceous plant species. Each aquatic habitat is set with a predefined *habitat capacity HC* (as mentioned in Section 4.4, *HC* regulates the aquatic mosquito population that the habitat can sustain and reflects the habitat heterogeneity to some degree). A total of 941 houses, each having a mean of five occupants, are also identified. These feature counts and their assigned capacity values are summarized in Table 10.2, in which the last column represents the assigned capacity per feature. Note that for wetland, which covers multiple cells in the northwest corner of the study area (see Fig. 10.1b), the same *HC* value is assigned to each cell.

10.5   SIMULATIONS AND SPATIAL ANALYSES

For each of the five vector control intervention scenarios of Baseline, $LSM_{Low} - ITNs_{Low}$, $LSM_{Low} - ITNs_{High}$, $LSM_{High} - ITNs_{Low}$, and $LSM_{High} - ITNs_{High}$ (see

[15]The *shapefile* format is a popular geospatial vector data format for GIS software; it is developed and regulated by the Environmental Systems Research Institute (Esri) [168] as an open specification for data interoperability among Esri and other GIS software products.

Section 10.3.2), 50 replicated simulation runs are performed and the average results are reported. Each simulation runs for 730 days (2 years) and reaches a steady state (equilibrium) at around day 50.[16] Interventions are applied on day 100 and continued up to the end of the simulation.

Initially, all simulations start with 1000 female adult mosquito agents (no male agents). Each female agent is assigned to a randomly selected aquatic habitat. The maximum daily range of movement for mosquito agents is set to 5 *cells per day*, which translates to $250\sqrt[2]{2}$ m. Biological aging (senescence) of the mosquitoes is assumed. The ABM implements age-specific mortality rates for the adult mosquitoes and the larvae (i.e., the probability of death for mosquito agents increases with their age).

10.5.1   Output Indices

As before, mosquito abundances have been used to generate the primary output index of the ABM (see Chapters 6, 8, and 9). However, the inclusion of GIS into the spatial model also allows us to explore other spatial indices by overlaying these on the entire landscape. These indices capture the spatial heterogeneity of various objects (aquatic habitats and houses) in the landscape. Some of these indices are generated as *cumulative aggregates* at the end of each simulation run and represent measures on a *per object* basis. The output indices are listed as follows:

1. Mosquito Abundance: It represents a spatial *snapshot* of the female adult mosquito population distribution at the end of simulations.
2. Oviposition Count per Aquatic Habitat: For each aquatic habitat x, it represents the *cumulative* number of female adult mosquitoes that have oviposited (laid eggs) in x, depicted spatially at the end of simulations by overlaying on top of the aquatic habitats.
3. Blood Meal Count per House: For each house y, it represents the *cumulative* number of blood meals successfully obtained by female adult mosquitoes in y, depicted spatially at the end of simulations by overlaying on top of the houses.

Note that for all output indices, the average measures of 50 replicated simulation runs are reported (in order to rule out any stochasticity effects; see Chapter 9 for details on replication). The spatial indices are sampled across all daily time steps throughout the entire simulations. The output maps are produced by overlaying the *averaged* indices on top of the relevant data layers.

All output indices are mapped using the graduated symbology. The graduated symbol renderer is one of the common renderer types used to represent quantitative information. Using a graduated symbols renderer, the quantitative values for the output indices are separately grouped into ordered classes, so that higher values cover larger areas on the map. Within a class, all features are drawn with the same symbol. Each class is assigned a graduated symbol from the smallest to the largest.

---

[16] All time units related to the simulation runs refer to *simulated time* as opposed to *physical time* or *wall clock time*.

10.5.2 Hot Spot Analysis

Using spatial statistics tools, hot spot analysis (spatial cluster analysis) is performed for all scenarios for the last two indices (*oviposition count per aquatic habitat* and *blood meal count per house*) in order to determine whether a specific value is statistically significant or not [19]. In hot spot analysis, if a higher value is surrounded by similar magnitude of other higher values, it is considered a hot spot (with 95% or 99% confidence intervals (CIs)). The cold spots are determined using the same principle. The values (or cluster of values) between the statistically significant hot spots and cold spots are considered as random samples of a distribution. The hot spot analysis tool calculates the *Getis-Ord Gi* statistic* (z-scores and p-values) for each feature in a data set [17]. z-Scores are measures of standard deviations and define the CIs (in this case, 95–99%). A p-value represents the probability that the observed spatial pattern was created by some random process.

The *null hypothesis* for pattern analysis essentially states that the expected pattern is just one of the many possible versions of complete spatial randomness. If the z-score is within the 95–99% CI or beyond, the exhibited pattern is probably too unusual to be of random chance, and the p-value will be subsequently small to reflect this. In this case, it is possible to reject the null hypothesis and proceed to determine the cause of the statistically significant spatial pattern. On the other hand, if the z-score lies below the 95% CI, the p-value will be larger, the null hypothesis cannot be rejected, and the pattern exhibited is more likely to indicate a random pattern. Thus, a high z-score and small p-value for a feature indicates a significant hot spot. Conversely, a low negative z-score and small p-value indicates a significant cold spot.

10.5.3 Kriging Analysis

Kriging, also known as *Gaussian process regression*, is a popular method of interpolation (prediction) for spatial data. It is an interpolation technique in which the surrounding measured values are weighted to derive a predicted value for an unmeasured location. Weights for the measured values depend on the distance between the measured points, the prediction locations, and the overall spatial arrangement among the measured points [173]. Various kriging techniques provide a framework for predicting values of a variable of interest at unobserved locations given a set of spatially distributed data, incorporating spatial autocorrelation and computing uncertainty measures around model predictions [62, 153].

In recent years, kriging has been extensively used in public health and epidemiology modeling for variable mapping to interpolate estimates of occurrence of a variable or risk of disease [61, 95, 305]. For example, de Carvalho Alves and Pozza characterized the spatial variability of common bean anthracnose using kriging and nonlinear regression models [139]. Alexeeff *et al.* evaluated the accuracy of epidemiological health effect estimates in linear and logistic regression when using spatial air pollution predictions from kriging and land use regression models [4]. For malaria modeling, the MAP [537] developed several Bayesian geostatistical kriging models for spatial prediction of *P. falciparum* prevalence, estimated human populations at risk, vector distribution, and so on, generating malaria maps of many endemic countries in sub-Saharan Africa [197, 248, 435].

The basic idea of kriging is to predict the value of a function at a given point by computing a weighted average of the known values of the function in the neighborhood of the point. To this end, kriging is closely related to the method of regression analysis. The data represent a set of observations of some variable(s) of interest, with some spatial correlation. Usually, the result of kriging is the expected value, referred to as the *kriging mean* and the *kriging variance* computed for every point within a region of interest. If kriging is done with a known mean, it is then called *simple kriging*. On the other hand, in *ordinary kriging*, estimating the mean and applying (simple) kriging are performed simultaneously.

Kriging uses semivariogram functions to describe the structure of spatial variability. A semivariogram is one of the significant functions to indicate spatial correlation in observations measured at sample locations and plays a central role in the analysis of geostatistical data using kriging. The effect of different semivariograms on kriging has also been a focus of interest in different branches of the literature (e.g., [223]). In this chapter, spatial analysis is conducted using ordinary kriging with circular semivariograms for all scenarios for all the output indices using ArcGIS 9.3 [18]. We note that similar analyses have also been conducted for other insects (e.g., for fig fly [51]).

10.6   RESULTS

In this section, we describe the results by categorizing them according to the output indices. For the output indices and scenarios (see Table 10.1), simulation results are presented with hot spot analysis and kriging analysis. To allow the viewers for an improved spatial analysis perspective and a better insight for the unmeasured locations on the maps, the kriged maps are presented right after the hot spot analysis maps. For clarity, houses and pit latrines are not shown in the output maps. Each scenario (in the output maps) represents the average results of 50 replicated simulations.

10.6.1   Mosquito Abundance

The mosquito abundance maps are shown in Fig. 10.3. These maps depict the *mosquito abundances* index, which represent a spatial snapshot of the female adult mosquito population distribution at the end of simulations. Figure 10.3a shows the abundance map for the baseline scenario (in which no intervention was applied). Figure 10.3b depicts the symbols used in the maps; it shows the village boundary, different types of aquatic habitats, and the graduated symbols for abundances. Note that for the aquatic habitats, the symbol sizes vary according to the assigned carrying capacities of the habitats (see Table 10.2). The graduated symbol sizes for abundances also vary depending on the magnitudes. Figure 10.3C–F show the abundance maps for the four different scenarios with control interventions LSM and ITNs having two coverage levels: $LSM_{Low} - ITNs_{Low}$, $LSM_{Low} - ITNs_{High}$, $LSM_{High} - ITNs_{Low}$, and $LSM_{High} - ITNs_{High}$, respectively. The corresponding kriged maps for mosquito abundance are illustrated in Fig. 10.4.

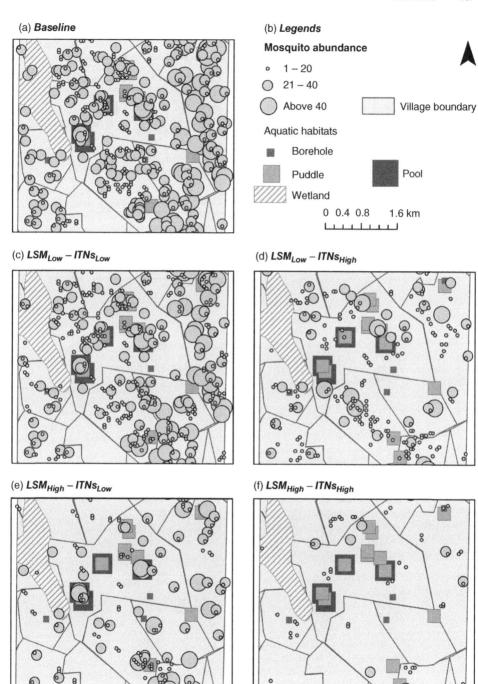

Figure 10.3 Maps for the *mosquito abundances* index. (a) Abundance map for baseline. (b) Legends: for clarity, houses and pit latrines are not shown. (c) Abundance map for $LSM_{Low} - ITNs_{Low}$. (d) Abundance map for $LSM_{Low} - ITNs_{High}$. (e) Abundance map for $LSM_{High} - ITNs_{Low}$. (f) Abundance map for $LSM_{High} - ITNs_{High}$. Used from Arifin *et al.* [20] under a Creative Commons Attribution 4.0 International License.

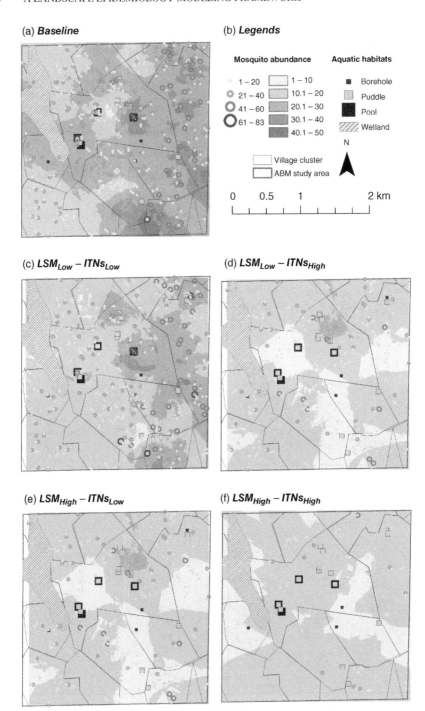

Figure 10.4   Kriged maps for the *mosquito abundances* index. (a) Kriged abundance map for baseline. (b) Legends. (c)–(f) The four intervention scenarios. Used from Arifin *et al.* [20] under a Creative Commons Attribution 4.0 International License.

As shown in Fig. 10.3, with increasing coverage levels of both interventions, the mosquito abundances are significantly reduced, as evident from the progressively lower number of "Above 40" symbols (which denote the highest abundances) in the series of figures. The changes are more clear and evident from the kriged maps (Fig. 10.4).

It is interesting to note that ITNs are more effective in reducing abundances than LSM (compare Fig. 10.3d and e as well as the kriged maps in Fig. 10.4d and e): covering 80% of the houses has more impact than removing a total of 80% different types of the aquatic habitats. This is partially due to the fact that the household-level complete coverage scheme prohibits a blood meal-seeking female mosquito to obtain a blood meal from any person in any house that is covered by ITNs.[17] As coverage of ITNs increases, more houses fall within the range of coverage and the probability of finding an unprotected human in another house (during the blood meal-seeking stage) decreases. Thus, with increasing coverage of ITNs, abundances are reduced more effectively.

The *low* (20%) coverage levels for both interventions do not produce significant reduction in abundances, as evident from the baseline and $LSM_{Low} - ITNs_{Low}$ maps (compare Fig. 10.3a and c). In general, higher abundances are observed near the pools (which have the highest carrying capacities) and in the northeast and the southeast portions of the map.

When either of the interventions has a *high* (80%) coverage level, abundances are significantly reduced, as evident from the $LSM_{Low} - ITNs_{High}$ and $LSM_{High} - ITNs_{Low}$ maps. For these two scenarios, the highest abundances observed are significantly lower than the baseline (compare Fig. 10.3d and e with Fig. 10.3a). However, for the $LSM_{Low} - ITNs_{High}$ scenario higher abundances do not always coincide with the spatial locations of aquatic habitats with higher carrying capacities, while for the other scenario this expected trend is observed for some cases.

Not surprisingly, when both interventions have *high* (80%) coverage levels, abundances are reduced to the lowest level, as evident from the $LSM_{High} - ITNs_{High}$ map shown in Fig. 10.3f. For this scenario, very few higher abundances are observed, which occur at greater distances from the spatial locations of aquatic habitats with higher carrying capacities, since most of them are eliminated by LSM.

10.6.2   Oviposition Count per Aquatic Habitat

Results for the *oviposition count per aquatic habitat* index are shown in Fig. 10.5. These maps depict the cumulative number of female adult mosquitoes that have oviposited (laid eggs) in the aquatic habitats, as well as the predicted hot spots and cold spots identified by hot spot analysis. For the five scenarios, oviposition counts for the aquatic habitats are placed into three ordered classes of 1–20,000, 20,001–50,000, and above 50,000 using the same quantitative scale and are shown using graduated symbols. Hot spots and cold spots are spatially clustered using two CI levels of 95 and 99%. The legends denote the color-coding for the classes, the hot spots, the cold spots, and the CIs. The corresponding kriged maps for oviposition counts are illustrated in Fig. 10.6.

---

[17] See Section 9.2.4 and Fig. 9.1 for the household-level complete coverage scheme used for ITNs.

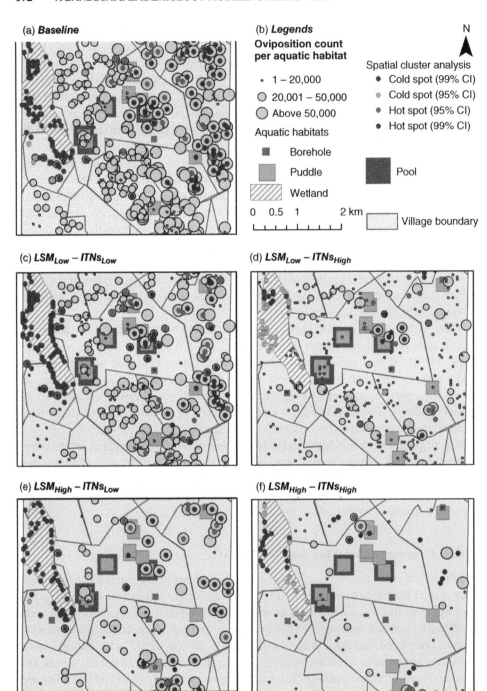

Figure 10.5 Maps for the *oviposition count per aquatic habitat* index. Oviposition counts are categorized using the same quantitative scale and are shown using graduated symbols. For clarity, houses and pit latrines are not shown. Hot spots and cold spots are spatially clustered. (a) Baseline. (b) Legends. (c)–(f) The four intervention scenarios. Used from Arifin *et al.* [20] under a Creative Commons Attribution 4.0 International License.

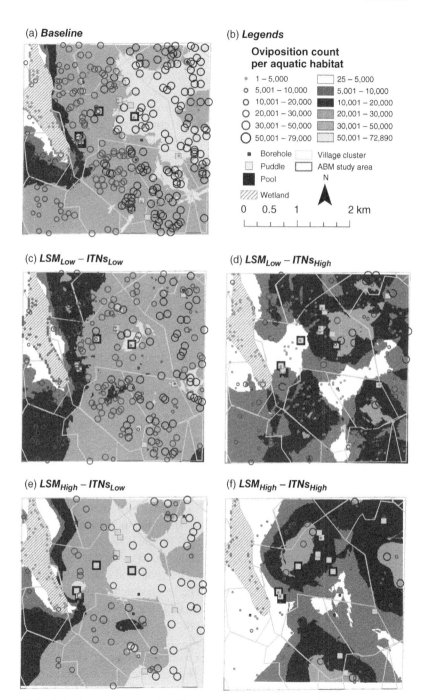

Figure 10.6 Kriged maps for the *oviposition count per aquatic habitat* index. (a) Baseline. (b) Legends. (c)–(f) The four intervention scenarios. Used from Arifin *et al.* [20] under a Creative Commons Attribution 4.0 International License.

Figure 10.5a shows a higher frequency of higher values for the *oviposition count per aquatic habitat* index in the baseline map. Significant number of these appears to be statistically significant, and hence considered as hot spots. Notable clustering of lower values can also be seen over the wetland area (where each cell is assigned a tiny *HC*), which are categorized as cold spots.

Figure 10.5c shows a drop in frequency of higher values in the $LSM_{Low} - ITNs_{Low}$ map for the same index, about half of which are considered as hot spots. In addition, more cold spots can be seen over the wetland area. Both of these results can be explained as the effects of *low* coverage levels for both interventions.

When either of the interventions has a *high* coverage level, frequencies of higher values are further reduced, as evident from the $LSM_{Low} - ITNs_{High}$ and $LSM_{High} - ITNs_{Low}$ maps in Fig. 10.5d and e, respectively. For the $LSM_{Low} - ITNs_{High}$ scenario, some moderate oviposition counts become statistically significant, fewer hot spots are detected, and most of the cold spots are eliminated from the wetland area. On the other hand, the $LSM_{High} - ITNs_{Low}$ scenario has higher frequencies of higher oviposition counts, hot spots, and cold spots. These observations confirm to our previous results (for abundances) that ITNs are more effective in reducing oviposition counts than LSM. As before, when both interventions have *high* coverage levels, frequencies of higher oviposition counts, hot spots, and cold spots are reduced to the lowest level, as evident from the $LSM_{High} - ITNs_{High}$ map shown in Fig. 10.5f.

Similar deductions can be made from the kriged maps presented in Fig. 10.6. For example, when both interventions are applied with higher coverages (Fig. 10.6f), areas with the lighter shades of gray representing the two highest levels of oviposition counts are simply nonexistent from the map, and the third lightest shades of gray is greatly diminished. This illustrates the drastic reductions in the oviposition counts.

10.6.3 Blood Meal Count per House

Results for the *blood meal count per house* index are shown in Fig. 10.7. These maps depict the cumulative number of blood meals obtained by female adult mosquitoes in the houses, as well as the predicted hot spots and cold spots identified by hot spot analysis. For the five scenarios, blood meal counts for the houses are placed into three ordered classes of 1–3000, 3001–9000, and above 9000 using the same quantitative scale and are shown using graduated symbols. Hot spots and cold spots are spatially clustered using two CI levels of 95 and 99%. The legends denote the color-coding for the classes, the hot spots, the cold spots, and the CIs. The corresponding kriged maps for blood meal counts are illustrated in Fig. 10.8.

The *blood meal count per house* index results show similar trends as observed for the *oviposition count per aquatic habitat* index results. Similar trends are also noticed from the kriged maps presented in Fig. 10.8. The baseline map possesses the highest frequencies of higher values, hot spots, and cold spots (Fig. 10.7a); all frequencies are reduced (with the introduction of a few cold spots in the lower left area) when both interventions have *low* coverage levels (Fig. 10.7c); ITNs (*high* coverage level) are more effective than LSM with further reduction in frequencies of higher values

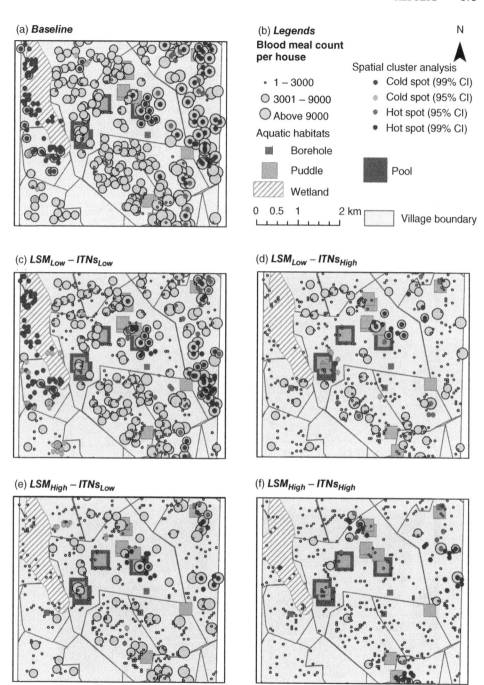

Figure 10.7 Maps for the *blood meal count per house* index. Blood meal counts are categorized using the same quantitative scale. For clarity, houses and pit latrines are not shown. Hot spots and cold spots are spatially clustered using two confidence intervals (CIs) of 95 and 99%. (a) Baseline. (b) Legends. (c)–(f) The four intervention scenarios. Used from Arifin *et al.* [20] under a Creative Commons Attribution 4.0 International License.

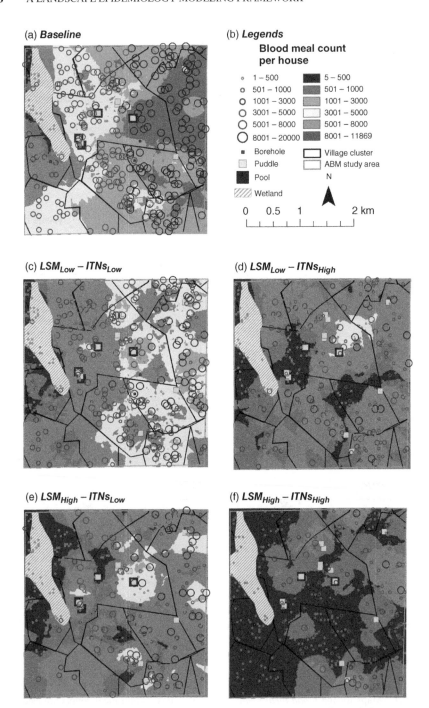

Figure 10.8 Kriged maps for all scenarios for the *blood meal count per house* index. (a) Baseline. (b) Legends. (c)–(f) The four intervention scenarios. Used from Arifin *et al.* [20] under a Creative Commons Attribution 4.0 International License.

(Fig. 10.7d and E); and very few higher values, hot spots, and cold spots remain when both interventions have *high* coverage levels (Fig. 10.7f). Interestingly, the $LSM_{Low} - ITNs_{High}$ map shows some cold spots in an area, where a few aquatic habitats with higher carrying capacities exist, and the $LSM_{High} - ITNs_{Low}$ map possesses very few cold spots. Similar trends are also observed in the corresponding kriged maps (Fig. 10.8).

In general, statistically significant higher values are detected over the northeast and the southeast portions of the maps as these portions contain more number of houses (hence more blood meal counts per house). This is also evident from the kriged maps. The central portions depict mostly random distribution of values that are not detected as hot spots.

10.7   DISCUSSION

This study has presented a landscape epidemiology modeling framework to integrate the simulation results from a spatial ABM of malaria-transmitting mosquitoes with a GIS, and then to apply spatial statistics techniques on the model outputs. Some of the key features, characteristics, and limitations of the framework are highlighted as follows.

10.7.1   Stochasticity and Initial Conditions

As we mentioned in Chapter 9, the ABM involves substantial stochasticity in the forms of probability-based distributions and equations. The mosquito agents' decisions and actions are often simulated using random draws from certain distributions. These sources of randomness are used to represent the diversity of model characteristics. To rule out any stochasticity effects introduced by these probabilistic events, 50 replicated simulation runs are performed for each simulation in each of the five scenarios and their aggregate measures are reported in the form of averages.[18]

To verify whether 50 replicated runs are enough for each simulation, we ran as many as 120 replicates of each simulation in the earlier phases of model development (to be specific, during the verification and validation (V&V) phases, as reported in Chapters 6 and 8). After analyzing the results, it became apparent that roughly 30 replicates were enough to rule out most issues regarding stochasticity, initial seed bias, bifurcation, and other chaos factors. We also verified that the average could be treated as a deterministic measure for the mosquito abundance outputs of the ABM.

The initial uniform random assignment of female agents to arbitrary aquatic habitats does not affect the current emerging outcomes of the ABM. This was previously ensured as part of the V&V studies of the ABMs by considering longer running times and with multiple initial random seeds to check for robustness [22, 23, 25]. In fact, this holds true for both cases of *with* and *without* the landscape approach, that is, when the simulations are run in spatial and nonspatial modes, respectively.

---

[18]Recall that 50 replicated runs were performed as well for each simulated landscape presented in Chapter 9.

10.7.2   Model Calibration and Parameterization

The proposed integration framework allows modelers for easy parameterizations of the model. For example, the arbitrary order of the different aquatic habitat types and the assigned *HC* per habitat can be readily changed to suit new scenarios and/or new areas of study. This, in turn, allows the ABM to produce scenario-specific outputs *without* the need for modifying the ABM itself. The simplicity in this scenario-based approach also allows modelers to feed different scenarios to the ABM using different capacities for various types of aquatic habitats without requiring to change the GIS data layers and other GIS features for future simulation runs.

In the ABM, the human population is modeled as static (i.e., humans do not move in space), all humans are assumed to be identical, and human mortality is not implemented. This may be one of the reasons for the unusually high blood meal counts per house (in the range of thousands). In the future, with the inclusion of explicit parasite population (as agents) and the availability of detailed demographic data of human populations and houses in Asembo, we plan to parameterize and calibrate the model to reflect a more realistic scenario for the specific region.

In general, robustness of a modeling framework depends on several factors, including the selection of appropriate model parameters and their respective values. This issue is closely related to various methodologies and techniques commonly used for V&V of ABMs such as calibration, parameter estimation, parameter fitting, and sensitivity analysis (see Chapters 7 and 8). For the current model, these may include the flight ability and perceptual ranges of mosquitoes, the habitat capacity of aquatic habitats, the detailed demographic data for human populations and houses, and so on. In the future, once the models are fully calibrated, we envisage the modeling framework to become *more robust*.

10.7.3   Emergence

As we described in Section 3.4, an important characteristic of an ABM is its capability to capture emergent phenomena resulting from the interactions of the individual agents from the bottom up (after the simulation reaches equilibrium or steady state). To this regard, our ABM exhibits the emerging spatial distribution of mosquito agents once the simulations reach equilibrium on or after day 50. The emergence is primarily governed by two factors: (1) the assigned carrying capacities of the aquatic habitats and (2) the spatial heterogeneity of the landscapes that translates to the distributions and densities of houses and aquatic habitats. In the simulations, the 50-day warm-up period ensures that the model has reached steady state and should not be treated as an absolute value. Each generation of the mosquitoes requires ≈ 15 days to become mature and it takes $\approx 2-3$ generations for the initial model to reach equilibrium. Thus, a 50-day warm-up period would have been sufficient in most cases. Note that the interventions (LSM and ITNs) are applied after day 100 and continued up to the end of the simulation. This longer period (100 days) also guards against oscillatory spikes in the abundance, which may occur due to several factors such as generation-to-generation oscillation tendency, density dependence and skip-oviposition effects, and short hiatus in egg laying (see Chapter 9 for details about the vector control interventions).

10.7.4   Complexity

In many complex systems, cause and effect relationships are usually not proportional to each other; as a result, manipulation attempts are often resisted, which may lead to an unexpected systemic shift or phase transition (the points of transitions are known as the so-called *tipping points* or *critical points*) [237]. In the spatial ABM, such tipping points may occur with certain combinations of the intervention parameters. For this study, the coverage levels of 0.2 and 0.8 were used for both interventions. They should be treated as representative sample points that resemble two points closer to the opposite ends of the 0.0–1.0 coverage continuum (hence, representing coverage levels on the two extremes of low and high, respectively). Earlier, we tested the ABM by running simulations with varying levels of coverages including 0.2, 0.4, 0.6, and 0.8, along with varying levels of repellence and mortality/insecticidal effect for the ITNs (see Chapter 9). Within these ranges and parameter settings, the simulations approached several tipping points with specific combinations of the three parameters. For example, in a landscape with high density of houses, 90% reductions in mosquito abundance were achieved with LSM coverage of 0.6, ITNs coverage of 0.87, and ITNs mortality of 0.5.

10.7.5   Data Resolution (Granularity)

The choice of spatial, temporal, and spectral resolutions determines the degree of precision, realism, and general applicability of the models [296]. Even with the recent rapid advances in computing power, these factors cannot always be maximized simultaneously. Although the resolution of the coordinates recorded in a modern GIS may now be of the order of only a few meters, the modeled resolution must be carefully decided so that it reflects the specific study, its objectives, and the objects being mapped: it should be sufficiently high to allow meaningful inferences to be made from the results but not too high to include irrelevant details.

As mentioned before, the spatial resolution (granularity) of the landscapes is chosen as 50 m × 50 m for this study. This selection is based on several factors, some of which include the spatial GIS data availability, the number of maximum cells that can be practically processed by the ABM (within bounded runtime), the limited flight ability and perceptual ranges of mosquitoes, and so on. The selected granularity may seem to be low (with a cell size of 50 m × 50m), particularly given the other assumptions on the distances that a mosquito agent can fly. In the future, with the availability of higher resolution spatial data and an advanced version of the ABM capable of processing multiple spatial nodes in parallel (e.g., using the message passing interface (MPI) technique), we plan to simulate landscapes with higher spatial resolution.[19]

---

[19]Note that the advanced individual-based model *EMOD*, presented in Chapter 11, is capable of processing multiple spatial nodes in parallel.

Due to the lack of detailed spatial data for aquatic habitats and demographic data for human populations and houses, arbitrary carrying capacities and occupants are assigned to the habitats and houses, respectively. However, the current study does ensure that the relative magnitudes of aquatic capacities follow the biological reality of the environment being modeled; for example, a pool cell possesses higher *HC* than a wetland cell, as described in Table 10.2. The flexible architecture of the modeling framework also provides an easy plug-in mechanism of such data from relevant future studies into the models.

Although in this pilot study we handled a comparatively smaller study area of ≈ 25 km² (which transforms to a 95 × 96 landscape of 50 m × 50 m cells for the spatial ABM), the methodology described here can be readily extended to include larger areas (e.g., the whole Asembo area). For the regions to be modeled, either real data can be used or synthetic/predicted data can be interpolated from a few point regions. To this end, kriging and/or other spatial analysis techniques can be used.

10.7.6   Spatial Analyses

In hot spot analysis, the higher frequency of cold spots for the oviposition counts and blood meal counts along the wetland may seem counterintuitive (see Figs. 10.5 and 10.7). This anomaly can be explained by considering two primary factors: (1) the distributions of and the relative distances between the two types of resources (houses and aquatic habitats) along the wetland and (2) the tiny carrying capacities assigned to each wetland cell (10 per cell, see Table 10.2). Both these indices (oviposition and blood meal counts) will have higher values depending on the successful completion of the cycles of alternate feeding and laying of eggs by adult female mosquito agents (the gonotrophic cycle). However, along the wetland (more noticeably along the western edge of the wetland, where a larger density of cold spots are present), despite the presence of a few nearby houses, the lack of any nearby higher capacity water bodies and the collective lower capacity (of the wetland cells and a few pit latrine cells, see Fig. 10.1c) prevent the female mosquitoes to complete their gonotrophic cycles. As a result, higher frequencies of cold spots are generated along the wetland for both indices. Also, in most cases, cold spots are absent along the southeast portion of the wetland since it is closer to both types of resources (in this case, large pools and houses). Eventually, this translates to the degree of ease with which adult female mosquitoes may find resources and can also be quantitatively measured by considering the *average travel time (ATT)* required by a female mosquito to complete each gonotrophic cycle.[20]

As the spatial distribution results show, there is a strong correlation between the *a priori* distribution of houses and aquatic habitats and the emerging distribution of hot and cold spots. Thus, in general, the hot spots of our output indices occur near the clusters of houses and aquatic habitats. Since there are 395 pit latrines distributed almost all over the study area (in fact, covering almost all the house clusters), in effect, there are indeed some aquatic habitats near almost every house-habitat cluster. Recall that the

---

[20]The *ATT* is inversely proportional to resource densities; for more details, see Section 6.6.

flight heuristics do not distinguish among the types of aquatic habitats (i.e., mosquito agents select the habitats randomly), and the agents do not engage in a directional flight during the simulations until and unless the aquatic habitats are found in the neighboring cells (see Section 6.4).

The strong spatial correlation, although not quantitatively measured in this study, is evident at some portions of the study area, where there are some houses with no aquatic habitat in the vicinity (i.e., without enough pit latrines nearby). For example, as shown in Fig. 10.1c, both the eastern portion of the southwest quadrant and most of the eastern edge of the wetlands portray two house clusters with very few or no aquatic habitats (including pit latrines) in the vicinity. As a consequence, these areas contain almost no hot spots, as depicted in the hot spot analysis results (see Figs. 10.3, 10.5, and 10.7), which hold true for both cases of *with* and *without* the mosquito control interventions.

For the entire study area, kriging analysis produces predicted values for unmeasured spatial locations, which are derived from the surrounding weighted measured values. Most of the spatial trends observed by the hot spot analysis are also visible in the kriging analysis results.

10.7.7   Habitat-based Interventions

In this study, habitats and houses were selected using random sampling for the vector control interventions. However, given the power of ABMs, other sophisticated, habitat-based strategies for interventions are also equally applicable. For example, latrines and boreholes for LSM, or a firewall of ITNs at the village boundary can be excellent choices to target first or in a limited-resource setting.

Some of the habitat-based strategies were investigated using targeted and nontargeted LSM in Chapter 9. The targeted interventions removed the aquatic habitats within 100, 200, and 300 m of surrounding houses, while the corresponding nontargeted interventions randomly removed the same number of habitats. As we described in Chapter 9, when LSM is applied in isolation, the results agreed with the findings of previous research that (1) LSM coverage of 300 m surrounding all houses can lead to significant reductions in abundance and (2) while targeting aquatic habitats to apply LSM, distance to the nearest houses can be an important measure. In the real world, similar research questions are currently being investigated with other interventions such as various types of spatial repellents (e.g., mosquito coils).

10.7.8   Miscellaneous Issues

As our key findings suggested, the availability of ecological resources (i.e., aquatic habitats and houses) and the relative distances between these distinct resource types are two crucial determinants for the female mosquitoes to complete their gonotrophic cycles. From the viewpoint of mosquito agents, these resources directly define landscape features such as spatial heterogeneity and host availability (in Chapters 6 and 9, we showed the importance of these factors for vector control using our spatial ABM and mentioned several other studies that demonstrated similar findings). Reduced availability of either type of these spatial resources would prolong the gonotrophic cycle of the female mosquito and potentially affect malaria transmission.

The *oviposition count per aquatic habitat* output index is designed to reflect the aquatic habitat heterogeneity in the landscapes. In this regard, alternative choices are also available (e.g., *eggs count per aquatic habitat*). However, the former is a better representative of habitat heterogeneity because it intrinsically considers the degree of ease with which mosquitoes can find the aquatic habitats (distance-based foraging), rather than merely focusing on the size or capacity of an aquatic habitat.

Although the modeling framework described in this chapter utilizes an ABM of malaria-transmitting mosquitoes, the approach is generally applicable to a wider range of other infectious VBD including dengue and yellow fever, provided that the disease epidemiology has already been modeled using some standard modeling method or technique (e.g., mathematical, agent-based). In addition to the three output indices used in this study, other widely used disease epidemiology variables such as incidence, prevalence, entomological inoculation rate (EIR), mean parasitaemia, sporozoite rate, and mortality rates can also be mapped and spatially analyzed using the current framework.

10.8   CONCLUSIONS

In this chapter, we presented a landscape epidemiology modeling framework, which integrates the outputs of simulation runs from our spatial ABM with a GIS. For an epidemiologically important study area in Kenya, we constructed three output indices and five landscape scenarios with varying coverage levels of two mosquito-control interventions, ran a total of 750 simulations for 2 years, and reported their average results. Using spatial analyses tools, we performed hot spot analysis for all scenarios in order to determine the statistical significance of the simulation results. We also applied ordinary kriging with circular semivariograms on the output indices. Hot spot analysis detected statistically significant hot spots and cold spots, and kriging analysis produced predicted values for unmeasured spatial locations for the entire study area.

The integration of epidemiological simulation-based results with the GIS-based spatial analyses techniques within a single modeling framework, as described in this chapter, can be useful to a variety of stakeholders such as simulation modelers, epidemiologists, disease control managers, and public health officials. It can also be a valuable tool for conducting various disease control activities such as exploring new biological insights, monitoring changes of key disease transmission indices and epidemiological landscapes, refining research questions and surveillance needs, and guiding resource allocation for further investigation. Although it utilizes an ABM of malaria-transmitting mosquitoes, the approach is generally applicable to a wider range of other infectious VBDs.

The framework showcased an ideal and useful application of the ABMs by advancing the *virtual, simulated* world of mosquito agents one step closer to the *real, malarious* world of mosquitoes. We conclude that similar integrated approaches, which are capable of combining knowledge from entomological, epidemiological, simulation-based, and geospatial domains, are required for the identification and analysis of relationships between various transmission variables, as demonstrated by this study. Eventually, such integration efforts may facilitate the Integrated Vector Management (IVM) agenda promoted by the World Health Organization (WHO) to achieve improved efficacy, cost-effectiveness, ecological soundness, and sustainability of disease and vector control activities.

In the next chapter, another advanced individual-based model (*EMOD*) is presented, which shows similar integration of knowledge from diverse but interconnected disciplines (e.g., M&S, epidemiology, and GIS) to derive insights and analyze the implications of simulation outputs for malaria eradication.[21]

---

[21] The *EMOD* individual-based model is contributed as a guest chapter from the Institute for Disease Modeling (IDM) [536].

11

THE EMOD INDIVIDUAL-BASED MODEL

PHILIP A. ECKHOFF AND EDWARD A. WENGER

Institute for Disease Modeling (IDM), Intellectual Ventures Management, LLC (IV), Bellevue, WA, USA

11.1 OVERVIEW

Mathematical modeling has been an important aspect of many of the largest-scale human endeavors for well over a century, ranging across finance, supply chain management, agriculture, military campaigns, and manufacturing [70, 93, 152, 213, 366, 527]. During the last century, it became established as a major aspect of disease control, perhaps most strikingly in the pioneering work of Macdonald in the 1950s [327]. The rise of timewise-exponentially more powerful electronic digital computing systems over the past half-century continues to provide crucial technical enablement for the spectacular flowering of mathematical modeling in myriad areas of human endeavor, including disease suppression.

This chapter explores many of the issues faced when modeling disease eradication in support of campaign design and execution, lays out model features required to address those issues, and then explains the basic approach of our family of models. Malaria was the initial target-disease of the present modeling development and malaria eradication simulation studies are among the model's most highly developed capabilities. While these capabilities are being extended to address other major sources of human morbidity and mortality, for example, polio, HIV-1, and tuberculosis, malaria is the exemplary disease for the purposes of the present chapter. In this chapter, the model implementation for malaria is explored in detail. Preliminary results for malaria

Spatial Agent-Based Simulation Modeling in Public Health:
Design, Implementation, and Applications for Malaria Epidemiology, First Edition.
S. M. Niaz Arifin, Gregory R. Madey and Frank H. Collins.
© 2016 John Wiley & Sons, Inc. Published 2016 by John Wiley & Sons, Inc.

patterns in Madagascar and combinations of interventions in a local setting demonstrate model capabilities for public health planning and informing the research agenda.

11.1.1   Motivation: Modeling of Malaria Eradication

Malaria is a serious public health problem throughout much of the developing world. Despite local elimination in many countries and significant reductions in malaria mortality over the past half-decade, there were over 200 million cases of malaria and over 650,000 deaths in 2010 due to malaria [560], with much of the burden borne by children in sub-Saharan Africa [508]. In addition to direct morbidity and mortality, missed school days among children and lost productivity in the workforce can slow economic growth in highly endemic countries [467].

In October 2007, Bill and Melinda Gates and WHO Director Margaret Chan announced a global campaign to definitively eradicate malaria throughout the world. Different countries and regions require different approaches for campaign success, as differences in climate, vector populations, ecology, and demographics limit the effectiveness of a one-size-fits-all program. A nation's decision for elimination is difficult to take in isolation from its neighbors and a global campaign can enable neighboring countries to coordinate efforts that benefit all [373]. Eradication is a global good, allowing resources spent on malaria to be shifted to other public health issues and reducing the burden on health systems in previously afflicted countries [190, 373].

For the malaria *Global Eradication* campaign recently commenced, there are many open questions of strategy and tactics, tools and methods, timing and durations; some of these are shared with the established Global Eradication campaign against polio and both campaigns are informed by the history of the successful Global Eradication campaign against smallpox, a third-century ago – as well as by the failed one against malaria, nearly a half-century ago. Modeling can assist in addressing existing issues and may even help shape the research agenda [5, 334], but the recently renewed focus on Global Eradication of infectious disease necessitates a reassessment of basic issues and consideration of model features-&-capabilities required to aptly address them. Modeling for Global Eradication is different from modeling for control – qualitatively so, in the Eradication endgame – and it's thus not surprising that new techniques and capabilities may be required for its apt support.

A *Monte Carlo* agent-based approach allows for both geographic scale and local resolution and tracks simulated individuals with detailed case histories and realistic infections. While such approaches are undeniably expensive in computing resources, they permit highly transparent (and thus overall reliable) embedding of model concepts and assumptions, moreover without significant compromises made to facilitate mathematical manipulations. Monte Carlo approaches provide results of known variability for a given number of samples, and thus variability in results can be "bought down" to whatever extent may be deemed necessary at an *a priori* known cost. If adequate computational resources are available, these advantages can be achieved. Computational efficiency may be improved through importance sampling strategies and a modular structure may be maintained so that ongoing research, for example, in molecular modeling, may continuously improve our understanding of population-level disease dynamics. The present approach is tightly focused on Eradication, with backward sensitivity analyses regarding attainment and maintenance of the Eradication state. Model-based simulations map out the region of campaign space for which durable Eradication has a high probability of success, moreover robust to the relevant uncertainties.

11.1.2   Questions that Arise in the Context of Malaria Eradication

Documented malaria control has existed since Empedocles the Greek reportedly stopped an epidemic by draining a swamp in the fifth century B.C.E. [458], but the most recent century experienced a dramatic increase in the scientific understanding of malaria and in the methods and tools available for its elimination. In the twentieth century, tools useful against malaria developed along many technological fronts as understanding of the disease, its ecology, and its transmission developed through the determined efforts of many scientists [555]. These tools include drugs such as chloroquine and artemisinin, better diagnostics, as well as vector control through insecticides, bed nets, house screening, larvicides, and land reclamation. The first set of questions posed to eradication modeling naturally center on currently existing interventions. What are the effects of currently existing interventions? What are the effects of combining interventions and what is the best way(s) to combine interventions into a campaign optimized for local conditions? Where is it possible to eliminate malaria when employing only currently existing interventions and at what costs? All these questions are important for planning and implementation, and modeling has an important role in each. The importance of site-specific modeling combined with detailed implementation of interventions was significantly advanced during the Garki Project in the 1970s [371].

New interventions under development may be necessary to complete the effort, and their potential uses can be illuminated by careful modeling. What are the possible effects of different interventions currently under development? What is the profile of new interventions that best complement extant interventions? What new types of intervention may be required for elimination in the most challenging transmission settings?

Campaigns are not static, monolithic entities but are necessarily quite dynamic in space and time. Elimination will not be achieved simultaneously everywhere and campaign timings may vary markedly from site to site. Indeed, several dozen countries are already working toward local elimination [373]. During a national or provincial campaign, the emphasis on various combinations of tools may be altered over time as disease prevalence and transmission change. The effects of varying campaign intensity, emphases, and tool choices over time can be most productively studied in models informed by and checked against "ground truth" from extant and future field trials and campaigns.

Campaigns are also dynamic due to finite durability of tools and to changes in disease transmission patterns in response to eradication efforts. Successful campaigns require sustained efforts replacing interventions that decay and switching tools that lose efficacy until success is achieved. Both peak and average blood concentrations of antimalarial drugs diminish in magnitude and antiparasite efficacy [73, 557, 559], and insecticide treatments lose efficacy as insecticide resistance develops. Drugs require repeated administration, insecticides repeated applications, and bed nets and screens maintenance. Because of the lack of durability of single interventions, durability of campaigns is critical. If the intense efforts required are stopped before the parasite is eliminated from vector and human reservoirs, or if the required surveillance and outbreak suppression postelimination are not maintained, the campaign will ultimately fail [122]. Finally, the development and spread of vector or pathogen resistance to a campaign material can be highly dependent on the intensity, duration, and quality of its use. Modeling must incorporate the durability of individual elements and their effective lifetimes for repeated use as a function of utilization, in order to ensure durability and sustainability of the combined campaign adequately far beyond the time required for success.

We cannot ignore the costs of different campaign designs, the benefits of success, or the consequences of failure. In a given setting, does a campaign exist that achieves the desired aims at an acceptable cost? If so, what are the different routes to elimination and the relative costs and robustness thereof? Before launching a campaign, modeling should inform the required costs, the probabilities of success, and even suggest the near- and far-term rewards of sustained success. Indeed, there can be severe consequences for failure: malaria epidemics imposed tremendous human costs in Sri Lanka and Madagascar following notable breaks in transiently attained control [436, 457].

Simulations of the impact and results of campaigns will have many sources of uncertainty, some minor, others possibly changing the outcome qualitatively. Uncertainty of outputs can be due to stochastic variation, variance in fits for model parameters, error in inputs such as population density or weather, defects in local campaign coverage, or even underlying model assumptions. Eradication modeling will investigate these sources and magnitudes of uncertainty transparently and support system-level analyses. Assumptions should be presented transparently and, if multiple assumptions are possible, modeling should address the effects of changing these assumptions. Many questions are addressed by past and current modeling efforts, which have made great contributions to our understanding of malaria, its transmission, and its elimination, but significant gaps remain. The open questions for modeling posed specifically by the malaria eradication campaign have also been well exposited through the MalERA collaboration [5, 334]. We now define capabilities required in eradication modeling, so as to inform rational campaign planning with careful treatment of near-elimination phenomena and quantitative results accompanied by sensitivity analyses. A summary of issues for eradication modeling is presented in Table 11.1.

11.1.3   Spatial Heterogeneity and Metapopulation Effects

Eradication modeling is driven by requirements for accurate representations of local conditions and capturing the effects of geographic scale and spatial heterogeneity while maintaining sufficient local resolution. Different regions exhibit diverse transmission

TABLE 11.1   Summary of Issues for Eradication Modeling

What are the effects of currently existing interventions?

What is the best setting-specific way to combine interventions into a campaign?

Where is it possible to eliminate infections using currently existing tools?

What toolset suffices to attain elimination everywhere?

What is the possible effect of different interventions under development?

What is the campaign intensity versus time profile required for a given setting?

How do underlying dynamics change in response to the campaign and what are the timescales involved?

How durable are the campaign and its specified set of tools, and how do these compare to the required duration?

Does a campaign exist that achieves elimination for acceptable costs in a given setting, and if so, what is it? What is the optimal campaign given the local constraints?

For a given campaign and setting, what is the probability of elimination as a function of time, and what are the sources and magnitude of uncertainty?

How robust is campaign success to stochastic variation as well as perturbations in system parameters such as weather, campaign coverage, intervention efficacy, and system latencies? How robust is campaign success to changing model assumptions?

What are the consequences of failure given a campaign design and setting?

characteristics: vector species and behavior, climate suitability and seasonality and intensity of transmission [130], and human factors of varying housing conditions, population densities, and innate resistance to infection. In the absence of interventions, climate variables can give good estimates of prevalence across areas with similar vector species [130]. With the vast availability of satellite and weather station data, local weather can be input with both the geographic scale and local resolution required for careful treatment of environmental effects on malaria. Models can be used to design campaigns robust against unexpected fluctuations about expected weather and microclimate.

Eradication modeling resolves the tactics and interventions that occur at the local scale. Mosquito and human populations mix locally [353], and vector control affects only mosquitoes that contact the particular intervention. Sufficient local resolution is here defined as adequately structuring the subsets of humans and mosquitoes that may come into contact during a simulation time step. Such local resolution also requires accurate population sizes for humans and mosquitoes. It is well known that the ratio of population sizes is critical [327, 353, 504], but elimination is a stochastic and discrete phenomenon and population sizes influence the probability of local infection fade-out as a function of time. The basic reproductive number R_0 [26] can be used to determine the steady state, but in the presence of a dynamic campaign that must be maintained, the system may not arrive at a steady state before the quasi-steady state changes.

As a side note, for airborne or sexually transmitted infections, the structure of the local transmission network may drive many aspects of disease dynamics. Childhood diseases often are coupled to school mixing, while other diseases may be driven primarily through family structure. The spread of sexually transmitted infections through any given population depends on the transmission network and its dynamics [177, 552], incorporating demographic heterogeneity in age, risk, and mixing.

Eradication modeling simulates broad geographic areas, since eradication is a global phenomenon and local elimination will not be attained simultaneously everywhere. Simulation of dynamics at any single location is insufficient to determine the path to elimination. People and mosquitoes are constantly moving from house to house, village to village, region to region, and nation to nation. Several nations were certified to have eliminated malaria, only to have malaria reestablished in them through importation of cases [122]. Well-connected areas can be more challenging for elimination, as seen along the Mexico–Guatemala border [133]. Large-scale persistence in spite of local fadeouts of infection has been studied in metapopulation models in general and spatial models of measles in particular [217]. Malaria fade-outs may be driven by local campaign tactics, but metapopulation phenomena require geographic-scale suppression for successful Eradication. Important work has defined receptivity and vulnerability of regions and nations [122], and similar principles apply among interconnected local settings within a single country or region. Like international migration, intranational migration poses difficulties for elimination but with several differences: migration rates can be higher and the same political and health authorities can have influence on both areas of interest.

Realistic migration links the local scale, where campaign tactics and human–mosquito mixing occur, to larger geographic scales, which serves to capture the effects of geographic heterogeneity on transmission and persistence. While finding accurate data on migration can be challenging, various groups have recently made progress using mobile phone data to inform and constrain migration rates within a country, with applications to malaria programs [556]. Migration can introduce new disease variants: chloroquine-resistant variants were most likely introduced to Madagascar from Comoros through the port of Mahajanga [361]. Local control efforts were heavily compromised and epidemics broke out in previously unaffected areas as soldiers returned home from the high-transmission conditions of trench warfare in World War I Italy [509]. Land disturbances and large-scale population movements produced an epidemic in post-World War I Russia near the Arctic Circle [416]. Tracking migrant populations across geography, rather than representing them as external inputs to single-location simulations, allows simulation of interventions targeted to mobile populations.

11.1.4 Implications for Model Structure

In addition to explicit spatial structure to address spatial heterogeneity, metapopulation effects, and human movement, other features may be required to address other questions raised by malaria eradication. These features are described below and each tends to fit well in an agent-based structure.

11.1.4.1 Modeling Individuals and Infections Immunity and previous exposure strongly influence the outcomes of new infections, and various individual hetero-geneities influence disease spread and response to interventions [504]. Studies in Kenya have shown that presence of anti-PfEMP1 antibodies is closely related to clinical response to new infections [87]. Whether an infection is symptomatic or asymptomatic can impact transmission [212]. Resolution of individuals is also essen-tial due to heterogeneity in migration rates that affect rate of spreading and variability in the immune response, as seen in malariatherapy patients [124, 331, 370, 417]. Heterogeneity in housing conditions can impact biting rates among individuals in the same local setting, and other factors such as body area can impact the vector biting rate [506]. There will also be variation in campaign access and individuals who miss the distribution or application of one intervention may be at higher risk of missing others. Existing modeling work illustrates that individual heterogeneities impact both transmission and intervention efficacy [10, 504].

Realistic models of single infections embed time-varying symptoms, probability of detection by various diagnostic tests, and infectivity, all of which may be influ-enced by individual heterogeneities. Together these allow a rich representation of patient-to-patient variability and provide a test bed for simulation of proposed new drugs and vaccines. Within-host modeling of single infections has a rich history and the variety of approaches has helped to define the research agenda for understanding the disease and examining effects of different aspects of the immune response [240, 331, 354, 370, 372]. Individual resolution with realistic single infections incorporates the effects of key latencies in malaria transmission and the shape of the duration distribution [469, 470, 505]. Latencies appear throughout malaria transmission and key human infection latencies include the liver stage, start of blood stage to detection or symptoms, a single cycle within the blood stage [476], and start of blood stage to infectivity to mosquitoes. At steady state or near a slowly varying endemic cycle, compartment models may capture dynamics without tracking these individual latencies, but in near-elimination circumstances, these latencies represent challenges for detection of cases and opportunities to quench an outbreak before any mosquitoes become infected or capable of infecting humans.

11.1.4.2 Modeling Mosquitoes Eradication modeling for malaria necessarily will involve study of detailed vector populations, with full weather-dependent latencies and vector behavior appropriate for the local setting. Latencies in the mosquito life cycle manifest in larval development, blood-feeding to oviposition [477], and successful completion of sporogony [215, 285, 503]. Just as in human infections, mosquito life-cycle latency effects are partially missed by compartment models based on ordinary differential equation (ODE). Around an endemic steady state, ODE-based models can account for the death of mosquitoes during the sporogony latency by decreasing the flux of mosquitoes from the susceptible to the infectious compartment to the number that would have survived sporogony [503], but instantaneous transport exists. Scaling up vector control could prevent any mosquitoes from becoming infectious and successfully transmitting due to latencies and finite populations and models can quantitatively estimate this effect. Finally, modeling mosquito populations for eradication requires accurate response to weather and climate. Through effects on availability of larval habitat, duration of larval development, adult mortality, and duration of sporogony, the adult vector population size and its capacity to transmit change in response to weather [148, 356]. Such effects also require accurate representations of the weather and climate data.

Details of mosquito behavior and ecology vary across species and can affect the impact of interventions. Different locations have different mixes of mosquito species, each with different ecological characteristics and behavior [286, 294]. Important variations include indoor versus outdoor feeding, time-of-day of feeding, larval breeding ecology, and host preference. Mosquito species breeding in more permanent bodies of water do not experience as large a dry season drop in population levels as do temporary pool breeders. Outdoor feeding and zoophily reduce the impact of insecticide-treated nets (ITNs) or indoor residual spraying (IRS), and the local mix of vector species can change over the course of a campaign emphasizing such means [205]. Nonlinear effects on transmission can result from this shift in species mix, and predicted campaign timelines can be affected by changes in observed tool effectiveness. Eradication modeling requires appropriate sufficiently accurate mix of local vectors, with characteristics informed by ground truth and local data.

11.1.4.3 Modeling Campaign Elements   Modeling eradication requires accurate and specific representation of campaign tools and use modalities. Key vector control tools include insecticide-treated bed nets [205, 500], IRS [112], and larval control [180]. The effects of vector behavior can have major impacts on the efficacy of interventions, such as the diminished effects of IRS and ITNs on outdoor feeding mosquitoes. Durability of individual nets is an issue [501], and durability of specific tools and changes in overall efficacy of the class of intervention in general due to development of resistance or vector behavior change must be accounted for. Drugs and vaccines may be key elements of elimination campaigns and modeling can guide their development and deployment. Vaccines have different possible modes, durations, and degrees of action and corresponding individual and population effects [429, 502, 516, 554]. Models for drugs can represent their antimalarial actions [557], drug resistance and its dynamic dependence on intensity, quality, and extent of use [73, 439], and implementation in a campaign [348, 390, 460].

Campaigns are dynamic and spatially structured, and modeling in support of rational planning of a campaign includes campaign structure and timing as well as logistics for distribution of campaign elements to targeted populations. It is easier to achieve coverage levels in some communities rather than others, depending on population densities, road access, health system access, and chosen distribution structure. Understanding existing healthcare structures is important in order to model the effects of case management [529], but also it is important to model the effect on coverage levels. A set of communities without sufficient campaign coverage could sustain an infectious reservoir that could spread to surrounding areas following lapses in campaign

TABLE 11.2   Summary of Features Desired for Eradication Modeling

---

Geographic scale combined with local resolution, linked by full migration

Individual case histories with heterogeneity and individual variability

Single individual-level infection realism

Detailed vector populations with full latencies and realistic responses to climate and weather

Vector control tools with effects dependent on vector population characteristics

Simulation of drug and vaccine actions, both for existing tools and those in development

Characterized durability of vector control tools

Effects of drug resistance and tracking spread of resistant strains

Dynamic effects, with accurate resolution of near-elimination phenomena

Modular design with software engineering oriented to ready reusability for other disease modeling projects

---

pressure. Healthcare systems are essential in monitoring for new cases in cleared or extremely low prevalence areas during the maintenance phase of the campaign [122], during which cases may present clinically more frequently after prolonged suppression [436, 457]. Modeling must also help inform costs for all phases of the campaign, including monitoring of cleared areas. Modeling can explore cost differences among different campaign designs, such as has been done for vaccine deployments [528]. A summary of features desired for eradication modeling is given in Table 11.2.

11.2   MODEL STRUCTURE

The Eradication endgame requirements of resolution, heterogeneity, individual case histories and single infection realism suggest the benefits of an agent-based approach, as has been implemented in earlier malaria models [179, 218, 502, 507]. We now walk through each aspect of the model and constructing model simulations.

11.2.1   Human Demographics and Synthetic Population

Each model study begins with construction of a geographic network of locations arranged in a node-edge graph (usually a regular grid, although the model's software does not require such regularity). The demographics, climate, and initial vector populations are input from file for each location, and if the chosen spatial resolution is sufficiently fine, these features vary smoothly across the grid. Migration connectivity is applied to the geography, with varying weights and transport modes connecting locations. Population distributions are generated from the GRUMP and GPW data sets from CIESIN at Columbia University [102, 103].

Once the geography is constructed, the simulation is populated with sample individuals, drawn from the local demographic distributions for age, gender, and risk factors. The sampling rate can be uniform, or it can vary so that sample particle density is uniform, or it can increase resolution in key segments of the population. Sampled individuals each receive a weight quantifying how many people that "particle" represents, which may support more statistically accurate accounting for human–mosquito mixing and reporting. Individuals can be heterogeneous in the mosquito biting rate that they endure, or in their various migration rates. Individuals are then randomly assigned infections with probability related to initial prevalence if known. If initial prevalence is not known, a moderate value is selected and the first part of the simulation is used as "burn-in". Which infection model is used can be selected for any given study, for example, whether the model is a full mechanistic intrahost model with antigenic variation and antigen-specific immunity, or one characterized by a draw from a duration distribution with simplified immunity features.

Each individual receives a weight W_i equal to the reciprocal of the sampling rate for that individual's characteristics. For example, if 20% of individuals are added to the simulation as sample particles, each has weight $W_i = 5$. Individuals can have different sampling rates weighted by age, location, local population density, or risk factors, which allows high-resolution sampling of key populations at a lower overall computational cost. If superinfection is included in the simulation, individuals each can have multiple infections, which combine to create a total infectiousness X_i, the rate at which contacts with the infectious individual become infected. This rate is then modified by natural characteristics of the infectious individual $Y_{i,transmit}$, which gathers factors such as acquired immunity or increased contact rate, and the transmission-reducing effects of interventions $Z_{i,transmit}$, which includes transmission-blocking vaccines, for example. The total infectiousness T of the local human population is then calculated as

$$T = \sum_i W_i X_i Y_{i,transmit} Z_{i,transmit} \tag{11.1}$$

For simulation of population density-independent transmission, individual infectiousness X_i includes the average contact rate of the infectious individual, so this total infectiousness is divided by the population P to get the force of infection $F_I = T/P$ for each individual in the population. The base rate of acquisition of new infections per person is then F_I, which can be modified for each individual i by their characteristics $Y_{i,acquire}$ and interventions $Z_{i,acquire}$. If an individual is completely immune, $Y_{i,acquire} = 0$, and a perfectly effective acquisition-blocking vaccine sets $Z_{i,acquire} = 0$. Heterogeneity in contact rate increases $Y_{i,transmit}$ for an infectious individual and increases $Y_{i,acquire}$ when determining if individual i acquires a new infection. Over a time step Δt, the probability of an individual i acquiring a new infection is then

$$P_{I,i} = 1 - \exp(-F_I Y_{i,acquire} Z_{i,acquire} \Delta t) \tag{11.2}$$

11.2.2   Vector Ecology

At each time step in the simulation constituting a specific model study, the vector populations are updated for the individual vector interactions with individuals, as well as the overall vector population dynamics [160]. Rainfall data for Madagascar were obtained from the Global Precipitation Climatology Centre [214] to generate gridded monthly averages to generate daily weather. Temperature data were obtained from ground station reports and NASA MODIS satellites. For spatial simulations, these data often need to be interpolated carefully to fill the landscape of interest [106].

For each species, the adult vector population dynamics in the absence of vector control will be driven by a time-dependent emergence of new adults from larval habitat. Different species occupy different characteristic habitats and these different habitats respond differently to rainfall, temperature, and humidity. *Anopheles gambiae* tends to breed in smaller temporary bodies of water, while *Anopheles funestus* is more often found in semipermanent bodies of water with emergent vegetation. As such, populations of *An. gambiae* tend to increase more rapidly after the start of the rainy season, and populations crash more rapidly once the rains stop, compared to *An. funestus*. For each species present, an appropriate function for the dynamics of available larval habitat must be selected and then fit to the recorded human biting rates for adult vectors in that location.

The EMOD model exhibits closed-loop egg laying – each new batch of eggs are laid after successful feeds by the adult females that night. Once hatched, aquatic development proceeds at a temperature-dependent rate to emergence. A mortality rate is imposed on the larval population and the progress of the cohort laid on a given day is incremented by the inverse of the days to emergence at that daily temperature. Once the cohort's progress reaches one, the surviving members of that cohort emerge.

After a short interval of delay, the newly emerged adults begin their life of feeding and egg laying. The adult dynamics are also affected by an adult mortality rate, which sets how the average number of days that an adult can expect to live. Adults that are infected by parasite-carrying humans as described below will go through another temperature-dependent latency [503] either as a cohort or as individually simulated mosquito agents until they are sporozoite positive and can infect susceptible humans. Finally, high temperatures can result in higher adult mortalities, and this phenomenon too is incorporated to the daily risk of dying.

11.2.3   Vector Transmission

The human population is then processed, with the probability distribution of outcomes for a feeding attempt on each sampled individual calculated based on their age, relative biting rate, and interventions such as bed nets. If the individual is infectious, the probabilities of passing on that infection to a mosquito and of the mosquito surviving the feeding event are calculated as well. The individual outcome distributions are then gathered into an overall outcome distribution, with individual contributions weighted by sampling weight and relative biting rate. Each vector population is then adjusted for mortality, successful feeds, and new infections. The success of an indoor biting attempt is then modified by the presence of individual interventions, such as bed nets or spatial repellents. This allows all individual heterogeneity arising from both vectors and humans in intervention coverage and compliance to be properly accounted. If a new infection occurs, a new Infection object is added to the individual's infection queue for processing. All individuals are then updated for the time step, with infections processed, immunity status updated, age and other factors updated, interventions aged and efficacies updated, and migration calculated, if applicable.

In a malaria simulation, the human population transmits infection to the local mosquito populations and acquires infection from mosquitoes, not from the human population. Therefore, simulation of the vector population occurs between the above-described steps of calculating the human population infectiousness and rate of new infections. An additional factor α_i represents the relative biting rate for that individual relative to the local population. $X_{i,transmit}$ is the probability that individual i infects a completely susceptible mosquito that survives a feed. The probability $P_{f,i}$ that individual i is sought by a human-feeding mosquito is then

$$P_{f,i} = \frac{\alpha_i W_i}{\sum\limits_i \alpha_i W_i} \tag{11.3}$$

Each feeding mosquito can then select an individual from the population and is infected while surviving the feed on an infectious individual with probability $X_i Y_{i,transmit}$, multiplied by the parameter for maximum probability of mosquito infection. The effect of interventions $Z_{i,transmit}$ is different for indoor and outdoor feeds as it includes the probability that the mosquito will survive the feed, which for an individual living in a house with IRS depends dramatically on whether the feed was indoor or outdoor. The distribution of outcomes for each individual are collected into the distribution of outcomes for the vector population. Further details of these calculations can be found in the paper describing the present vector model [160] and calculation of human infectivity $X_{i,transmit}$ can be done through a variety of methods and models.

An individual is infected by attempted infectious bites with a probability $bY_{i,acquire} Z_{i,acquire}$, in which b is the probability of successful infection by a bite on a completely susceptible, nonimmune individual [503]. $Z_{i,acquire}$ depends on whether the infectious bites are attempted indoors or outdoors. Infectious bites are distributed among the population according to the relative biting rates and total available human hosts, and if N_f Nf infectious mosquitoes attempt to feed in a given time step, an individual's rate of new infections is then

$$R_i = N_f \frac{\alpha_i}{\sum\limits_i \alpha_i W_i} bY_{i,acquire} Z_{i,acquire} \tag{11.4}$$

Note that the individual's sampling weight W_i does not influence the number of infectious bites received, just the individual's relative cross section for infecting mosquitoes. For indoor and outdoor bites, there will be two infection rates that have different N_f and $Z_{i,acquire}$ and are then summed. An individual's probability of infection in a time step Δt is then $1 - \exp(-R_i \Delta t)$.

The feeding cycle with its possible outcomes is depicted in Fig. 11.1 and the full calculations for the outcomes can be found in [160].

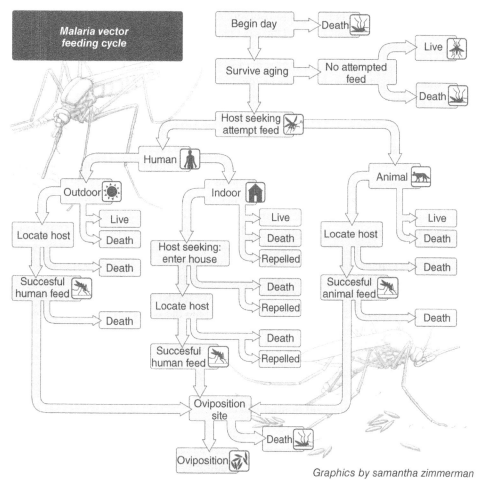

Figure 11.1   The EMOD model of the mosquito feeding cycle with outcomes. By Eckhoff [160], used under a Creative Commons Attribution 4.0 International License.

11.2.4   Within-Host Disease Dynamics

The Monte Carlo framework supports use of detailed individual state spaces and single infection models. Phenomena such as the probabilistic outcome for gametocyte transmission from a human to a mosquito during a single blood feed are modeled and statistical mechanics exhibit how these microinteractions affect the whole [161]. Development of immunity depends on exposure and immunity to a broad spectrum of antigens, as seen in field studies [87] and implemented in the model [162]. Exciting new discoveries are continuing to be made on many disease-suppression fronts, but most models do not have the physiological specificity that would enable the incorporation of such new knowledge. A Monte Carlo approach with microsolvers for low-level outcomes makes it feasible to incorporate gracefully detailed individual models for infection and immunity into even a continental or global-scale model study. Validation of models is pursued by building microsolvers with applicable data sets and then comparing the system-level outputs to data sets that did not enter into model construction.

A new infection receives an incubation period and an infectious period from specified distributions and a counter tracks the full latency, which is possible when simulating individual particles. After the incubation period, the counter for the infectious period begins, during which time the infection contributes to the individual's infectiousness X_i. Note that the sampling weight W_i is not included in the probability of acquiring a new infection. Sample particles are simulated as single individuals; their weighting W_i is used to determine their effects upon the rest of the simulation.

After the incubation period in the liver, merozoites emerge and begin invading red blood cells. Successfully parasitized red blood cells go through a 48-hour latency, whereupon they release 16 merozoites to invade other red blood cells. This destruction of red blood cells, expression of novel antigens, and release of parasite by-products creates a powerful inflammatory response that has some antiparasite effects [514]. Beyond the innate immune response, an adaptive immune response develops to the specific antigens expressed on the infected red blood cell's membranes. As a result of this adaptive immune pressure, the parasite has developed the ability to change the adhesive proteins through a set of 50–60 PfEMP-1 variants. We model this switching process and the innate and adaptive responses in order to compute the within-host dynamics of the parasite population, the duration of infection, and the dynamics of the sexual-stage gametocytes driven by the infected red blood cell cycle. Further details and equations are available [161].

11.2.5 Human Migration and Spatial Effects

There is a well-understood virtue to modeling and to understanding the effects of geography. The Monte Carlo framework provides a platform into which to incorporate diverse geographic inputs and their corresponding implications. Realistically represented migration of humans and mosquitoes links spatial scales and allows study of Eradication as a regional and global event. Simulation results are examined for persistent features that can be validated against current data such as prevalence maps from Malaria Atlas Project [232]. Other qualitative features affecting campaign success can be discerned in campaign space, the many-dimensional state-space of intervention coverage in space and time. Areas requiring greater intensity of Eradication-directed effort become clearly visible.

For spatially distributed simulations, mixing of individuals or individuals and vectors occurs locally, but each location can affect other cells through migration of individuals or vectors. Persistence can occur even if the overall level of intervention coverage drops the average R_0 below one, since areas with gaps in coverage can sustain transmission that can then return to cleared areas if pressure is diminished. Simulation of the migration that knits the different spatial scales is described below.

Each grid cell has a list of other cells to which it is connected, with each edge i having a rate r_i given as probability for a given person making that migration per day as well as a defined mode of transportation. Modes of transportation can be local, longer-distance road or train travel, air travel or sea travel, and system sensitivities to each mode of migration can be studied by scaling factors x_{local}, $x_{regional}$, x_{air}, x_{sea}. Each location then has a total rate of migration $R_{migration}$ summed over all edges:

$$R_{migration} = \sum_{i,local} x_{local} r_i + \sum_{i,regional} x_{regional} r_i + \sum_{i,air} x_{air} r_i + \sum_{i,sea} x_{sea} r_i$$

Heterogeneity in individual migration rates is incorporated by a rate adjustment $k_{migration}$ for each individual's heterogeneous propensities to travel, and the waiting time for each individual's next migration is calculated as a random number drawn from an exponential distribution with parameter $R_{migration}$. The destination for the next migration is calculated by a uniform random number that determines the edge traveled by each migration edge's contribution to the total rate. For each successive edge i, $x_{type} r_i$ is added to an indexed sum creating a cumulative probability function when divided by $R_{migration}$. The inverse function of this distribution maps from the unit interval to a destination.

The diffusiveness of migration is changed through three separate models. In fully diffusive migration, upon arrival in the new destination, an individual's next migration is determined by the rate and destination array of the new location. If round trips are incorporated into the simulation, then with a certain probability the individual will return to the original location after an exponentially distributed waiting time that depends on the mode of transportation of the first migration, and migration is sub-diffusive. In waypoint migration, individuals have a home location and can migrate outward in a longer-distance, multiple-step migration but return home by retracing their outward trip.

Rather than have every human within the area of interest represented as a particle in the simulation, a subset with stochastically chosen features may represent the whole. The population does not need to be sampled uniformly, as some individuals are more important to malaria transmission than others; importance sampling is performed as described below. Each sampled individual receives a sampling weight that determines its contributions to both collective infectivity and statistical outcomes, and this sampling weight is the reciprocal of the adjusted sampling rate for that individual.

Certain individuals drive disease transmission more than others and different sampling rates are required for accuracy in different areas. A highly populated city on a plateau with rare malaria transmission does not need the same proportional sampling of individuals as a more sparsely populated rural setting with intense malaria transmission. The sampling strategy necessarily depends on desired outputs and the required resolution: for example, if severe outcomes among children is a key output, then children can be sampled at a higher rate compared to the population as a whole. Sampling strategies can be tested to whatever degrees may be sufficient for attainment of the desired accuracy by increasing sampling until local changes in sampling strategy are not significantly affecting the model output of interest, such as the estimate of campaign success. A Monte Carlo approach also provides statistically assured error bounds on model results for the ensemble of trajectories and more model runs can be added at a priori known costs until error bounds are satisfactorily small.

11.2.6 Stochastic Ensembles

In summary, an initial set of individuals are added to the simulation represented as sample particles; these particles can be removed for death or downsampling and such particles can be added for births or when splitting an existing particle. The current state then transitions to the next state according to probability distributions that depend on the current state. For instance, the number of mosquitoes with maturing oocysts at a later state depends on the current ensemble of human gametocyte counts, individual biting rates, and individual interventions such as nets that modulate biting rate. The future parasite counts of a single individual's current infections depend on the individual's inflammatory and adaptive immune responses, the current parasite count, and the expressed parasite surface antigens. The change in inflammatory and adaptive immune responses in turn depend on the expressed parasite surface antigens [87].

By maintaining the set of sampled individuals, a realistic ensemble of case histories is maintained. At the end of a time step, spatial and simulation average data are collected and reported. Eradication campaigns are modeled as a composition of events, such as bed net distributions, IRS treatments, administered medications, vaccination events, or other intervention possibilities. If an event occurs at a given time step, the intervention distribution occurs and the number distributed is updated along with the estimated cost. After completing one instance corresponding to particular initial and boundary conditions, the simulation can be rerun with a new set of sampled individuals, for example, in support of variance estimation. Many probabilistic paths are computed and the ensemble of trajectories from the current state to the Eradication state defines a path integral formulation for Eradication.

Backward sensitivity analysis is then possible for the Eradication state. Many simulation paths reach Eradication, but the key question is not only what paths reach Eradication, but the sensitivity of this outcome to perturbations. If a trajectory goes to zero, what was the probability of this outcome? If certain model features are perturbed slightly, for example, modeled environmental temperatures are slightly higher, then how does that affect the probability of Eradication? These questions can be answered within this framework and each proposed campaign has a distribution of probabilistic outcomes for analysis. Stochastic variability can become increasingly important in near-elimination conditions. Model results can present stochastic variability as well as sensitivities to inputs, model parameters, and campaign coverages and efficacies, with special focus on the sensitivity of outputs of interest such as the probability of fade-out. One way to display results for sensitivity is through a plot showing the transition of behavior, for example, from a high probability of fade-out to a low probability of fade-out, over several dimensions of parameters. Such displays, which are here termed separatrix plots, can be overlaid with associated costs or probabilities of other events. The separatrix algorithm uses an ensemble of binary simulation outcomes (e.g., true only if eradication is achieved) to estimate the probability of success as a function of the study parameters [298]. The algorithm iterates between two main steps: the first uses kernel smoothing to perform the estimation with the available simulation results and the second uses an experiment design procedure to select several new configurations to simulate. The algorithm can be configured to explore globally or focus computational effort on identifying regions of the study space for which the success probability is near a desired level.

Our approach is not only interested in best parameter fits; instead, the overarching issue that we pose is what campaign design will have a high probability of Eradication success across the full space of parameter sensitivity, model architecture, and campaign logistics uncertainties. It is possible in general to "engineer around uncertainty" by accepting higher campaign costs: successful campaigns in the past succeeded in spite of significant remaining unknowns, the smallpox one being exemplary in the Global Eradication context. This modeling approach puts a price tag on this trade-off. The parameters in the present model are based on low-level phenomena with real-world measurables. If the uncertainty in a given parameter is high and the system is sensitive to it, it may be more cost-effective overall to do direct experiments to reduce the uncertainty, rather than to campaign-engineer around its extant magnitude.

11.3   RESULTS

In this section, we present some results of three sets of simulations run on varying geographical scale: a village, a district (the Garki District), and an island country (Madagascar).

11.3.1   Single-Village Simulations

The transmission setting based on Namawala, Tanzania, which was used in [160] to explore the effects of transmission intensity, vector behavior, intervention coverage, and intervention efficacy, is reexplored to study the effects of combinations of more potentially orthogonal interventions, namely vector control through IRS and a transmission-blocking vaccine. The climate and weather data are input, along with the age distribution of the local population. There is no spatial structure explored in this example, so only a single node location is initiated. The vector population includes *An. gambiae*, *Anopheles arabiensis*, and *An. funestus*, with *An. arabiensis* feeding indoors 50% of the time and the other species modeled to take every feed indoors. Each population expands and contracts according to its fitted model of vector larval dynamics. IRS is modeled with 80% coverage repeated every year and an efficacy of 0.7. The transmission-blocking vaccine has an initial efficacy of 0.8 exponentially decaying with a time constant of 4 years, with mass distribution every 5 years. The IRS campaign has 80% coverage with 70% killing efficacy for indoor resting feeds and is repeated every year. The prototype transmission-blocking vaccine is mass distributed every 5 years with 80% coverage, reducing transmission by 80% with a 4-year decay time constant. Adding interventions adds variability to the simulation, with the transmission-blocking vaccine providing an additional reduction in transmission of over a factor of 2, which would be difficult for further interventions targeting

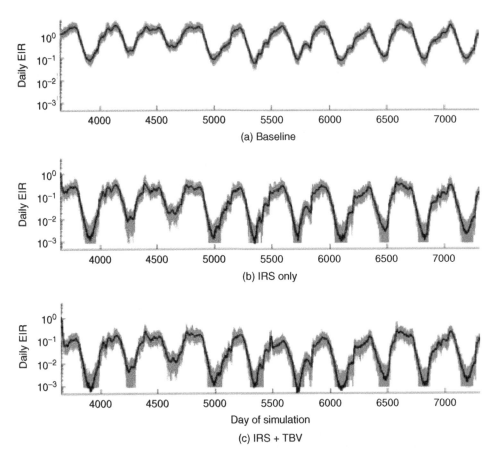

Figure 11.2   Simulation of Namawala, Tanzania, as described in [160], shows changes in EIR due to seasonal variations at baseline (a), with IRS (b), and with IRS and a transmission-blocking vaccine (c). Adding interventions adds variability to the simulation, with the transmission-blocking vaccine providing an additional reduction in transmission of over a factor of 2, which would be difficult for further interventions targeting indoor feeding to achieve on top of IRS. By Eckhoff [160], used under a Creative Commons Attribution 4.0 International License.

indoor feeding to achieve on top of IRS. The effects on entomological inoculation rate (EIR), the rate of infectious bites per person, can be seen in Fig. 11.2. Such a model platform can be used to explore potential product profiles and their effects in different transmission settings and as components of different intervention combinations. Other combinations of vector control, transmission blocking, and more in Namawala are explored as well [163].

11.3.2   Spatial Simulations: Garki District

In the early 1970s, intense malaria control efforts were organized in the Garki District in Nigeria to see what combination of vector control and drug treatments might be

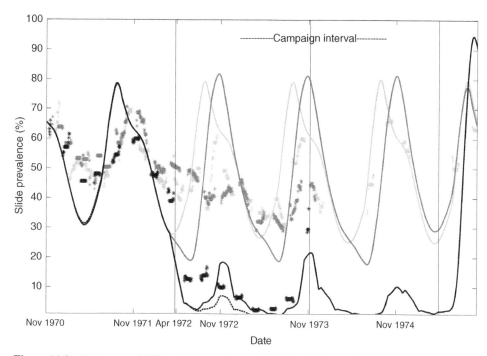

Figure 11.3 Outcomes of different intervention combinations in the Garki District [163]. The light gray is baseline, the dark gray adds in IRS, the dark line is with infrequent drug campaigns, and the dark dashed line with frequent drug campaigns. The dots are field data from the Project. © 2013 AJTMH. Reprinted, with permission, from [163].

necessary in a high-transmission region [371]. One of the notable features of this district is that baseline EIR ranged from 18 infectious bites per person per year in Rafin Marke up to over 100 infectious bites per person per year in Sugungum, and the mix of vector species compositions varied as well. The Project also was spatially heterogeneous in its application of an IRS spraying schedule, IRS plus occasional drug distributions, or IRS plus frequent drug distributions.

We start by fitting a model to an average Garki location of intermediate transmission intensity and matching the effects of each of the levels of Project activity as seen in Fig. 11.3 [163]. We then also created local models for the range of villages in the study [163]. These can then be knit together in a spatial pattern with migration as described above. Alternatively, each can be run independently with an importation rate of new infections. This importation rate can be tuned to match the level expected from the prevalence in surrounding areas. The EMOD model supports both spatially coupled simulation and explicit rates of import.

11.3.3 Madagascar

Recent modeling efforts have focused on Madagascar, since it exhibits many of the climate regions of interest for a Global Eradication campaign against the human-infecting

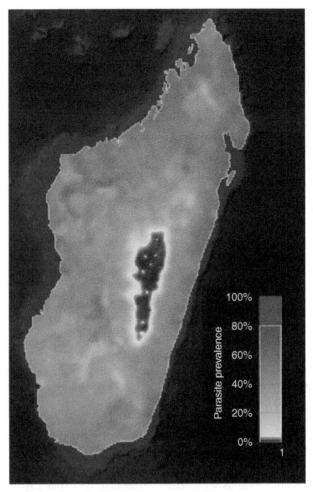

Figure 11.4   Modeled distribution of detected prevalence in Madagascar. This can be compared to estimates for prevalence from the Malaria Atlas Project [232].

species of *Plasmodium*, has a large spatial extent, and is an island. The simulated prevalence patterns for microscopy-based detection of the blood-stage parasite correspond to spatial patterns in the surveys in the Malaria Atlas Project [232], as shown in Fig. 11.4. These studies were not fitted to the MAP data, but rather demographic, climate, and vector data were inputted as best estimates to the model, which was simulated in the absence of interventions, and the spatial prevalence data are used for postvalidation. Vector populations simulated include *An. gambiae* ss, *An. arabiensis*, and *An. funestus*, with a stronger, more transient response to rainfall for *An. gambiae* sl compared with *An. funestus*. Maps of simulated average vector populations and sporozoite rates

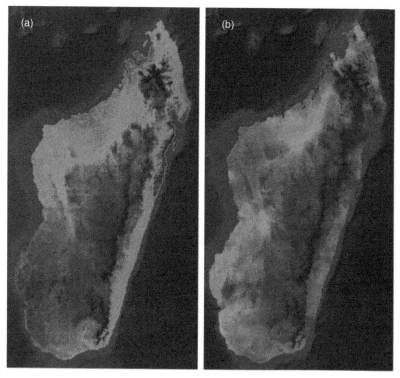

Figure 11.5   Modeled vector population density distributions in Madagascar. (a) Adult vector distribution averaged daily over a simulated 3-year period. (b) Sporozoite rates for all local *Anopheles* averaged over the same period. Average rates are highest in tropical wet and dry climate zones due to the high rates at the end of the wet season, when the average age of the vector population increases without a large influx of emerging mosquitoes.

show spatial patterns that are salient in planning national-scale campaigns as depicted in Fig. 11.5. Separatrix plots display the transition from a region of low probability of success to a region with high probability of success, if it exists. These are powerful tools for quantitatively understanding the Eradication-pertinent effects of varying intervention coverages and efficacies and for understanding the impact of uncertain inputs such as migration rates. Separatrix plots of the modeled probability of successful Eradication in Madagascar are shown in Fig. 11.6. For a uniformly distributed and maintained campaign, scaling migration rates does not significantly affect campaign outcomes, although this could change for a more spatiotemporally patterned campaign. Several simplifying assumptions are made to illustrate the use of such tools: all mosquitoes are set to feed indoors and bed nets have overly high efficacies at killing vectors. With realistic vector populations on Madagascar and current bed net efficacies, a bed net campaign alone is insufficient to interrupt transmission.

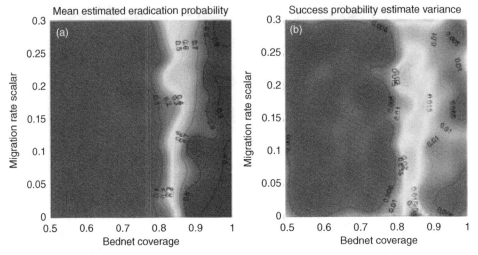

Figure 11.6   (a) Separatrix plots of the modeled probability of successful Eradication in Madagascar, showing the division of the high probability of success region separated from the low probability of success region. (b) The estimate variance. The two parameters shown here are ITN coverage and a linear scaling of migration rates. In these simulations, all vectors are indoor feeders and bed nets have perfect efficacy and do not decay. For realistic vector populations including outdoor biting, bed nets alone are insufficient for elimination and must be combined with other interventions. Increasing migration rates given broadly uniform high coverage spreads out the transition from low probability of success to high probability of success.

11.4   DISCUSSION

Rational campaign design for the Global Eradication of an infectious disease such as malaria requires new modeling tools beyond what may be necessary or sufficient for its local control. Key issues for eradication modeling are examined in this chapter, and the features likely required to address these issues are reviewed. Simple models provide insight into the contributing effects of different individual phenomena and campaign elements, but such model structures necessarily omit some interdependences of various system features. For example, modeling the effects of vector control without spatial structure, species-specific effects, and second-order population impacts may not accurately capture the disease-related phenomena with fidelity sufficient to support time-efficient, reliable local elimination.

A more comprehensive set of modeling tools is necessary for rational planning of reasonably optimal Eradication campaigns. Local elimination requires careful resolution of near-Eradication dynamics, when discrete disease latencies and discrete individuals become important and steady states become irrelevant. In such circumstances, spatial mixing and spatial heterogeneity ever more severely limit the effectiveness of simplified continuous modeling as a single population characterized by a basic infection reproductive number R_0. Merely reducing this single-population reproductive number below replacement does not ensure that the real-world heterogeneous community will ever experience sustained elimination, even though the single-population asymptotic limit is zero. All such issues may be addressed through careful analyses of larger spatial simulations, which serve to eliminate innately troublesome "edge effects". Quantitative estimates of timing and effort required for disease elimination on larger spatial and temporal scales requires all the above features, simultaneously interacting.

Such modeling studies improve with improving field data and data access, with the vector maps of *Anopheles* vectors being assembled by Malaria Atlas Project providing a fine continuing example [235]. This modeling framework provides a powerful toolset for an Eradication campaign planner by combining diverse data ranging from vector behavior, vector species distributions, climate and weather, to detailed malaria infection data such as individual-specific antibody effects on infected red blood cells in support of evaluating various Campaign strategies and tactics.

We continue to develop a Monte Carlo agent-based approach to satisfy these requirements for new Global Eradication campaign-supporting modeling tools. A sample set of individuals populates a broad geography with location-specific climate, demography, and migration connectivity. In the case of vector-borne diseases such as malaria, individuals mix with the vector populations locally, but migration allows parasites to be carried throughout the simulation study. Possible campaigns are implemented-in-simulation within the model, and the probabilities of Eradication are calculated, along with the sensitivities to different parameters, as well as to data and model structural uncertainties. Campaign costs can be tracked for both materials and operations, which allows comparison of costs and the probability and robustness of Eradication for different potential campaign designs. The model can be extended to all pertinent modes of infectious disease transmission, that is, it is not restricted to vector-borne diseases and is intended to support possible Global Eradication campaigns directed against many types of pathogens.

For specificity and to enhance clarity, we have employed Eradication of malaria to illustrate the principles of computer-based modeling to Eradication campaigns, and we have already-good and swiftly growing reason to believe that they may be generally applicable to a wide variety of Eradication campaigns directed against other infectious diseases. Other major infectious diseases are treated fundamentally similarly in the model, albeit presently at less mature stages of model development and in manners specialized to each particular disease and its causative pathogen. It is planned to eventually include Eradication campaign-support quality models for all infectious diseases of potential Eradication interest.

We utilize a variety of model architectures and approaches from compartmental modeling to individual-based approaches within this overall study of infectious disease Eradication. Compartmental models can provide significant computational savings for applicable model state spaces, and a variety of analytical approaches can also produce useful results. Reduced state-space models can be easier to understand and cheaper to reduce variance, so simplifications are sought when additional model complexity is not necessary for the question at hand. The more complicated models are used in parallel to understand the effects of assumptions embedded in simple models and to answer questions that require such detail. Realization of such detailed individual-based stochastic modeling presents challenges of design and implementation, but it may become a valued tool for those professionally concerned with infectious disease suppression, in addition to Eradication campaign planners. It requires extended cooperation and collaboration, because it must be driven by high-quality local data, both to initiate realistic model simulations and to provide real-time "midcourse corrections" during campaigns. Assumptions and sensitivities must be rigorously explored and exposed, and cost-effectiveness of different campaign plans and designs objectively evaluated. Modular design of the model provides a key enablement of such capabilities and facilitates repurposing for other diseases. When these several distinct features are carefully combined in model studies, they will contribute to refining key issues for research, development of new tools, and rational design of both the structure and execution of Eradication campaigns. The most successful campaigns may be those that can best utilize disease surveillance, data management and communications, modeling based on near-real-time data, and low-latency responses via apt supply chain management.

APPENDIX A

ENZYME KINETICS MODEL FOR VECTOR GROWTH AND DEVELOPMENT

A.1 OVERVIEW

This appendix describes the theoretical background on the enzyme kinetics model used by the core model and the ABMs to regulate the growth and development of mosquito vectors.[1] Since mosquitoes are *poikilothermic*, temperature is a critical variable in the growth and development kinetics of *Anopheles gambiae*, and hence in malaria epidemiology modeling.[2] Temperature is one of the most influential parameters that can affect the rates of growth and development of malaria mosquitoes. For instance, in the range of 18–26°C, a change of only 1°C in temperature can change a mosquito's life span by more than a week [148]. Understanding this theoretical background is thus crucial to select the appropriate temperature model for the mosquito agents in the ABMs.

The organization of this appendix is as follows: Section A.2 discusses some recent works on stochastic thermodynamic models. Section A.3 discusses the origin of historical models for organism development, including the Arrhenius plots and the Arrhenius equation. The Eyring equation Eq. (A.3) is derived next. Concepts of Gibbs free energy, entropy, and enthalpy are then sequentially incorporated into the equation, yielding the final form of the Eyring equation Eq. (A.6).

---

[1] The core model and the ABMs were presented in Chapters 4–6.
[2] A *poikilotherm* is a plant or animal whose internal temperature varies along with that of the ambient environmental temperature.

Spatial Agent-Based Simulation Modeling in Public Health:
Design, Implementation, and Applications for Malaria Epidemiology, First Edition.
S. M. Niaz Arifin, Gregory R. Madey and Frank H. Collins.
© 2016 John Wiley & Sons, Inc. Published 2016 by John Wiley & Sons, Inc.

Section A.4 discusses the model developed by Sharpe and DeMichele [488], deriving Eq. (A.10) as the final equation of development for this model. Section A.5 discusses the nonlinear regression model derived by Schoolfield *et al.* [483]. Starting with Eq. (A.10) from Section A.4, it reformulates the model using nonlinear regression. Section A.6 discusses the model developed by Depinay *et al.* [148] and concludes with the major findings that are directly affected by temperature.

A.2 STOCHASTIC THERMODYNAMIC MODELS

Sharpe and DeMichele developed a stochastic thermodynamic model of poikilothermic development from the Eyring equation, assuming multiple activity states of the underlying developmental control enzymes [488]. However, the model was not well suited for nonlinear regression. To alleviate this, Schoolfield *et al.* used nonlinear regression techniques in describing a new formulation of the Sharpe and DeMichele model [483]. Their model was partly based on Hultin's formulation [255], and discussed biological and graphical interpretation of the model parameters, illustrating regression suitability with a typical data set.

Depinay *et al.* presented a model simulating the *Anopheles* population dynamics by incorporating biological and environmental variables [148]. The model used the enzyme kinetics model derived by Sharpe and DeMichele [488] and the simplified form derived by Schoolfield *et al.* [483]. It was based on absolute reaction rate kinetics of enzymes for the temperature-dependent developmental rates of eggs, larvae, and pupae and the duration of the gonotrophic cycle. It focuses on two abiotic factors (temperature and moisture) and three biotic factors (nutrient competition, predation or death by disease, and dispersal).

Bayoh and Lindsay examined the influence of temperature on the survival of larval stages (larvae and pupae) of *An. gambiae* Giles *sensu stricto* and subsequent adult production [55]. They observed groups of 30 mosquitoes in laboratory at constant temperatures ($10-40\,^{\circ}\mathrm{C}$) from the first instar until death or metamorphosis of the last individual.

A.3 POIKILOTHERMIC DEVELOPMENT MODELS

Among numerous empirical formulations of organism development, the following two are more relevant to poikilothermic development [488]:

1. The day-degree or temperature summation model:
   - Proposed by Candolle [138] and Reibisch [449]
   - Approximates observed values within certain temperature limits
   - Assumes that the rate of development is proportional to temperature: $k = b(T - T_a)$, where k is the rate of development, b is a constant, T is the absolute temperature, and T_a is the temperature at the developmental zero.

2. The nonlinear temperature inhibition model:
   - Derived by Johnson and Lewin [266] for high temperatures and by Hultin [255] for low temperatures
   - Describes the inhibiting effect of either high or low temperatures on organism development.

Sharpe and DeMichele's model comprised a linear response in mid-temperature ranges and nonlinear temperature inhibition (as modeled by the above two formulations) in high- and low-temperature ranges [488]. To deduce the formula for the transition rate constant, it used the Arrhenius equation and the Eyring equation, as well as the concepts of entropy and enthalpy. However, the last two originate from the concept of the Gibbs free energy, which is described as follows.

A.3.1   Log-Linear Models

A log-linear model is a mathematical model that takes the form of a function whose logarithm is a first-degree polynomial function of the model's parameters, making it suitable for (possibly multivariate) linear regression. Log-linear models postulate a linear relationship between the independent variables and the logarithm of the dependent variable. As shown in the following, the temperature-dependent rate equations are usually plotted using the log-linear models. Specifically, Eq. (A.2) explains why these equations bear the log-linear values in the ordinate axis and inverse temperature values in the abscissa.

A.3.2   The Arrhenius Model

Temperature governs the rate of a chemical reaction. In 1889, Swedish scientist Svante Arrhenius first provided a physical justification and interpretation for this. The Arrhenius plots and the Arrhenius equation, both named after him, are used to define this relationship quantitatively. At higher temperatures, the probability that two molecules will collide is higher. This higher collision rate results in a higher kinetic energy, which has an effect on the activation energy of the reaction. The activation energy is the amount of energy required to ensure that a reaction happens.

The extent of temperature inhibition on the rates of chemical reactions can be shown by an Arrhenius plot. An Arrhenius plot displays the logarithm of kinetic constants ($\ln(k)$, ordinate axis, where k is the rate constant) plotted against inverse temperature ($1/T$, abscissa). For a single rate-limited thermally activated process, an Arrhenius plot gives a straight line, from which the activation energy and the preexponential factor can both be determined. The original Arrhenius equation is as follows:

$$k = A\mathrm{e}^{\frac{-E_a}{RT}} \tag{A.1}$$

where k is the rate constant, A is the preexponential factor, E_a is the activation energy, R is the gas constant, and T is the absolute temperature. Taking natural logarithm to

Eq. (A.1) yields

$$\ln(k) = \ln(A) - \frac{E_a}{R}\left(\frac{1}{T}\right) \tag{A.2}$$

Thus, in an Arrhenius plot, the value of the "y-intercept" corresponds to $\ln(A)$, and the gradient of the line equals to $-E_a/R$. The gradient $(-E_a/R)$ represents the fraction of the molecules present in a gas that have energies equal to or in excess of activation energy at a particular temperature. The ordinate axis $(\ln(k))$ denotes the specific growth rate $(time^{-1})$ and the abscissa $1/T$ ($°K^{-1}$) denotes the reciprocal absolute temperature.

Other terms of interest are interpreted as follows:

- The preexponential factor, A: A constant of proportionality that describes a number of factors such as the frequency of collision between and the orientation of the reacting particles (often taken as constant across small temperature ranges)
- The activation energy, E_a: This is the minimum energy needed for the reaction to occur, expressed in joules per mole
- The gas constant, R: This comes from the *Ideal gas law* that relates the pressure, volume, and temperature of a particular number of moles of gas: $pV = nRT$, where p, V, and n are the absolute pressure, volume, and amount of substance (usually measured in moles) of the gas, respectively; R is the gas constant (8.314472 joules per $°K$ per mole) and T is the absolute temperature.

Thus, the Arrhenius equation Eq. (A.2) shows the effect of a change of temperature on the rate constant and thus on the rate of the reaction. For example, if the rate constant doubles the rate of the reaction would also almost double.

A.3.3 The Eyring Equation

The Eyring equation, developed in 1935 by Henry Eyring, is trivially equivalent to the Arrhenius equation Eq. (A.2) and relates the reaction rate to temperature. The basic form of the equation is

$$k = \frac{k_B T}{h} e^{-\frac{\Delta G^{\ddagger}}{RT}} \tag{A.3}$$

where k is the rate constant, k_B is Boltzmann's constant ($1.3806504(24) \times 10^{-23}$ J/$°K$), h is Planck's constant ($6.62606896(33) \times 10^{-34}$ Js), $\Delta G^{\ddagger}$ is the Gibbs energy of activation (the Gibbs free energy), R is the gas constant, and T is the absolute temperature.

To determine whether a reaction will occur or not, both enthalpy and entropy changes are important. The Gibbs free energy establishes a relationship between enthalpy and entropy and hereby accommodates them into the Eyring equation Eq. (A.3).

A.3.4 The Gibbs Free Energy, Entropy, and Enthalpy

The *Gibbs free energy*, developed in the 1870s by the American mathematician Josiah Willard Gibbs, is a thermodynamic potential that measures the *useful* or process-initiating work obtainable from an isothermal, isobaric thermodynamic system. It is the maximum amount of nonexpansion work that can be extracted from a closed system and can be attained only in a completely reversible process. When a system changes from a well-defined initial state to a well-defined final state, the Gibbs free energy, $\Delta G^{\ddagger}$, equals the work exchanged by the system with its surroundings, less the work of the pressure forces, during a reversible transformation of the system from the same initial state to the same final state [431]. The term *free* was attached to mean *available in the form of useful work* for systems at constant pressure and temperature. The Gibbs free energy is defined as

$$G = U + pV - TS$$

which is the same as

$$G = H - TS \tag{A.4}$$

where U, p, V, T, S, and H denote internal energy (in joule), pressure (in pascal), volume (in m^3), temperature (in $°$K), entropy (in joule per $°$K), and enthalpy (in joule), respectively.

Entropy is the quantitative measure of disorder in a system. It measures how much of the energy of a system is potentially available to do work and how much of it is potentially manifest as heat. The concept comes from thermodynamics and *the second law of thermodynamics* can be stated as follows: *In any closed system, the entropy of the system will either remain constant or increase.* It is also (imprecisely) known as *disorder, chaos, randomness*, and so on. In an isothermal process, the change in entropy (ΔS) is the change in heat (δQ) divided by the absolute temperature (T):

$$\Delta S = \frac{\delta Q}{T}$$

The SI unit of entropy is joule per $°$K.

Enthalpy is a thermodynamic property of a thermodynamic system. It can be used to calculate the heat transfer during a process taking place in a closed thermodynamic system under constant pressure (isobaric process). The enthalpy change ΔH is equal to the change in the internal energy of the system and the work that the system has done on its surroundings. The change in enthalpy under such conditions is the heat absorbed by a chemical reaction [571].

A.3.5   Incorporating Entropy and Enthalpy into Eyring Equation

For constant temperature (T), Eq. (A.4) can be written as

$$\Delta G = \Delta H - T\Delta S \tag{A.5}$$

Free energy change is the net driving force of a chemical reaction—it determines whether the reaction will be spontaneous or not. Thus, once ΔG is calculated,

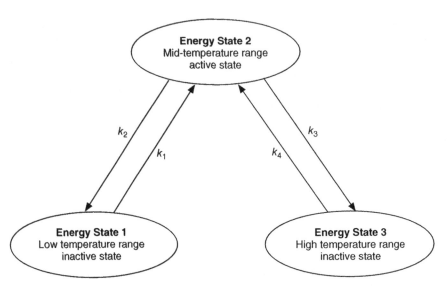

Figure A.1 Energy states of the kinetic model (redrawn from [488]). The directed arrows indicate possible transitions. *Energy State 1* predominates at low temperatures. *Energy State 2* represents the active enzyme configuration and predominates over the mid-temperature range. *Energy State 3* predominates at high temperatures.

spontaneity can be predicted as follows: If $\Delta G < 0$, the reaction is spontaneous. If $\Delta G > 0$, the reaction is nonspontaneous. If $\Delta G = 0$, the reaction is at equilibrium.

Replacing ΔG from Eq. (A.5) into Eq. (A.3) yields

$$
\begin{aligned}
k &= \frac{k_B T}{h} e^{-\frac{\Delta H^{\ddagger} - T \Delta S^{\ddagger}}{RT}} \\
&= \frac{k_B T}{h} e^{\left(\frac{\Delta S^{\ddagger}}{R} - \frac{\Delta H^{\ddagger}}{RT} \right)} \\
&= \frac{k_B T}{h} e^{\frac{\left(\Delta S^{\ddagger} - \frac{\Delta H^{\ddagger}}{T} \right)}{R}}
\end{aligned}
$$

Thus, for each possible transition (see Figure A.1) k_i, for $i = 1, 2, 3, 4$, we get

$$
k_i = \frac{k_B T}{h} e^{\frac{\left(\Delta S^{\ddagger} - \frac{\Delta H^{\ddagger}}{T} \right)}{R}} \tag{A.6}
$$

A.4 THE SHARPE AND DeMICHELE MODEL

From the Eyring–Gibbs equation Eq. (A.6), Sharpe and DeMichele derived a stochastic thermodynamic model of poikilothermic development.

A.4.1   Energy States

To calculate the probability that the control enzyme is in an active state, [488] defined three energy states and possible transitions between them (see Figure A.1):

- *Energy State 1*: Predominates at low temperatures
- *Energy State 2*: Represents the active enzyme configuration; predominates over the mid-temperature range
- *Energy State 3*: Predominates at high temperatures.

Other important assumptions made by the model are as follows:

- At any temperature, the probability of being in any specific form is less than one and the cumulative probability of being in energy State 1, 2, or 3 is equal to one.
- The probability that the enzyme molecule at any given temperature T can move from State 1 directly to State 3 is negligible; therefore, to move from State 1 to State 3 and vice versa, the enzyme must pass through State 2.
- Transitions between states are randomly distributed with a mean transition rate specified by the form of the Eyring-Gibbs equation Eq. (A.6), with transition rate constants k_i.

A.4.2   Exponential Distribution of Transition Times

If no transition between states of the enzyme occurred during time interval Δt, the probability of a transition occurring in the next time interval is not changed. Thus, the time between transitions becomes *exponentially distributed*. This implies that the probability of a transition occurring during a very short time interval Δt is $k_i \Delta t$. As Δt becomes infinitely small ($\Delta t \to 0$), the probability of more than one transition occurring during the time interval becomes infinitely small. Therefore, the probability of no transitions occurring during Δt becomes approximately $\{1 - k_i \Delta t\}$.

A.4.3   Probability Calculations

The probability of the enzyme being in State 1 at time $t + \Delta t$, $P_1(t + \Delta t)$, can be calculated by summing up the probability of being in State 1 at time Δt (i.e., $(1 - k_1 \Delta t)$) and the probability of moving from State 2 to State 1 at time Δt:

$$P_1(t + \Delta t) = P_1(t)(1 - k_1 \Delta t) + P_2(t)k_2 \Delta t$$

Rearranging, we get the rate of change of the probability of being in State 1:

$$\frac{P_1(t + \Delta t) - P_1(t)}{\Delta t} = -k_1 P_1(t) + k_2 P_2(t)$$

Taking the limit as $\Delta t \to 0$,

$$\frac{dP_1(t)}{dt} = -k_1 P_1(t) + k_2 P_2(t)$$

Similarly, the rates of change of the probability of being in States 2 and 3 become

$$\frac{dP_2(t)}{dt} = k_1 P_1(t) - (k_2 + k_3)P_2(t) + k_4 P_3(t)$$

$$\frac{dP_3(t)}{dt} = k_3 P_2(t) - k_4 P_3(t)$$

For steady-state conditions, all rates of change become 0; thus, equating $\frac{dP_i(t)}{dt} = 0$ for $i = 1, 2, 3$, and then solving for P_2, we get

$$P_2 = \frac{1}{1 + \frac{k_2}{k_1} + \frac{k_3}{k_4}}$$

Substituting the Eyring-Gibbs equation Eq. (A.6) for k_1, k_2, k_3, k_4 yields

$$P_2 = \frac{1}{1 + \frac{\frac{k_B T}{h} e^{\frac{(\Delta S_2^\ddagger - \Delta H_2^\ddagger/T)}{R}}}{\frac{k_B T}{h} e^{\frac{(\Delta S_1^\ddagger - \Delta H_1^\ddagger/T)}{R}}} + \frac{\frac{k_B T}{h} e^{\frac{(\Delta S_3^\ddagger - \Delta H_3^\ddagger/T)}{R}}}{\frac{k_B T}{h} e^{\frac{(\Delta S_4^\ddagger - \Delta H_4^\ddagger/T)}{R}}}}$$

$$= \frac{1}{1 + \frac{e^{\frac{(\Delta S_2^\ddagger - \Delta H_2^\ddagger/T)}{R}}}{e^{(\Delta S_1^\ddagger - \Delta H_1^\ddagger/T)/R}} + \frac{e^{\frac{(\Delta S_3^\ddagger - \Delta H_3^\ddagger/T)}{R}}}{e^{\frac{(\Delta S_4^\ddagger - \Delta H_4^\ddagger/T)}{R}}}} \quad (A.7)$$

At equilibrium in a given temperature, only the differences in entropy of activation and enthalpy of activation need be considered. For all the three states, these terms are defined in Table A.1. Using these activation terms, Eq. (A.7) can be further simplified as

$$P_2 = \frac{1}{1 + e^{\frac{(\Delta S_L - \Delta H_L/T)}{R}} + e^{\frac{(\Delta S_H - \Delta H_H/T)}{R}}} \quad (A.8)$$

TABLE A.1   Entropy and Enthalpy of Activation

Parameter	Definition	Applies to
ΔS_L	Difference in entropy of activation	State 1 and State 2
ΔH_L	Difference in enthalpy of activation	State 1 and State 2
ΔS_H	Difference in entropy of activation	State 2 and State 3
ΔH_H	Difference in enthalpy of activation	State 2 and State 3

TABLE A.2 Enzyme, Reaction, and Rate Constant

Parameter	Definition
ϵ_c	Total concentration of the control enzyme
$\Delta S_A^{\neq}$	Entropy of activation of the reaction
$\Delta H_A^{\neq}$	Enthalpy of activation of the reaction
k_2'	Rate constant for development

P_2 represents the probability that the developmental enzyme will be in the active state and thus affect the developmental process.

To calculate the rate of development, Sharpe and DeMichele [488] define four additional terms, which we describe in Table A.2. The last term, k_2', assumes no enzyme inactivation and is described by the Eyring–Gibbs equation Eq. (A.6). Then, the rate of development, R_D, becomes

$$R_D = \epsilon_c k_2' P_2$$

Substituting for k_2' from Eq. (A.6) and P_2 from Eq. (A.8):

$$R_D = \frac{\epsilon_c \dfrac{k_B T}{h} e^{(\Delta S_A^{\neq} - (\Delta H_A^{\neq}/T)/R}}{1 + e^{(\Delta S_L - \Delta H_L/T)/R} + e^{(\Delta S_H - \Delta H_H/T)/R}} \qquad (A.9)$$

The unknown thermodynamic constants ϵ_c and $\Delta S_A^{\neq}$ can be summarized by ϕ, where

$$\phi = \Delta S_A^{\neq} + \ln\left(\frac{k_B \epsilon_c}{h}\right)$$

Taking the exponential,

$$e^{\phi} = \frac{e^{\Delta S_A^{\neq}} k_B \epsilon_c}{h}$$

Replacing e^{ϕ} in Eq. (A.9),

$$R_D = \frac{T * e^{\frac{(\phi - \Delta H_A^{\neq}/T)}{R}}}{1 + e^{\frac{(\Delta S_L - \Delta H_L/T)}{R}} + e^{\frac{(\Delta S_H - \Delta H_H/T)}{R}}} \qquad (A.10)$$

which is the final equation for development.

A.5 THE SCHOOLFIELD *ET AL.* MODEL

The original formulation of Sharpe and DeMichele is not well suited for nonlinear regression, which is needed to fit any kinetic model to observed growth and development rate. The model derived by Schoolfield *et al.* [483] uses nonlinear regression techniques. It also discusses the biological and graphical interpretations of the parameters.

The model starts from Eq. (A.10) by denoting the mean development rate at temperature T as $r(T)$:

$$r(T) = \frac{T * e^{\frac{(\phi - \Delta H_A^{\neq}/T)}{R}}}{1 + e^{\frac{(\Delta S_L - \Delta H_L/T)}{R}} + e^{\frac{(\Delta S_H - \Delta H_H/T)}{R}}} \qquad (A.11)$$

It defines three new thermodynamic parameters to replace three parameters in Eq. (A.11): $\rho_{(25°C)}$, $T_{1/2_L}$, and $T_{1/2_H}$.

$\rho_{(25°C)}$ relates the standard reference temperature (25°C) at which most poikilotherms experience little low or high temperature enzyme inactivation. 25°C is used as a standard reference temperature in many scientific disciplines. $\rho_{(25°C)}$ is defined as

$$\rho_{(25°C)} = 298 * e^{\frac{(\phi - \Delta H_A^{\neq}/298)}{R}}$$

where ϕ, $\Delta H_A^{\neq}$, and R are as defined before. Solving for ϕ, we get

$$\phi = \frac{\Delta H_A^{\neq}}{298} + R * \ln \frac{\rho_{(25°C)}}{298} \qquad (A.12)$$

Substituting ϕ from Eq. (A.12) into the numerator of Eq. (A.11), the new numerator becomes

$$T * e^{\frac{\left(\frac{\Delta H_A^{\neq}}{298} + R*\ln \frac{\rho_{(25°C)}}{298} - \frac{\Delta H_A^{\neq}}{T} \right)}{R}}$$

$$= T * e^{\frac{\Delta H_A^{\neq}}{298R}} * \frac{\rho_{(25°C)}}{298} e^{\frac{R}{R}} * e^{-\frac{\Delta H_A^{\neq}}{TR}}$$

$$= \frac{T * \rho_{(25°C)}}{298} * e^{\frac{\Delta H_A^{\neq}}{R} \left(\frac{1}{298} - \frac{1}{T} \right)} \qquad (A.13)$$

$T_{1/2_L}$ and $T_{1/2_H}$ were defined by Hultin [255] as the ratio of difference in enthalpy to difference in entropy at low- and high-temperature inactivation, respectively:

$$T_{1/2_L} = \frac{\Delta H_L}{\Delta S_L}$$

$$T_{1/2_H} = \frac{\Delta H_H}{\Delta S_H}$$

Solving for ΔS_L and ΔS_H,

$$\Delta S_L = \frac{\Delta H_L}{T_{1/2_L}}$$

$$\Delta S_H = \frac{\Delta H_H}{T_{1/2_H}}$$

Replacing ΔS_L and ΔS_H into the denominator of Eq. (A.11), the new denominator becomes

$$1 + e^{\frac{\Delta H_L}{R}\left(\frac{1}{T_{1/2L}} - \frac{1}{T}\right)} + e^{\frac{\Delta H_H}{R}\left(\frac{1}{T_{1/2H}} - \frac{1}{T}\right)} \tag{A.14}$$

Assembling the new numerator and denominator from Equations (A.13) and (A.14) into Eq. (A.11), we get

$$r(T) = \frac{\rho_{(25°C)}\frac{T}{298}e^{\frac{\Delta H_A^{\ddagger}}{R}\left(\frac{1}{298} - \frac{1}{T}\right)}}{1 + e^{\frac{\Delta H_L}{R}\left(\frac{1}{T_{1/2L}} - \frac{1}{T}\right)} + e^{\frac{\Delta H_H}{R}\left(\frac{1}{T_{1/2H}} - \frac{1}{T}\right)}} \tag{A.15}$$

which is the final form of the modified equation.

A.6   DEPINAY *ET AL.* MODEL

Depinay et al. [148] present a model simulating the *Anopheles* population dynamics by incorporating biological and environmental variables. The model focuses on two abiotic factors (temperature and moisture) and three biotic factors (nutrient competition, predation or death by disease, and dispersal). In this appendix, only the effect of temperature is discussed.

In this model, the mosquito life cycle has four stages: three immature stages (egg, larva, and pupa) occurring in a water body and then the mature stage (flying adult). An adult female disperses from the water body and begins a cycle that is maintained throughout the rest of her life, alternating between obtaining a blood meal and ovipositing in a water body.

Temperature is included as a critical regulator of growth and development within each stage, in determining the end of one stage and the beginning of the next, and in regulating the length of the gonotrophic cycle. The model uses the enzyme kinetics model derived by Schoolfield et al. (see Section A.5) to realize the temperature-dependent developmental rates of eggs, larvae, and pupae, and the duration of the gonotrophic cycle, with the basic assumption that poikilothermic development is regulated by a single *control enzyme*, whose reaction rate determines the development rate of the organism.

A.6.1   Cumulative Development

The model directly uses Eq. (A.15) to define $r(T_{t_k})$, the developmental rate per hour at temperature T (°K), where T_{t_k} is the mean temperature (°K) over the time interval k. All other parameters of Eq. (A.15) are defined as above.

At time step t_n of $t_0, t_1, \cdots, t_n$, the development within each of the four stages, during the time step $\Delta t_k = t_k - t_{k-1}$ is defined by

$$d_k = r(T_{t_k}) * \Delta t_k \tag{A.16}$$

The cumulative development (of each of the three immature stages and the length of the adult gonotrophic cycle) depends only on temperature. For each time step t_n, it is defined as

$$CD(t_n) = \sum_{k=1}^{n} d_k \qquad (A.17)$$

with d_k defined as in Eq. (A.16).

To allow variability (10%) in the cumulative development time, a normal random variable G is defined. A stage is considered completed and the next stage begins when

$$CD(t) > CD_f = 1 + G(0, 0.1) \qquad (A.18)$$

The model uses Eq. (A.15) to produce three curves by varying the equation parameters. They find that all three curves provide similar fits to the *An. gambiae* relevant published data and select the middle one for further analysis.

However, as noted by the authors, these different curves have important implications for vector population dynamics and reinforce the need for more data for these species, particularly at the temperature extremes (low and high). Since any number of curves might fit the data, in order to fit an optimal curve, more data for the extreme temperatures is needed.

The thermal death point for *An. gambiae* is 40°C, which is the reported temperature in most small pools. To model the effect of varying water temperature on mortality, the model considers a daily larval mortality of 10, 50 and 100% for a maximum water temperature rise of 1, 2, and 3 °C, respectively, above the thermal death point.

A.6.2   Results

As an example run, the model simulates over a 20-month period on a small cluster of six houses, each with five residents, and a total of three oviposition sites: a semipermanent pool P_1 and two temporary pools P_2 and P_3. Each female mosquito chooses at random among oviposition sites and among houses and residents at different points in her gonotrophic cycle. Temperature inputs were obtained from data on Kilifi, on the coast of Kenya.

The first set of simulations consist of 300 eggs and 10 adults, with all six houses but only pool P_1 present. It considers the stochastic effect allowed in the cumulative development time, length of the initial gonotrophic cycle, and number of eggs oviposited per female. The resulting *An. gambiae* adult abundance (mean) curve shows similarities to several published trends in the literature, specifically in that there are relatively low levels of mosquitoes throughout the year, with fluctuations due to competition and/or predation and several high peaks in short time intervals.

To analyze the effects of temperature, two additional temperature curves, one with 2°C increase and the other with 2°C decrease in the actual temperatures, are used. It reveals that

- with increasing temperature, the level and number of peaks are increased, and the egg-to-adult development time is shortened, thus producing more mosquitoes
- the 2°C rise increases *An. gambiae* adult abundance by 15% and the 2°C drop decreases it by 17% overall.

At the end, the model admits temperature as an important factor for the adult abundance curve and, particularly, to the occurrence of the initial peak after a drought period (simulated in the 20-month period), which might be critical for control purposes.

A.7   SUMMARY

In this appendix, we described the effect of temperature on the growth and development kinetics of *An. gambiae*. We discussed some recent stochastic thermodynamic models, including the origin of historical models for organism development, the Arrhenius plots, and the Arrhenius equation. We derived the Eyring equation Eq. (A.3) from the Arrhenius equation and incorporated the concepts of Gibbs free energy, entropy, and enthalpy into the Eyring equation.

We then discussed the Sharpe and DeMichele [488] model, and the nonlinear regression model derived by Schoolfield *et al.* [483]. Lastly, we discussed the Depinay *et al.* [148] model, analyzed the effects of temperature, and concluded with the major findings of the model.

APPENDIX B

FLOWCHART FOR THE ABM

B.1 FLOWCHART FOR THE AGENT-BASED MODEL (ABM)

In this appendix, we present the detailed flowchart for a specific version of the ABM implementation, which is developed following the specification of the core model. The core model was presented in Chapter 4. The ABM and its spatial extension were presented in Chapters 5 and 6, respectively.

In the flowchart, the labeled circles (e.g., "A") and pentagons (e.g., "P1") indicate pointers for easy navigation, the rectangles indicate regular instruction(s), and the diamonds indicate decision-making instruction(s). All parameters are defined in Chapter 4 and most of the parameters are initialized as specified in Table 4.2.

The life cycle of mosquito agents in the ABM, which consists of *aquatic* and *adult* phases, is depicted in Fig. 4.1. The *aquatic* phase consists of three aquatic stages: *Egg (E)*, *Larva (L)*, and *Pupa (P)*. The *adult* phase consists of five adult stages: *Immature Adult (IA)*, *Mate Seeking (MS)*, *Blood Meal Seeking (BMS)*, *Blood Meal Digesting (BMD)*, and *Gravid (G)*.

Spatial Agent-Based Simulation Modeling in Public Health:
Design, Implementation, and Applications for Malaria Epidemiology, First Edition.
S. M. Niaz Arifin, Gregory R. Madey and Frank H. Collins.
© 2016 John Wiley & Sons, Inc. Published 2016 by John Wiley & Sons, Inc.

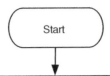

Start

Initialize parameters

- Ambient temperature, $T = 30$
- Probability of a female adult to find a human host, $P_{FindHost} = 25\%$
- Probability of finding a blood meal, $P_{FindBMS} = 100\%$
- Probability of a female adult to find an aquatic habitat, $P_{FindHabitat} = 25\%$
- Fecundity in the first gonotrophic cycle:
  $mean = 170$, $standard\ deviation = 30$
- Habitat sampling weight, $w = 1, 2,$ or 3
- Combined seasonality factor, $r = 1.0$
- Baseline daily mortality rate (DMR), $\alpha = 0.1$
- Exponential mortality increase with age, $\beta = 0.04$
- Degree of mortality deceleration, $S = 0.1$
- Number of initial adults = 1000
- Number of aquatic habitats = 5

Initialize agent lists
- List of all aquatic habitats: aquaticHabitatList
- List of all adult mosquitoes: *adultsList*
- List of all eggs in the system: *eggsList*
- List of all larvae in the system: *larvaeList*
- List of all pupae in the system: *pupaeList*

Initialize system
- Create aquatic habitats with varying habitat capacities
- Create global timer variables for simulation (e.g., tick count)
- Create 1000 initial adult mosquito agents, all female

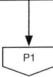

P1

Step 1: Kill existing adults

- Build a hash to construct and save adult age-groups
- Each bucket in the hash represents one age-group
- For each bucket, keys are ages of mosquitoes, values are indices of adultsList
- Iterate *adultsList* and save each mosquito-9index to the correct age-group
- Iterate over each *age-group*, one at a time

Any age-group left?   no → P2

yes

Kill adults from this age-group by Daily mortality rate (DMR)

- For an age-group, DMR_{Adult} depends on population size of the adult age-group
- HMR_{Adult} denotes the corresponding hourly mortality rate
- Calculate number of adults to kill (*toKill*) from this age-group:

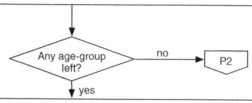

$$DMR_{Adult}(Age) = \frac{\alpha \times e^{Age \times \beta}}{1 + \frac{\alpha \times S}{\beta}(e^{Age \times \beta} - 1)}$$

$$HMR_{Adult}(Age) = 1 - (1 - DMR_{Adult}(Age))^{\frac{1}{24}}$$

- for *toKill* times do:
  – get a random index (of adult mosquito) from this age-group
  – if duplicate (i.e. the adult mosquito already dead), get a random index again, continue until unique
  – mark the adult mosquito as 'dead'

- Now actually kill those adult mosquitoes marked above as 'dead'
- Use an iterator to iterate over *adultsList*, removing the 'dead' ones

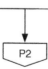

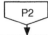

P2

Step 2a: Kill eggs and pupae
- Eggs are kept globally in eggsList; pupae are kept globally in pupaeList
- Calculate number of eggs and pupae to kill:

$$DMR_{Egg|Pupa} = 0.1$$

$$HMR_{Egg|Pupa} = 1 - (1 - 0.1)^{\frac{1}{24}} = 0.00438$$

$$toKill_{Eggs} = HMR_{Egg} \times size(EggList)$$

$$toKill_{Pupae} = HMR_{Pupa} \times size(pupaeList)$$

- for *toKill* times do:
  - get a random index (of egg) from *eggsList*
  - if duplicate (i.e., the egg already dead), get a random index again, continue until unique
  - mark the egg as 'dead'
- Now actually kill those eggs marked above as 'dead'
- Use an iterator to iterate over *eggsList*, removing the 'dead' ones
- Adjust global *eggsCount* by decrementing *tokill*
- Repeat the above for pupae

Step 2b: Kill larvae from all aquatic habitats

A → Any aquatic habitat left? — no → P4

yes

Kill larvae from this aquatic habitat aH
- Build a hash to construct and save larvae age-cohorts
- Each bucket in the hash represents one age-cohort of larvae
- For each bucket, keys are ages of larvae, values are indices of aHLarvaeList
- Iterate aHLarvaeList and save each larva-index to the correct age-cohort
- Calculate biomass and one-day equivalent larval population N_e:

$$Biomass = N_{Egg} + N_e + N_{Pupa}$$

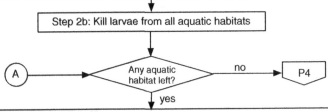

$$N_e = \sum_{Age_{Cohort} = 0}^{max} Age_{Cohort} \times N_{Larvae\,PerCohort}$$

- Iterate over each age-cohort, one at a time

Any age-group left? → A

yes

P3

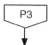

Kill larvae from this age-group
- DMR_{Larva} depends on population size of the larva age-cohort
- Capacity of this aquatic habitat: HC
- Using N_e, calculate number of larvae to kill (*toKill*) from this age-cohort:

$$DMR_{Larva}(AgeCohort) = \alpha \times e^{\frac{N_e}{AgeCohort \times HC}}$$

$$HMR_{Larva}(AgeCohort) = 1 - (1 - DMR_{Larva}(AgeCohort))^{\frac{1}{24}}$$

$$toKill = HMR_{Larva}(Age_{Cohort}) \times size(aHLarvaeList\ (AgeCohort))$$

- for *toKill* times do:
  - get a random index (of larva) from this age-cohort
  - if duplicate (i.e. the larva already dead), get a random index again, continue until unique
  - mark the larva as 'dead'

- Now actually kill those larvae marked above as 'dead'
- Use an iterator to iterate over a*HLarvaeList*, removing the 'dead' ones
- Also remove those larvae from the global larvae list, *larvaeList*

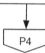

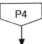

P4

Step 3a: Process existing eggs

for each *egg* in *eggsList* do:
    if egg.wait == 0:
- get the aquatic habitat a*H* the *egg* is in
- increment *larvaeCount* of aH by 1
- decrement *eggCount of* aH by 1
- add (this new larva) to global list larvaList & also to *aHLarvaeList*
- remove *egg* from the list *eggsList*
- change stage to L, set *wait* to 0
- set *cumulativeLarvalstageDelay* to 0

Step 3b: Process existing larvae

for each *larvae* in *larvaeList* do:
    if larvae.*wait* == 0:
- use mean larval development rate $r(T)$8to update cumulative larval delay CD_{larva}:

$$r(T) = T \times 0.000305 - 0.003285$$

$$CD_{larva} = \sum_{i=0}^{n} r(T)_i \times 24$$

- if $CD_{larva} >=$ larvalstageDelay:
    change stage to P,
    set CD_{larvae} to 0

- get the aquatic habitat a*H* the larva is in
- increment *pupaeCount* of aH by 1
- decrement *larvaeCount of* aH by 1
- add this new pupa to global list *pupaeList*
- remove from the list *larvaeList* & also from aHLarvaeList
- Change stage to L
- Set wait to 1

P5

Step 3c: Process existing pupae

for each *pupa* in *pupaeList* do:
  if pupa.*wait* == 0:
    • get the aquatic habitat *aH* the pupa is in
    • decrement *pupaeCount* of aH by 1
    • add (this new adult) to global list *adultsList*
    • remove pupa from the list *pupaeList*
    • Change stage to IA
    • Set pupa *wait* to $Incubation_{Egg}(T)$:

$$Incubation_{Egg}(T) = -0.9 \times T + 61$$

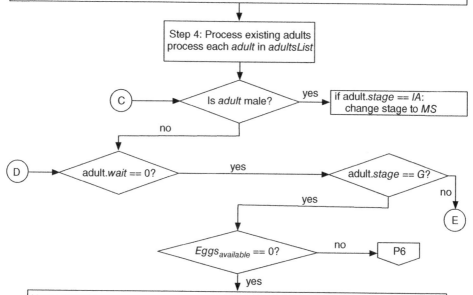

Step 4: Process existing adults
process each *adult* in *adultsList*

Is *adult* male? — yes → if adult.*stage* == *IA*: change stage to *MS*

C

no

D → adult.*wait* == 0? — yes → adult.*stage* == G?

no → E

yes

$Eggs_{available}$ == 0? — no → P6

yes

New oviposition:
  • For successive gonotrophic cycles, generate $Eggs_{max}$ with mean 170 and standard deviation 30:

$$Eggs_{Max}(gcn) = \begin{cases} N(170,30) & : gcn = 1 \\ 0.8 \times Eggs_{Max}(gcn - 1) & : gcn > 1 \end{cases}$$

  • Set $Eggs_{avilable} = Eggs_{max}$
  • Try to lay $Eggs_{avilable} = eggs$

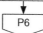

P6

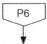

Lay eggs

set $Eggs_{laid} = 0$

for i = 1 to w times do:
($Eggs_{available} = Eggs_{available} - Eggs_{laid}$

if ($Eggs_{available}$ == 0: goto P7

- select an aquatic habitat aH at random
- use one-day equivalent larval population N_e and habitat sampling weight w to calculate biomass and $Eggs_{Potential}(gcn, w)$:

$$Biomass = N_{Eggs} + N_e + N_{Pupae}$$

$$Eggs_{Potential}(gcn,w) = Eggs_{Max}(gcn) \times \left(1 - \frac{Biomass}{w * HC}\right)$$

if ($Eggs_{available}$ >= $Eggs_{Potential}$) $Eggs_{laid} = Eggs_{Potential}$
else $Egg_{laid} = Eggs_{available}$

- lay $Eggs_{laid}$ number of eggs in this aquatic habitat:
  for (j = 0; j < $Eggs_{laid}$; j++):
  - create the egg, attach to this aquatic habitat
  - calculate $Incubation_{Egg}(T)$:

  $$Incubation_{Egg}(T) = -0.9 \times T + 61$$

  - set egg $wait = Incubation_{Egg}(T) + Hatch_{Egg}(T)$
  - add the egg to $eggList$
- increment aH.eggsCount by $Eggs_{laid}$

Update egg-count of the female:
  if $Eggs_{available}$> 0:
    $Eggs_{available} = Eggs_{available} - Eggs_{laid}$
    – force the female to stay in G stage for another day: set wait = 1

  else:
    set $Eggs_{available}$ to 0

P7

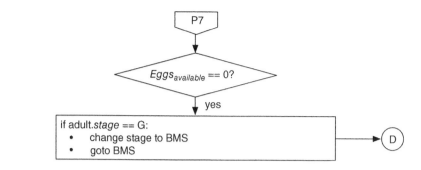

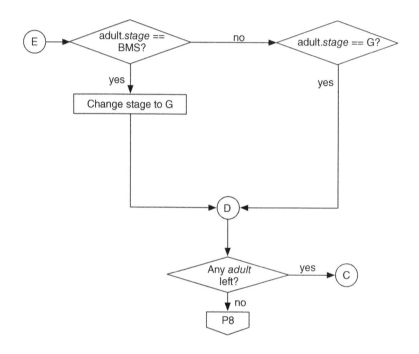

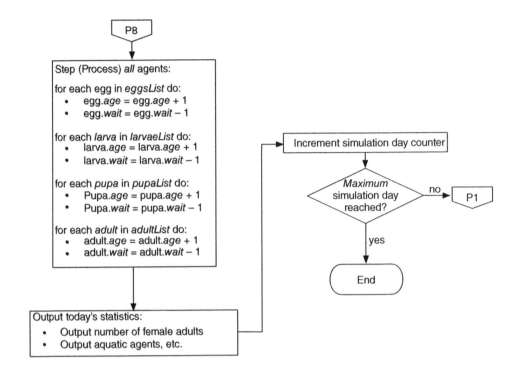

APPENDIX C

ADDITIONAL FILES FOR CHAPTER 10

In this appendix, we present some additional figures for Chapter 10, which describe the landscape epidemiology modeling framework. These figures were created while processing the geographic information system (GIS) data layers and extracting the study area (see Fig. 10.1). The GIS data layers were eventually converted into XML format and then fed as inputs to the spatial ABM for the landscape epidemiology modeling framework simulations (for other details, see Chapter 10). These figures are presented to help the reader/modeler in grasping a deeper understanding of the GIS processing steps (Figs. C.1–C.6).

Spatial Agent-Based Simulation Modeling in Public Health:
Design, Implementation, and Applications for Malaria Epidemiology, First Edition.
S. M. Niaz Arifin, Gregory R. Madey and Frank H. Collins.
© 2016 John Wiley & Sons, Inc. Published 2016 by John Wiley & Sons, Inc.

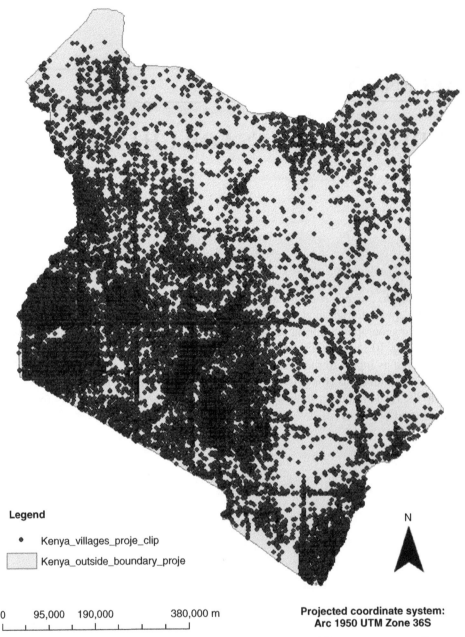

Legend

• Kenya_villages_proje_clip

Kenya_outside_boundary_proje

0   95,000   190,000   380,000 m

Projected coordinate system:
Arc 1950 UTM Zone 36S

N

Figure C.1 Clipped eater sources for Kenya. The figure shows different water source features, including rivers, wetlands, and other types of water points, clipped within Kenya.

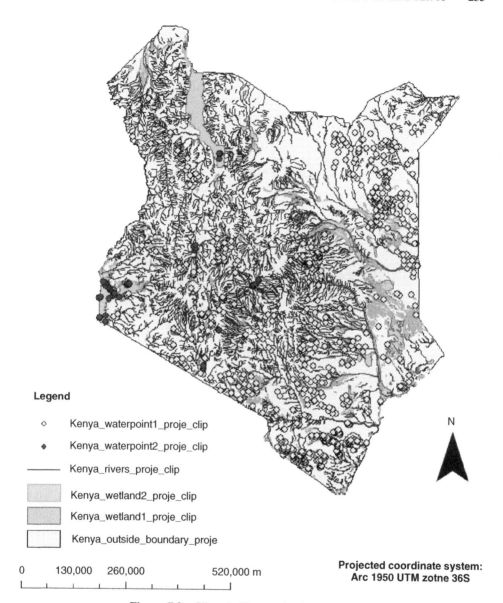

Legend

○   Kenya_waterpoint1_proje_clip

◆   Kenya_waterpoint2_proje_clip

———   Kenya_rivers_proje_clip

Kenya_wetland2_proje_clip

Kenya_wetland1_proje_clip

Kenya_outside_boundary_proje

0   130,000   260,000   520,000 m

**Projected coordinate system:
Arc 1950 UTM zotne 36S**

Figure C.2   Clipped village projections for Kenya.

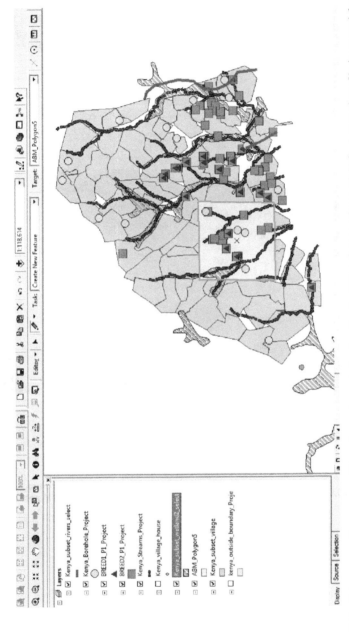

Figure C.3 Polygon creation process. The polygon is created using the ArcGIS software release 10 [16]. A new shapefile is created for the desired polygon. The boundary for the polygon is created in the editing mode and the area of the polygon is calculated using the *Calculate Areas* tool. Finally, the polygon area is highlighted in the editing mode.

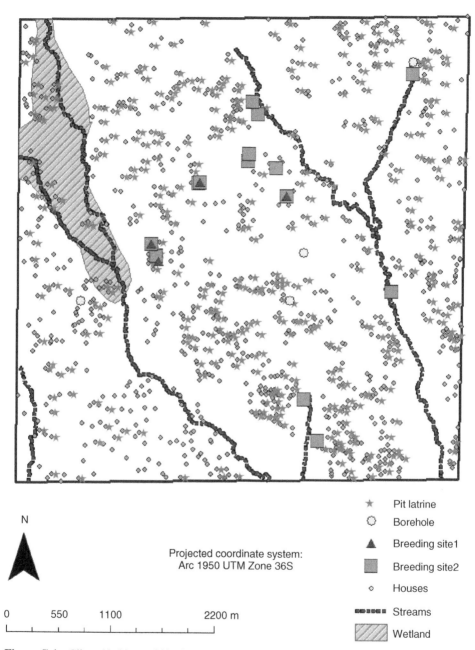

N

Projected coordinate system:
Arc 1950 UTM Zone 36S

0   550   1100   2200 m

★ Pit latrine

○ Borehole

▲ Breeding site1

■ Breeding site2

◇ Houses

Streams

Wetland

Figure C.4 Clipped habitats within the selected polygon. A new shapefile is created for the desired polygon. The boundary for the polygon is created in the editing mode and the area of the polygon is calculated using the *Calculate Areas* tool using the ArcGIS software release 10 [16]. Finally, the polygon area is highlighted in the editing mode.

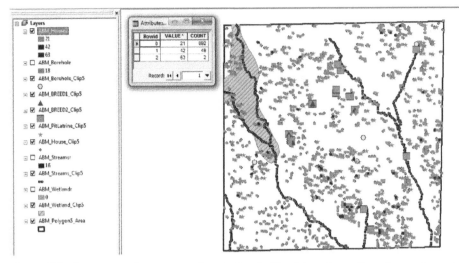

Figure C.5 Data conversion to raster format, Part 1. The figure shows the values and counts of house features in the attribute table after the raster conversion. From these attributes, the counts of features per grid cell are generated.

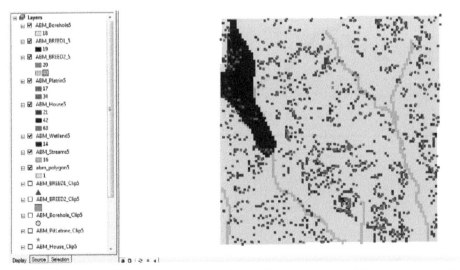

Figure C.6 Data conversion to raster format, Part 2. The figure shows all features converted into the raster format within the polygon area for the ABM. The interpretation of each *ID* (as supplied by the ABM) for each feature and count of features per grid cell are also linked.

APPENDIX D

A POSTSIMULATION ANALYSIS MODULE FOR AGENT-BASED MODELS

D.1 OVERVIEW

Agent-based models (ABMs) can produce large volumes of textual output, potentially in the range of hundreds of gigabytes. In most cases, these outputs contain inherent logical structures that can be naturally expressed in terms of abstract mathematical notions such as graphs and relations. Moreover, the simulation user is often interested in visualizing these structures in the forms of data plots, time-series analysis, visual graphs, and the like. To understand the simulation results and patterns exhibited by the agents, it is crucial to be able to effectively analyze this voluminous textual output, and to produce the desired visualization with ease. Appropriate analysis and visualization also play important roles in verification and validation (V&V) of ABMs. However, simulation modelers often invest the majority of their resources (time and money) on model development and programming, with little attention paid to analysis of simulation output data [309].

In this appendix, we present the design and implementation of a software module called *P-SAM* (which stands for *Postsimulation Analysis Module*). It was created to analyze and visualize postsimulation outputs generated by ABMs, with special emphasis on biological simulation models.[1] P-SAM is written in the Perl programming language

[1]Portions of this appendix appeared in Arifin *et al.* [24]; results have been reported in Kennedy *et al.* [276] and Lane-deGraaf *et al.* [306]. We would like to thank our colleagues Drs. Ryan C. Kennedy, Kelly E. Lane-deGraaf, Agustin Fuentes, Hope Hollocher, and Paul Brenner for their collaboration and support.

Spatial Agent-Based Simulation Modeling in Public Health:
Design, Implementation, and Applications for Malaria Epidemiology, First Edition.
S. M. Niaz Arifin, Gregory R. Madey and Frank H. Collins.
© 2016 John Wiley & Sons, Inc. Published 2016 by John Wiley & Sons, Inc.

[539] and differs from conventional statistical computation software by emphasizing the visualization part that arises from the interaction between abstract entities present in the textual output, with the goal to automate postsimulation analysis tasks for ABMs.

Analyzing large volumes of textual output poses the challenges of huge memory and runtime requirements. To alleviate these, P-SAM uses the technique of serialization (see Section D.4). It builds the visualization structures as soon as the output data is available and then writes them to files in specific formats (e.g., the dot format for visual graphs). This allows the user to load the structures from files in minimal amount of time and thereby increases the response time. The major strengths of P-SAM lie in allowing visualization of certain network structures and saving those structures for further analysis. For example, a *pathogen transmission graph* (see Section D.5.4) allows the user to visually track the transmission record of a pathogen. This is particularly helpful with respect to the validation and interpretation of simulation output.

As a case study, we also describe the application of P-SAM to a biological simulation model named *LiNK* that analyzes the spread of disease among macaque monkeys in the Indonesian island of Bali. Reported results [276, 306] indicate the importance of using P-SAM to perform V&V of the LiNK model by allowing internal validity checking and tracing the model entities.

We envision P-SAM to be useful to other types of ABMs that produce large volumes of textual output. These may include different types of agents (e.g., humans, mosquitoes, monkeys) present in biological models that simulate, for example, the spread of diseases. P-SAM is specially suited for these types of simulations since it can be used to identify the exact chains of transmission, to check whether any transmission link exists between multiple agents, and so on.

The organization of this appendix is as follows: Section D.2 presents a brief review on simulation output analysis, describing statistical analysis and other visualization and analysis tools in general. Section D.4 briefly discusses the LiNK Model and the P-SAM architecture. Section D.5 describes some of the analysis and visualization results performed by P-SAM on LiNK, Section D.6 briefly analyzes P-SAM performance with respect to LiNK, and Section D.7 concludes.

D.2 SIMULATION OUTPUT ANALYSIS: A REVIEW

In this section, we discuss some of the previous works involving simulation output analysis. We begin with statistical analysis and describe its limitations when used as the single tool of analysis. We then point to relevant literature that describes historical reasons for inadequate and inappropriate cases of output data analyses. Some recent works on visualization and analysis tools are also discussed.

D.2.1 Statistical Analysis

There are well-known statistical software tools that focus on conventional statistical analysis. These can be used to analyze and visualize (to some extent) the simulation output. For example, Simulink [496] is an environment for multidomain simulation and model-based design for dynamic and embedded systems. It provides an interactive graphical environment and a customizable set of block libraries to design, simulate, implement, and test a variety of time-varying systems, including communications, controls, signal processing, video processing, and image processing. R [445] is a popular language and environment for statistical computing and graphics. It provides a wide variety of statistical and graphical techniques that include linear and nonlinear modeling, classical statistical tests, time-series analysis, classification, clustering, and so on. SPSS (Statistical Package for the Social Sciences) [512] is another widely used package for statistical analysis in social science. It is used by market researchers, health researchers, survey companies, government, education researchers, marketing organizations, and others. The base software includes descriptive statistics (cross tabulation, frequencies, ratio statistics, etc.), bivariate statistics (means, t-test, ANOVA, correlation), nonparametric tests, prediction for numerical outcomes (linear regression), prediction for identifying groups (factor analysis, cluster analysis), and so on. STATPerl [513] is a free statistical software based on Perl, packaged with source codes for various statistical analysis and an inbuilt Perl interface. Users can add new analysis and edit existing ones.

However, as noted in [309], simulation studies that rely solely on a few statistical estimates for output analysis run the risk of making erroneous inferences about the system, because the statistical estimates, based on random variables, may have large variances. Law [307] described several historical reasons of why output data analyses have not been conducted in an appropriate manner and presented a survey of statistical analyses for simulation output data of a single simulated system, concluding with a discussion of how developments in simulation languages, computer graphics, and computer execution speed may affect the future of output analyses.

With regard to output analysis, Law [309] categorized simulations as *terminating* (a simulation for which there is a natural event that specifies the length of each run) and *nonterminating* (a simulation with no such natural event; also called *steady-state* simulation), and discussed statistical analysis methods for both categories. He concluded by listing three pitfalls in output analysis: analysis involving formulae-based runs that assume independence and hence might result in gross underestimation of variances and standard deviations, failure to have a warm-up period for nonterminating simulation analysis, and failure to determine the statistical precision of output statistics by the use of a confidence interval.

Law [310] presented techniques for building valid and credible simulation models and discussed the difficulty in using formal statistical techniques to validate simulation models. In particular, he described the limitation of classical statistical tests to conduct a specific form of validation, known as *results validation*, which compares the model and system output data with those from the corresponding real-world system. Since the output processes of real-world systems and simulations are nonstationary (the distributions of the successive observations change over time) and autocorrelated (the observations in the process are correlated with each other), classical statistical tests based on independent, identically distributed (IID) observations are not directly applicable [307, 310].

Goldsman [208] emphasized simulation output analysis to be one of the most important aspects of any simulation study, pointing out to some of the issues and techniques relevant to conducting valid analysis. Seila [487] reviewed some methods for analyzing data produced by simulations for estimating parameters of stationary output processes. The techniques include some variations of the batch means method, sequential methods, standardized time-series estimators, methods based upon Hoeffding's inequality, quantile estimation, and multivariate estimation methods.

D.2.2   Visualization and Analysis Tools

Bell and O'Keefe [58] showed the usefulness of VIS (Visual Interactive Simulation), which is a simulation methodology for experimental analysis that allows users to suspend the execution of the simulation model, change one or more parameters and resume model execution with the help of a graphic display. To examine the effectiveness of VIS to model experimentation, they performed a task-based behavioral experiment with 51 subjects, provided with VIS, to solve a case study based around the allocation of trucks in a mining operation. Results showed that the subjects performed worse relative to a known solution obtained through detailed formal experimentation but performed well compared to solutions they provided prior to use of the model, and the use of animated display was not associated with correct solutions but was associated with more efficient use of the VIS. They suggested the need for improvement in the design of interaction within the VIS software.

Kurkowski *et al.* [304] discussed an open-source (C++ and OpenGL-based) visualization and analysis tool, named iNSpect (interactive NS-2 protocol and environment confirmation tool), for use with NS-2 (the Network Simulator 2) wireless simulations. They emphasized the need of a visualization tool to understand the large amount of data produced during network simulations. Describing the default (existing) tool called NAM (Network Animator), they showed how its limitations necessitated iNSpect for wireless simulations and how iNSpect handled three areas of NS-2 based simulation research: (1) validation of the mobility model's output and the node topology, (2) validation of new versions of the NS-2 simulator itself, and (3) statistical and visual analysis of the results of NS-2 simulations.

The Stanford Microarray Database (SMD) [147] provides a wide array of web-accessible tools for processing, analyzing, visualizing, and sharing microarray data in a research environment. The users, having access to data from thousands of microarrays, need effective tools to locate microarrays of interest. To accomplish this, SMD provides two different search forms (*basic* and *advanced*) to find relevant data. The users are presented with a variety of flexible options that allow them to find data based on specific researcher who entered the microarray data, keywords, text searches of experiment descriptions or pregrouped selections of microarrays.

Gollub *et al.* [209] described how SMD serves as a resource for the entire scientific community, by making its source code open and providing full public access to data published by SMD users, along with many tools to explore and analyze those data. They discussed, for example, a data visualization tool, named *Array Color*, that provides a simplified view of the ratio data for a given microarray, allowing the user to quickly examine the microarray. In addition to the graphical display, the Array Color tool provides simple analysis of variance (ANOVA) calculations. Hubble *et al.* [253] described their implementation of the GenePattern microarray analysis software package into the SMD code base that provides access to many new analysis tools and allows users to directly integrate and share additional tools through SMD.

The OpenScience project [538] hosts numerous open-source software packages with simulation analysis and visualization tools to be used in versatile scientific domains. These include Packmol for molecular dynamics (MD) simulations, AGM Build for interactive model preparation for MD simulations, Scilab for numerical computations and relevant simulation, OpenFOAM (Field Operation and Manipulation), and so on. A list of the popular projects can be found at [538].

Simbios, the NIH Center for physics-based simulation of biological structures [494], provides infrastructure and software to help biomedical researchers. SimTK, the Simbios biosimulation toolkit [495], provides a collection of technologies to build Simbios applications for a wide variety of domains, ranging from molecules to whole organisms. The major biological projects include RNA folding, protein folding, myosin dynamics, neuromuscular dynamics, and cardiovascular dynamics.

D.3 THE LINK MODEL

P-SAM was initially developed for a GIS-aware ABM named LiNK (initially named *LiNKStat* that stands for *Statistics builder for LiNK*). In this section, we briefly discuss LiNK.[2]

LiNK is an interdisciplinary project between the Departments of Computer Science, Biological Sciences, and Anthropology at Notre Dame. It models pathogen transmission among long-tailed macaque monkeys on Bali, Indonesia. Macaques on Bali exist in distinct populations: within temple sites and dispersing (roaming). LiNK models each population separately while offering the capability for appropriate macaques to move between populations. It aims to address specific research questions such as the potential rates and routes of pathogen transmission in macaques across the island and the impact of the pathogen life history parameters on this transmission, paying careful attention to the role of landscape on pathogen transmission. Further information is available in the literature [276] and online [318].

The model consists of a display of Bali with temple sites and macaques, along with a display of the contents of the temples. LiNK can simulate a wide array of pathogens through various pathogen parameters, such as infectivity, virulence, and latency. Macaques are simulated as agents, with each macaque having its own properties (e.g., location, sex, age). They can also move through their environment, interact with other macaques, transmit pathogens, reproduce, and die. The LiNK ABM is coded in Java with the Repast simulation toolkit [452], and the visualizer is written

[2]For details on the LiNK model, see, for example, Kennedy *et al.* [276], Lane-deGraaf *et al.* [306], and [318].

in OpenMap [395]. The user is provided with multiple model and pathogen parameter options. The basic components of the model, abridged and rewritten from [276], are described below.

D.3.1   Agents, Interface, and Pathogens

The model includes macaques as agents. Each macaque has its own properties such as location, sex, age, natal temple, and infection status. Macaques move in accordance to their surrounding environment and males have the ability to enter and leave temples. LiNK can support thousands of agents.

Macaques have the ability to move through their environment, interact with other macaques, reproduce, and die. Movement is dictated by their surrounding environment as macaques query their neighborhood and move appropriately. Macaques within a temple move randomly, with no GIS influence. All macaques have the ability to transmit pathogens when within a specified distance of one another. Reproduction is handled by allowing female macaques to produce offspring, with inherited traits, after they reach a specified age. As macaques age, they have a higher probability of dying. Researchers interact with the model through a control panel that allows them to tweak the simulation parameters. Once the parameters are set, the user can begin running the simulation.

LiNK simulates a wide array of pathogens through the incorporation of several pathogen parameters. These include *infectivity* (how infectious the pathogen being modeled is), *virulence* (the proximity a macaque must be to another to have the ability to transmit a pathogen), *latency* (how long a macaque takes to become symptomatic after becoming infected), *acquired immunity* (the amount of time a macaque is immune to contracting a pathogen after having been previously infected), *clearance time* (the amount of time a macaque takes to be cleared of a pathogen), and *natural resistance* (the proportion of macaques that are immune to a given pathogen).

D.3.2   Space and Time

The macaques move about on 2-*D* grids that represent temple sites and the island. The island grids are extrapolated from GIS data, at a customized granularity. A grid cell has sides of roughly 100 m, leading to over 1 million possible locations. Each grid is called a layer. LiNK simulates a total of eight layers: cities, forests, lakes, rice fields, rivers, roads, temples, and the actual island (called coast). These eight layers are melded together and use the same coordinate system. The coast and temple layers are mandatory, while the rest can be turned on or off. One time step in the simulation correlates to 12 real-world hours. The desired accuracy is obtained by coupling this with the grid cells.

D.3.3   Verification and Validation

As described in Chapter 7, V&V refers to a collection of techniques to determine whether an ABM is an accurate representation of the real system. The LiNK model was developed in conjunction with domain experts from multiple fields and has undergone extensive face validation, both through its display and evaluation of its output. The use of P-SAM enabled checking for its internal validity and to trace its entities. More real-world data are currently being collected to perform additional V&V of LiNK.

D.4   P-SAM ARCHITECTURE

The core P-SAM architecture (see Fig. D.1) consists of two programs called the *writer* and the *reader*. The *writer* first serializes the simulation output; then, the *reader* builds the interactive visualization structures. Both of them are described below.

D.4.1   The Writer

The *writer* analyzes and serializes the simulation output. *Serialization*, also known as *deflating* or *marshalling* an object, is the process of converting a data structure or object into a sequence of bits so that it can be stored in a file, a memory buffer, or transmitted across a network connection link to be rebuilt later in the same or another environment. When the resulting series of bits is reread according to the serialization format, it can be used to create a semantically identical clone of the original object. The opposite operation, i.e., extracting a data structure from a series of bytes, is called *deserialization*.

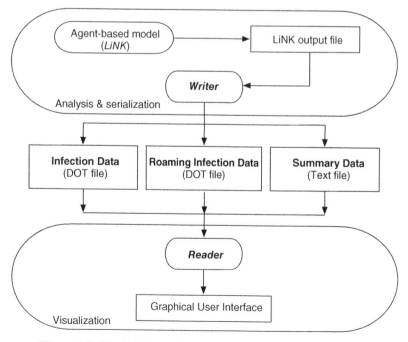

Figure D.1   The P-SAM architecture. Updated from Arifin *et al.* [24].

Several available Perl modules provide serialization mechanisms (e.g., *FreezeThaw*, *Data::Dumper*, *Storable*). However, for LiNK, we chose to use the *Graph* module due to the following reasons:

- The pathogen transmission pattern of LiNK can be most naturally expressed with the notion of a (mathematical) graph structure.
- *Graph* allows the recorded information to be easily saved and later retrieved for visualization.

The *writer* takes the LiNK file as its input (produced as output from the LiNK simulation) and serializes it (after analysis) into three separate files: *Infection Data*, *Roaming Infection Data*, and *Summary Data*. The first two are written in the DOT format, which is a plain-text graph-description language to describe graphs usable by both humans and computer programs. DOT allows hierarchical or layered drawings of directed graphs. The last one records the summary information about the LiNK file and the P-SAM processing.

D.4.2 The Reader

Once analysis and serialization are complete, the *reader* allows visualization by building the Graphical User Interface (GUI). It *reads* in the aforementioned serialized DOT files and projects the information into the *Infection Statistics* and *Roaming Infection Statistics* tabs for *Infection Data* and *Roaming Infection Data*, respectively (see Section D.5).

D.4.3 Advantages of Using Perl

Both the *writer* and the *reader* are written in Perl [539] and hence offer the following advantages:

Portability: Perl does not use system-specific features and maintains the portability of an interpreted language while achieving nearly the speed of a compiled language. Thus, P-SAM can be run on any platform.

String Processing and Regular Expression Support: The major processing task of P-SAM is to handle large volumes of textual output from the LiNK simulation. This is the most compelling reason of choosing Perl, which has highly versatile regular expression support, seamlessly integrated into the language.

Reusable Code Repository: P-SAM uses several Perl extension modules (see Table D.1) from CPAN [125], which has a huge collection of free and reusable Perl code. Use of these modules ensures tested error-free code, avoiding the need to reinvent the wheel.

TABLE D.1 Perl Extension Modules Used

Module	Purpose
Tk/Tcl	To provide access to the Tk library and build the Graphical User Interface
Graph	To create abstract graph data structures and use the corresponding graph algorithms
GraphViz	To visualize the graphs generated by Graph
Devel::Size	To report the memory usage of the graphs and the GUI
Devel::NYTProf	To profile the source code (both statement profiling and subroutine profiling)
Devel::Profile	To profile the source code (basic profiling)

D.5 POSTSIMULATION ANALYSIS AND VISUALIZATION

P-SAM works on relations defined by the user. The user identifies different relations involving relevant entities (e.g., agents) in the simulation output file and specifies how much satellite data should accompany each relation. P-SAM then builds the visualization structures separately for each type of relations and outputs those in the form of visual graphs, data plots, and so on. Also, structures that require more time and memory to be built can be saved in different formats (e.g., image files, relational database records). The visualization process enables the user to visually analyze the following features built from the simulation output. LiNK uses a unique naming convention for each macaque with natal temple number concatenated with an id concatenated with a gender identifier.

D.5.1 Infection Statistics

An infection event occurs when a macaque transmits the pathogen to another macaque *inside* a temple, allowing self-transmission. The *Infection Statistics* tab, shown in Fig. D.2, depicts all the initially infected macaques (top left) and the macaques that did not infect any other macaque (top right) in the course of the whole simulation. It lists all macaques that took part in infection events (the leftmost vertical list), and populates the bottom-left frame with details of *all* infection events, listing the time step, infected macaque and the temple where each event took place. To allow interactive probing, when the user clicks on an individual macaque on the vertical list, it dynamically populates the bottom-right frame with details of all infection events for the macaque.

D.5.2 Roaming Infection Statistics

A roaming infection event occurs when a macaque transmits the pathogen to another macaque *outside* the temples, allowing self-transmission. Each roaming infection event is accompanied by location information, such as the latitude and longitude, as well as

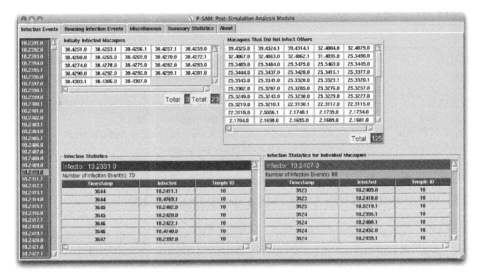

Figure D.2   P-SAM Infection Statistics tab. Used from Arifin *et al.* [24].

the landscape in which the infection took place, such as in *City*, *Forest*, *Rice Field*, *River*, *Road*, and *Coast*.

The *Roaming Infection Statistics* tab, shown in Fig. D.3, is similar to the *Infection Statistics* tab, except it does not contain any initially infected macaques (as roaming). It lists all macaques that took part in roaming infection events (the leftmost vertical list), and populates the top frame with details of *all* roaming infection events, listing the time step, infected macaque, temple, latitude, longitude, and landscape. When the user clicks on an individual macaque on the vertical list, it dynamically populates the bottom frame with details of all roaming infection events for the macaque.

D.5.3   Birth and Death Statistics

In a birth event, a mother macaque gives birth to an infant. A death event records the time, place, and cause of deaths. LiNK simulates three different causes of deaths: aging, dispersal, and pathogen. The birth and death events are listed under the *Miscellaneous* tab, as shown in Fig. D.4. It depicts all birth events with the corresponding time steps (left), and all death events with the corresponding time steps, causes of deaths and the location temple (right).

D.5.4   Pathogen Transmission Graphs

The major strengths of P-SAM lie in allowing visualization of certain network structures and saving those structures for further analysis (e.g., by direct printing). A *pathogen transmission graph* is an example of one such network structure that allows the user to visually track the transmission record of pathogen. This is particularly helpful with respect to the validation and interpretation of simulation output.

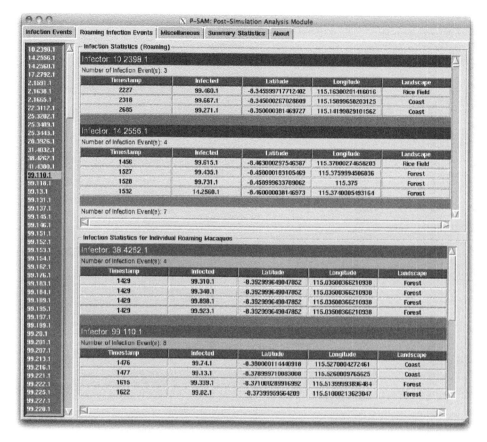

Figure D.3   P-SAM Roaming Infection Statistics tab. Used from Arifin *et al.* [24].

Figure D.5 shows an example of a pathogen transmission graph with nodes representing macaques and edges representing infection events. The topmost node (27.2969.0) is parsed as a female macaque with temple 27 as its natal temple and 2969 as its id. Infection events are listed with the time step and location where the infection occurred. Starting at the top, macaque 27.2969.0 infected macaque 27.2775.0 at time step one, in temple 27. Macaque 27.2775.0 went on to infect three other macaques (infecting macaque 27.2753.0 twice at time steps 11 and 12), and was also reinfected by macaque 27.2870.1. Autoinfection (reinfecting oneself) is possible, as indicated by macaques 27.2863.0 and 27.2805.1.

D.5.5   Summary Statistics

The *Summary Statistics* tab (see Fig. D.6) lists summary information about the input file (from LiNK) and the P-SAM processing events. The *Input/Output Statistics* frame (top left) lists several original parameters from the LiNK file, including acquired immunity, clearance time, virulence, infectivity, random seed, and initially infected temples.

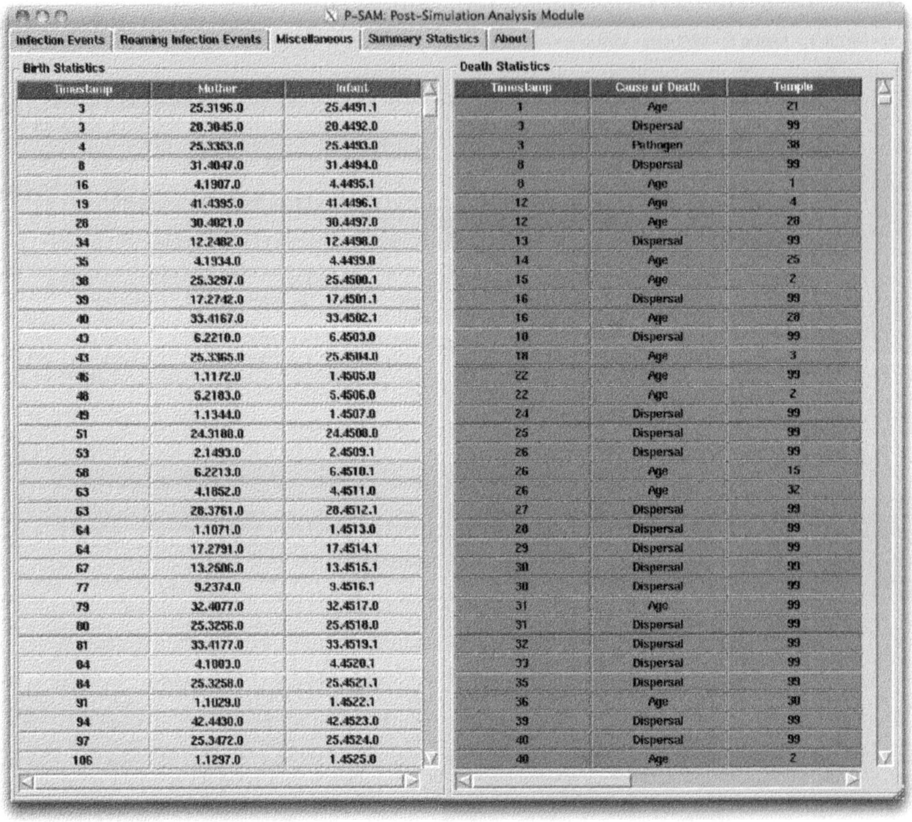

Figure D.4 P-SAM birth and death statistics tab. Used from Arifin *et al.* [24].

The *Line count and Event Statistics* frame (top right) lists various useful information obtained after P-SAM finishes processing the LiNK file. These include the counts for initially infected macaques, infections, roaming infections, the total number of infected macaques (separately at temples and as roaming), and the totl number of infected males and females. It also summarizes the total number of death events, categorized by the cause of death with separate counts. The *Temple Statistics* frame (bottom left) summarizes the number of unique infections occurring at *each* temple. The *Runtime and Memory Statistics* frame (bottom right) reports the memory and runtime consumed by P-SAM.

D.6 P-SAM PERFORMANCE

LiNK output files can reach sizes in the tens or hundreds of gigabytes, with terabytes of uncompressed output data generated so far. This poses P-SAM with challenges of

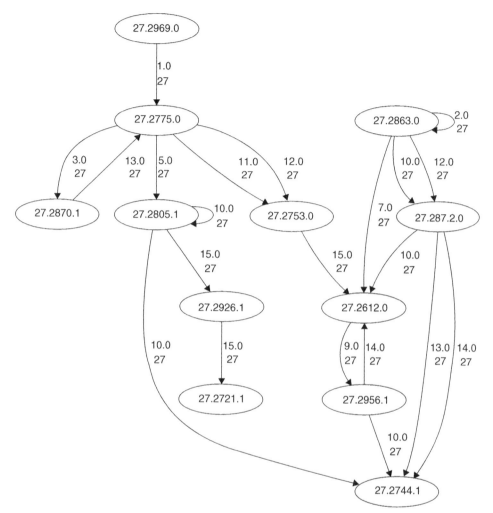

Figure D.5 Example of a *pathogen transmission graph*. Nodes represent macaques and edges represent infection events. Loops represent autoinfection. Used from Arifin *et al.* [24].

large memory and runtime requirements. Using serialization, P-SAM alleviates some of these issues by building the visualization structures as soon as the data is available and then writing them to files for later retrieval. This allows the user to load the structures from files in minimal time and thereby increases the response time.

P-SAM runtime is dominated by the number of infection events and their degree of proliferation in the original LiNK simulation. In collaboration with CRC [104] at the University of Notre Dame, we achieved some performance improvements by working iteratively over *three* major phases. As evident from Fig. D.7, the runtime scales best (with respect to input file sizes) in *Phase 3*. This was done primarily by profiling and code optimization, which are described below.

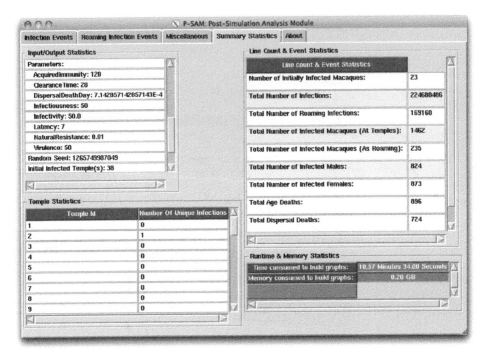

Figure D.6   P-SAM Summary Statistics tab. Used from Arifin *et al.* [24].

D.6.1   Profiling

Software profiling is a form of dynamic program analysis that investigates a program's behavior using information gathered as the program executes with the purpose of determining which sections of a program to optimize (i.e., to increase its overall speed, decrease its memory requirement). A profiler is a performance analysis tool that measures the frequency and duration of function calls and collects extensive performance data.

We use two different profilers, Devel::Profile and Devel::NYTProf, both available at CPAN [125]. The use of two profilers enables us to compare the profiles and identify hotspots with increased confidence. Devel::Profile is a simple profiler that collects information about the execution time and about the subroutines in the code. This information can be used to determine the duration and calling frequency of the subroutines. Devel::NYTProf is a powerful feature-rich profiler and is the fastest reported so far. It offers profiling with finer granularity, that is, per-line statement profiling, per-subroutine statement profiling, per-opcode profiling, and per-block statement profiling. It can perform inclusive and exclusive timing of subroutines with submicrosecond resolution and generate richly annotated, cross-linked html reports.

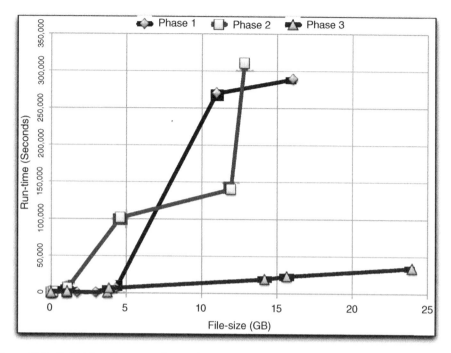

Figure D.7   P-SAM performance. For each phase, the seven data points represent average values of output files, obtained by varying parameter settings of the LiNK model. The same seven sets of parameters are used for all phases. *Phase 1* bypasses the GUI. *Phase 2* eliminates unnecessary existence checks for *infection* hash used in the *Writer*, thus reducing search penalties for *macaque* nodes in the hash. Finally, *Phase 3* optimizes some hash operations using sets. Used from Arifin *et al.* [24].

D.6.2   Code Optimization

Profiling is a useful tool for optimizing code, but it can only point to the potential location of the problem and not actually resolve those. Since most programs spend most of the execution time in a few small hotspots, after the hotspots are identified by profiling, certain optimization techniques can help improve the performance. For Perl, the combination of logic sequence and generated bytecode may have drastic effect on performance. To partially minimize this, several checks and practices may be helpful [80]. These include using references for large arrays and hashes, avoiding excessive function calls in loops, using short circuit logic, and so on.

After analyzing the profiles, we eliminate unnecessary existence checks for *infection* and *roaming infection* hashes used in the *Writer*. This greatly reduces the search penalties for *macaque* nodes in the graphs (which are stored as hashes). We also replace some hash operations using sets, which provide faster subroutines for operations such as *set union* and *set intersection*.

Once P-SAM is fully checked against these, we were able to perform more complex, multirun analysis involving large data sets with improved runtime. This, in turn, allowed the simulation (LiNK) users to further validate and refine their model and to use it to help better predict the real-world behavior being simulated.

D.7 CONCLUSION

In this appendix, we described a software module, called P-SAM, which was developed for simulation output analysis and visualization. We demonstrated its application to a biological simulation model named LiNK [318], which produces voluminous textual outputs (in the range of hundreds of gigabytes). We showed how P-SAM can analyze and visualize logical structures (e.g., pathogen transmission graphs) inherent in LiNK outputs, thus helping V&V of the model by allowing internal validity checking as well as tracing the model entities. We also described the P-SAM architecture, its major strengths, and how it copes with the huge memory and runtime requirements. While P-SAM was used for the LiNK model, the general architecture can be modified and/or extended to suit other ABMs.

REFERENCES

1. L. Aarons, M. O. Karlsson, F. Mentré, F. Rombout, J.-L. Steimer, A. van Peer, et al. *European Journal of Pharmaceutical Sciences*, 13(20):115–122, 2001.

2. N. Achee, M. Bangs, R. Farlow, G. Killeen, S. Lindsay, J. Logan, S. Moore, M. Rowland, K. Sweeney, S. Torr, L. Zwiebel, and J. Grieco. *Malaria Journal*, 11(1):164, 2012.

3. M. S. Alber, M. A. Kiskowski, J. A. Glazier, and Y. Jiang. On cellular automaton approaches to modeling biological cells. In *Mathematical Systems Theory in Biology, Communications, Computation, and Finance*, pages 1–39. Springer, 2003.

4. S. E. Alexeeff, J. Schwartz, I. Kloog, A. Chudnovsky, P. Koutrakis, and B. A. Coull. *Journal of Exposure Science and Environmental Epidemiology*, 2014, doi:10.1038/jes.2014.40:1 - 7.

5. P. L. Alonso, G. Brown, M. Arevalo-Herrera, F. Binka, C. Chitnis, F. Collins, O. K. Doumbo, B. Greenwood, B. F. Hall, M. M. Levine, K. Mendis, R. D. Newman, C. V. Plowe, M. H. Rodróguez, R. Sinden, L. Slutsker, and M. Tanner. *PLoS Med*, 8(1):e1000406, 2011.

6. N. Amek, N. Bayoh, M. Hamel, K. Lindblade, J. Gimnig, F. Odhiambo, K. Laserson, L. Slutsker, T. Smith, and P. Vounatsou. *Parasites & Vectors*, 5(1):86, 2012.

7. E. Amouroux, S. Desvaux, and A. Drogoul. Towards virtual epidemiology: an agent-based approach to the modeling of h5n1 propagation and persistence in north-vietnam. In *Intelligent Agents and Multi-Agent Systems*, pages 26–33. Springer, 2008.

8. L. An. *Ecological Modelling*, 229:25–36, 2012.

9. G. An, Q. Mi, J. Dutta-Moscato, and Y. Vodovotz. *Wiley Interdisciplinary Reviews: Systems Biology and Medicine*, 1(2):159–171, 2009.

10. R. M. Anderson and R. M. May. *Mathematical Medicine and Biology*, 1(3):233–266, 1984.

Spatial Agent-Based Simulation Modeling in Public Health:
Design, Implementation, and Applications for Malaria Epidemiology, First Edition.
S. M. Niaz Arifin, Gregory R. Madey and Frank H. Collins.
© 2016 John Wiley & Sons, Inc. Published 2016 by John Wiley & Sons, Inc.

11. A. A. Angehrn. *Interfaces*, 23(3):3–16, 1993.

12. Anopheles. Wikipedia. Website, 2015. URL http://en.wikipedia.org/wiki/Anopheles. Accessed April, 2015.

13. Anopheles Mosquitoes. Centers for Disease Control and Prevention (CDC). Website, 2015. URL http://www.cdc.gov/malaria/about/biology/mosquitoes/index.html. Accessed April, 2015.

14. K. Antelman. *College & Research Libraries*, 65(5):372–382, 2004.

15. AnyLogic: Multimethod Simulation Software. Website. URL http://www.anylogic.com/. Accessed April, 2015.

16. ArcGIS Desktop. *Release 10*. Environmental Systems Research Institute (ESRI), Redlands, CA, 2011. Accessed April, 2015.

17. ArcGIS Desktop: Release 10. ESRI 2011. Website. http://www.esri.com/. URL http://www.esri.com/. Accessed April, 2015.

18. ArcGIS Desktop: Release 9.3. Website. http://www.esri.com/. URL http://www.esri.com/. Accessed April, 2015.

19. ArcGIS: Hot Spot Analysis (Getis-Ord Gi*) (Spatial Statistics). 2014. URL http://resources.esri.com/. Accessed April, 2015.

20. S. M. N. Arifin, R. R. Arifin, D. de A. Pitts, M. S. Rahman, S. Nowreen, G. R. Madey, and F. H. Collins. *Land*, 4(2):378–412, 2015.

21. S. M. N. Arifin and G. R. Madey. Verification, validation, and replication methods for agent-based modeling and simulation: lessons learned the hard way! In *Concepts and Methodologies for Modeling and Simulation*, Chapter 10, pages 217–242. Springer, 2015.

22. S. M. N. Arifin, G. J. Davis, S. J. Kurtz, J. E. Gentile, and Y. Zhou. Divide and conquer: a four-fold docking experience of agent-based models. In *Winter Simulation Conference (WSC)*, December 2010.

23. S. M. N. Arifin, G. J. Davis, and Y. Zhou. Verification & validation by docking: a case study of agent-based models of *Anopheles gambiae*. In *Summer Computer Simulation Conference (SCSC)*, July 2010.

24. S. M. N. Arifin, R. C. Kennedy, K. E. Lane, A. Fuentes, H. Hollocher, and G. R. Madey. P-SAM: a post-simulation analysis module for agent-based models. In *Summer Computer Simulation Conference (SCSC)*, July 2010.

25. S. M. N. Arifin, G. J. Davis, and Y. Zhou. Modeling space in an agent-based model of malaria: comparison between non-spatial and spatial models. In *Proceedings of the 2011 Workshop on Agent-Directed Simulation*, pages 92–99, 2011.

26. S. M. N. Arifin, G. J. Davis, and Y. Zhou. *International Journal of Agent Technologies and Systems*, 3(3):17–34, 2011.

27. S. M. N. Arifin, R. R. Arifin, D. de Alwis Pitts, and G. R. Madey. Integrating an agent-based model of malaria mosquitoes with a geographic information system. In The 25th *European Modeling and Simulation Symposium (EMSS)*, September 2013.

28. S. M. N. Arifin, G. R. Madey, and F. H. Collins. *Malaria Journal*, 12(1):290, 2013.

29. S. M. N. Arifin, Y. Zhou, G. J. Davis, J. E. Gentile, G. R. Madey, and F. H. Collins. *Malaria Journal*, 13(1):424, 2014.

30. J. L. Aron and R. M. May. The population dynamics of malaria. In *The Population Dynamics of Infectious Diseases: Theory and Applications*, pages 139–179. Springer, 1982.

31. W. B. Arthur, S. N. Durlauf, and D. A. Lane. *The Economy as an Evolving Complex System II*, volume 28. Addison-Wesley Reading, MA, 1997.

32. R. Axelrod. *Journal of Conflict Resolution*, 24(1):3–25, 1980.

33. R. Axelrod. *The Evolution of Cooperation*. Basic Books, 1984.

34. R. Axelrod. Advancing the Art of Simulation in the Social Sciences. Working papers, Santa Fe Institute, 1997.

35. R. Axelrod. Advancing the art of simulation in the social sciences. In *Simulating Social Phenomena*, pages 21–40. Springer, 1997.

36. R. M. Axelrod. *The Complexity of Cooperation: Agent-Based Models of Competition and Collaboration*. Princeton University Press, 1997.

37. R. Axtell, R. Axelrod, J. M. Epstien, and M. D. Cohen. *Computational and Mathematical Organization Theory*, 1:123–141, 1996.

38. R. Bagni, R. Berchi, and P. Cariello. *Journal of Artificial Societies and Social Simulation*, 5(3), 2002.

39. O. Balci. How to assess the acceptability and credibility of simulation results. In *Proceedings of the 21st Conference on Winter Simulation*, pages 62–71. ACM, 1989.

40. O. Balci. *Annals of Operations Research*, 53(1):121–173, 1994.

41. O. Balci. Principles and techniques of simulation validation, verification, and testing. In *Proceedings of the 27th Conference on Winter Simulation*, pages 147–154, Washington, DC, 1995. IEEE Computer Society.

42. O. Balci. Verification, validation and accreditation of simulation models. In *Proceedings of the 29th Conference on Winter Simulation*, pages 135–141, Washington, DC, 1997. IEEE Computer Society.

43. O. Balci. *Winter Simulation Conference*, 1:41–48, 1998a. ISSN: 0743-1902.

44. O. Balci. *Verification, Validation, and Testing*, pages 335–393. Wiley; Co-published by Engineering & Management Press, New York [Norcross, GA], 1998b.

45. O. Balci. Verification, validation, and certification of modeling and simulation applications: verification, validation, and certification of modeling and simulation applications. In *Proceedings of the 35th conference on winter simulation: driving innovation*, pages 150–158. Winter Simulation Conference, 2003.

46. O. Balci. Quality assessment, verification, and validation of modeling and simulation applications. In *Proceedings of the 2004 Winter Simulation Conference*, volume 1. IEEE, 2004.

47. O. Balci, R. E. Nance, J. D. Arthur, and W. F. Ormsby. Improving the model development process: expanding our horizons in verification, validation, and accreditation research and practice. In *Proceedings of the 34th Conference on Winter Simulation: Exploring New Frontiers*, pages 653–663. Winter Simulation Conference, 2002.

48. S. C. Bankes. *Proceedings of the National Academy of Sciences of the United States of America*, 99(Suppl. 3):7199–7200, 2002.

49. J. Banks, J. Carson, and B. Nelson. *Prentice-Hall international series in industrial and systems engineering*, 1996.

50. C. L. Barrett, K. R. Bisset, S. G. Eubank, X. Feng, and M. V. Marathe. EpiSimdemics: an efficient algorithm for simulating the spread of infectious disease over large realistic social networks. In Proceedings of the 2008 ACM/IEEE Conference on Supercomputing, IEEE Press, 2008.

51. M. P. Batistella Pasini, A. Dal'Col Lúcio, and A. Cargnelutti Filho. *Pesquisa Agropecuária Brasileira*, 49(7):493–505, 2014.

52. M. Batty. Agent-based pedestrian modelling. In *Advanced Spatial Analysis: The CASA Book of GIS*, P. A. Longley and M. Batty, editors, pages 81–108. ESRI Press: Redlands, CA, 2003.

53. M. Batty, J. DeSyllas, and E. Duxbury. *International Journal of Geographical Information Science*, 17(7):673–697, 2003.

54. A. L. Bauer, C. A. Beauchemin, and A. S. Perelson. *Information Sciences*, 179(10):1379–1389, 2009.

55. M. N. Bayoh and S. W. Lindsay. *Medical and Veterinary Entomology*, 18(2):174–179, 2004.

56. L. M. Beck-Johnson, W. A. Nelson, K. P. Paaijmans, A. F. Read, M. B. Thomas, and O. N. Bjørnstad. *PLoS ONE*, 8(11), 11 2013.

57. J. C. Beier. *Annual Review of Entomology*, 43(1):519–543, 1998.

58. P. C. Bell and R. M. O'Keefe. *Management Science*, 41(6):1018–1038, 1995.

59. S. E. Bellan. *PLoS ONE*, 5(4):e10165, 2010.

60. J. Benavides, P. D. Walsh, L. A. Meyers, M. Raymond, and D. Caillaud. *PLoS ONE*, 7(2):e31290, 2012.

61. O. Berke. *International Journal of Health Geographics*, 3(1):18, 2004.

62. N. Best, S. Richardson, and A. Thomson. *Stat Methods Med Res*, 14(1):35–59, 2005.

63. K. Beven and A. Binley. *Hydrological Processes*, 6(3):279–298, 1992.

64. L. Bian. *Ecological Modelling*, 159(2–3):279–296, 2003.

65. Bill & Melinda Gates Foundation. Website. URL http://www.gatesfoundation.org/. Accessed April, 2015.

66. Biostatistics. Website, 2015. URL http://biostatistics.oxfordjournals.org/. Accessed April, 2015.

67. L. G. Birta and G. Arbez. *Modelling and Simulation*. Springer, 2007.

68. J. F. Bithell. *Statistics in Medicine*, 19(17–18):2203–2215, 2000.

69. B.-C. Björk, P. Welling, M. Laakso, P. Majlender, T. Hedlund, and G. Guðnason. *PLoS ONE*, 5(6):e11273, 2010.

70. F. Black and M. Scholes. *Journal of Political Economy*, 81:637–659, 1973.

71. N. Bolloju, M. Khalifa, and E. Turban. *Decision Support Systems*, 33(2):163–176, 2002.

72. E. Bonabeau. *Proceedings of the National Academy of Sciences of the United States of America*, 99(Suppl. 3):7280–7287, 2002.

73. M. F. Boni, D. L. Smith, and R. Laxminarayan. *Proceedings of the National Academy of Sciences of the United States of America*, 105(37):14216–14221, 2008.

74. T. R. Bonnell, R. R. Sengupta, C. A. Chapman, and T. L. Goldberg. *Ecological Modelling*, 221(20):2491–2500, 2010.

75. G. Booch. *Object Oriented Analysis & Design with Application*. Pearson Education India, 2006.

76. M. K. Boulos, A. V. Roudsari, and E. R. Carson. *Journal of Biomedical Informatics*, 34(3):195–219, 2001.

77. H. L. Bowen. *Malaria Journal*, 12(1):36, 2013.

78. G. E. Box and N. R. Draper. *Empirical Model-Building and Response Surfaces*. John Wiley & Sons, 1987.

79. W. A. Brock and S. N. Durlauf. *The Review of Economic Studies*, 68(2):235–260, 2001.

80. M. C. Brown. *Perl: The Complete Reference*. Osborne/McGraw-Hill, second edition, 2001.

81. B. N. Brown, I. M. Price, F. R. Toapanta, D. R. DeAlmeida, C. A. Wiley, T. M. Ross, T. D. Oury, and Y. Vodovotz. *Mathematical Biosciences*, 231(2):186–196, 2011.

82. D. G. Brown, R. Riolo, D. T. Robinson, M. North, and W. Rand. *Journal of Geographical Systems*, 7(1):25–47, 2005.

83. J. S. Brownstein, H. Rosen, D. Purdy, J. R. Miller, M. Merlino, F. Mostashari, and D. Fish. *Vector Borne and Zoonotic Diseases*, 2(3):157–164, 2002.

84. L. Bruce-Chwatt. *Bulletin of the World Health Organization*, 32(3):363–387, 1965.

85. L. Bruce-Chwatt and J. de Zulueta. *The Rise and Fall of Malaria in Europe: A Historico-Epidemiological Study*. Oxford University Press, 1980.

86. T. Bui and J. Lee. *Decision Support Systems*, 25(3):225–237, 1999.

87. P. C. Bull, B. S. Lowe, M. Kortok, C. S. Molyneux, C. I. Newbold, and K. Marsh. *Nature Medicine*, 4(3):358–360, 1998.

88. N. Bullen, G. Moon, and K. Jones. *Social Science & Medicine*, 42(6):801–816, 1996.

89. R. M. Burton. *Computational & Mathematical Organization Theory*, 9(2):91–108, 2003.

90. A. Buscarino, L. Fortuna, M. Frasca, and V. Latora. *EPL (Europhysics Letters)*, 82(3):38002, 2008.

91. K. M. Carley. *Simulation Modelling Practice and Theory*, 10(5–7):253–269, 2002.

92. K. M. Carley, D. B. Fridsma, E. Casman, A. Yahja, N. Altman, L.-C. Chen, B. Kaminsky, and D. Nave. *IEEE Transactions on Systems, Man and Cybernetics, Part A: Systems and Humans*, 36(2):252–265, 2006.

93. R. Carmona and N. Touzi. *Mathematical Finance*, 18(2):239–268, 2008.

94. C. Carpenter and L. Sattenspiel. *American Journal of Human Biology*, 21(3):290–300, 2009.

95. F. Carrat and A.-J. Valleron. *American Journal of Epidemiology*, 135(11):1293–1300, 1992.

96. R. Carter. *Vaccine*, 19(17–19):2309–2314, 2001.

97. R. Carter and K. N. Mendis. *Clinical Microbiology Reviews*, 15(4):564–594, 2002.

98. L. Cassettari, R. Mosca, and R. Revetria. *Mathematical Problems in Engineering*, 2012:17, 2012, doi:10.1155/2012/463873.

99. J.-C. Castella, T. N. Trung, and S. Boissau. *Ecology and Society*, 10(1):27, 2005.

100. F. Castiglione, F. Pappalardo, M. Bernaschi, and S. Motta. *Bioinformatics*, 23(24):3350–3355, 2007.

101. C. J. Castle and A. T. Crooks. Principles and concepts of agent-based modelling for developing geospatial simulations. In *CASA Working Paper 110*. UCL Centre for Advanced Spatial Analysis, 2006, http://discovery.ucl.ac.uk/3342/ Accessed November, 2015.

102. C. U. Center for International Earth Science Information Network (CIESIN) and C. I. d. A. T. (CIAT). Gridded population of the world version 3 (gpwv3), 2005. URL http://sedac.ciesin.columbia.edu/gpw.

103. C. U. Center for International Earth Science Information Network (CIESIN), I. F. P. R. I. (IFPRI), T. W. Bank, and C. I. d. A. T. (CIAT). Global rural-urban mapping project (grump), alpha version, 2004. URL http://sedac.ciesin.columbia.edu/gpw.

104. Center for Research Computing (CRC). University of Notre Dame. Website. URL http://researchcomputing.nd.edu/. Accessed April, 2015.

105. Centers for Disease Control and Prevention (CDC). Website, 2015. URL http://www.cdc.gov/malaria/. Accessed April, 2015.

106. G. Chabot-Couture, K. Nigmatulina, and P. Eckhoff. *PLoS ONE*, 9(4):e94741, 2014.

107. H. Chen, U. Fillinger, and G. Yan. *The American Journal of Tropical Medicine and Hygiene*, 75(2):246–250, 2006.

108. X. Chen, J. W. Meaker, and F. B. Zhan. *Natural Hazards*, 38(3):321–338, 2006.

109. X. Chen and F. B. Zhan. *Journal of the Operational Research Society*, 59(1):25–33, 2008.

110. A. Chervenak, R. Schuler, C. Kesselman, and S. Koranda. *International Journal of High Performance Computing and Networking*, 5(3):124–134, 2008.

111. N. Chiabaut and C. Buisson. Replications in stochastic traffic flow models: incremental method to determine sufficient number of runs. In *Traffic and Granular Flow '07*, pages 35–44. Springer, Berlin Heidelberg, 2009.

112. N. Chitnis, J. Hyman, and J. Cushing. *Bulletin of Mathematical Biology*, 70(5):1272–1296, 2008.

113. N. Chitnis, T. Smith, and R. Steketee. *Journal of Biological Dynamics*, 2(3):259–285, 2008.

114. N. Chitnis, D. Hardy, and T. Smith. *Bulletin of Mathematical Biology*, 74:1098–1124, 2012.

115. N. Chitnis, A. Schapira, T. Smith, and R. Steketee. *The American Journal of Tropical Medicine and Hygiene*, 83(2):230–240, 2010.

116. M. Chouaibou, F. Simard, F. Chandre, J. Etang, F. Darriet, and J. Hougard. *Malaria Journal*, 5:77, 2006.

117. K. Christensen and Y. Sasaki. *Journal of Artificial Societies and Social Simulation*, 11(3):9, 2008.

118. T. Churcher, E. Dawes, R. Sinden, G. Christophides, J. Koella, and M.-G. Basanez. *Malaria Journal*, 9(1):311, 2010.

119. K. C. Clarke, S. L. McLafferty, and B. J. Tempalski. *Emerging Infectious Diseases*, 2(2):85, 1996.

120. A. Clements and G. Paterson. *Journal of Applied Ecology*, 18(2):373–399, 1981.

121. R. C. Cockrell, S. Christley, E. Chang, and G. An. *PLoS ONE*, 10(3):e0122192, 2014.

122. J. M. Cohen, D. L. Smith, A. Vallely, G. Taleo, G. Malefoasi, and O. Sabot. Holding the line. In *Shrinking the Malaria Map*, Book Section 3, pages 40–60. The Global Health Group: UCSF Global Health Sciences, San Francisco, CA, 2009.

123. H. Collins. *Changing Order: Replication and Induction in Scientific Practice*. University of Chicago Press, 1992.

124. W. E. Collins and G. M. Jeffery. *The American Journal of Tropical Medicine and Hygiene*, 61(Suppl. 1):4–19, 1999.

125. Comprehensive Perl Archive Network (CPAN). Website. URL http://www.cpan.org/. Accessed April, 2015.

126. Computational Social Science Society of the Americas (CSSSA). 2015. URL https://computationalsocialscience.org/. Accessed May, 2015.

127. T. H. Cormen, C. E. Leiserson, R. L. Rivest, and C. Stein. *Introduction to Algorithms*. McGraw-Hill, second edition, 2001.

128. N. R. Council. Assessing the reliability of complex models: mathematical and statistical foundations of verification, validation, and uncertainty quantification, 2012.

129. F. Cox. *Parasites & Vectors*, 3(1):5, 2010.

130. M. Craig, R. Snow, and D. Le Sueur. *Parasitology Today*, 15(3):105–111, 1999.

131. Creative Commons. 2015. URL https://creativecommons.org/. Accessed May, 2015.

132. C. M. Croner, J. Sperling, and F. R. Broome. *Statistics in Medicine*, 15(18):1961–1977, 1996.

133. M. Cueto. *Journal of Latin American Studies*, 37(03):533–559, 2005.

134. F. Dangendorf, S. Herbst, R. Reintjes, and T. Kistemann. *International Journal of Hygiene and Environmental Health*, 205(3):183–191, 2002.

135. P. Davidsson, L. Henesey, L. Ramstedt, J. Törnquist, and F. Wernstedt. *Transportation Research Part C: Emerging Technologies*, 13(4):255–271, 2005.

136. E. Dawes, T. Churcher, S. Zhuang, R. Sinden, and M.-G. Basanez. *Malaria Journal*, 8(1):228, 2009.

137. R. J. Dawson, R. Peppe, and M. Wang. *Natural Hazards*, 59(1):167–189, 2011.

138. A. de Candolle. *Géographie Botanique Raisonée*, page 606. Masson, Paris, 1885.

139. M. de Carvalho Alves and E. A. Pozza. *Applied Geomatics*, 2(2):65–72, 2010.

140. M. C. de Castro and B. H. Singer. *Journal of Archaeological Science*, 32(3):337–340, 2005.

141. L.-F. B. De Châteauneuf. *Rapport sur la Marche et les Effets du Choléra-Morbus dans Paris et les Communes Rurales du Departement de la Seine, Année 1832*. Impr. Royale, 1834.

142. A. L. de Espíndola, C. T. Bauch, B. C. T. Cabella, and A. S. Martinez. *Journal of Statistical Mechanics: Theory and Experiment*, 2011(05):P05003, 2011.

143. M. J. De Lepper, H. J. Scholten, and R. M. Stern. *The Added Value of Geographical Information Systems in Public and Environmental Health*, volume 24. Kluwer, Springer Science & Business Media, 1995.

144. S. De Marchi and S. E. Page. *Annual Review of Political Science*, 17:1–20, 2014.

145. M. L. C. Degli Atti, S. Merler, C. Rizzo, M. Ajelli, M. Massari, P. Manfredi, C. Furlanello, G. S. Tomba, and M. Iannelli. *PLoS ONE*, 3(3):e1790, 2008.

146. L. Dematté and D. Prandi. *Briefings in Bioinformatics*, 11(3):323–333, 2010.

147. J. Demeter, C. Beauheim, J. Gollub, T. Hernandez-Boussard, H. Jin, D. Maier, J. C. Matese, M. Nitzberg, F. Wymore, Z. K. Zachariah, P. O. Brown, G. Sherlock, and C. A. Ball. *Nucleic Acids Research*, 35(Suppl. 1):D766–D770, 2007.

148. J. Depinay, C. Mbogo, G. Killeen, B. Knols, J. Beier, J. Carlson, J. Dushoff, P. Billingsley, H. Mwambi, J. Githure, A. Toure, and F. E. McKenzie. *Malaria Journal*, 3(1):29, 2004.

149. D. Dery, C. Brown, K. Asante, M. Adams, D. Dosoo, S. Amenga-Etego, M. Wilson, D. Chandramohan, B. Greenwood, and S. Owusu-Agyei. *Malaria Journal*, 9:314, 2010.

150. Development of a European Multimodel Ensemble system for seasonal to inTERannual prediction (DEMETER). Website. URL http://www.ecmwf.int/research/demeter/. Accessed April, 2015.

151. W. G. Dewald, J. G. Thursby, and R. G. Anderson. *The American Economic Review*, 76(4):587–603, 1986.

152. K. Dietz and J. Heesterbeek. *Mathematical Biosciences*, 180(1–2):1–21, 2002.

153. P. Diggle, R. Moyeed, B. Rowlingson, and M. Thompson. *Applied Statistics*, 51:493–506, 2002.

154. K. Dow and S. L. Cutter. *Natural Hazards Review*, 3(1):12–18, 2002.

155. W. R. Dowdle. *Bulletin of the World Health Organization*, 76(Suppl. 2):22, 1998.

156. C. Drakeley, D. Schellenberg, J. Kihonda, C. Sousa, A. Arez, D. Lopes, J. Lines, H. Mshinda, C. Lengeler, J. Schellenberg, M. Tanner, and P. Alonso. *Tropical Medicine & International Health*, 8:767–774, 2003.

157. R. M. D'Souza, M. Lysenko, S. Marino, and D. Kirschner. Data-parallel algorithms for agent-based model simulation of tuberculosis on graphics processing units. In *Proceedings of the 2009 Spring Simulation Multiconference*, page 21. Society for Computer Simulation International, 2009.

158. D. D. Dudenhoeffer, M. R. Permann, and M. Manic. CIMS: a framework for infrastructure interdependency modeling and analysis. In *Proceedings of the 38th Conference on Winter Simulation*, pages 478–485. Winter Simulation Conference, 2006.

159. B. Ebbell. *The Papyrus Ebers: the Greatest Egyptian Medical Document*. Levin & Munksgaard, 1937.

160. P. Eckhoff. *Malaria Journal*, 10(1):303, 2011.

161. P. Eckhoff. *PLoS ONE*, 7(9):e44950, 2012.

162. P. A. Eckhoff. *Malaria Journal*, 11:419, 2012.

163. P. Eckhoff. *The American Journal of Tropical Medicine and Hygiene*, 88(5):817–827, 2013.

164. B. Edmonds and D. Hales. *Journal of Artificial Societies and Social Simulation*, 6:4, 2003.

165. P. Elliott, J. C. Wakefield, N. G. Best, and D. J. Briggs, editors. *Spatial Epidemiology: Methods and Applications*. Oxford University Press, 2000.

166. N. N. Emmanuel, N. Loha, M. O. Okolo, and O. K. Ikenna. *Asian Pacific Journal of Tropical Disease*, 1(3):247–250, 2011.

167. T. Emonet, C. M. Macal, M. J. North, C. E. Wickersham, and P. Cluzel. *Bioinformatics*, 21(11):2714–2721, 2005.

168. Environmental Systems Research Institute (Esri). 2015. URL http://www.esri.com/. Accessed May, 2015.

169. Epidemiological Modeling. (EMOD). Website, 2015. URL http://intellectualventureslab.com/. Accessed April, 2015.

170. B. Epstein. Agent-based modeling and the fallacies of individualism. In *Models, Simulations, and Representations*, pages 115–144. Routledge, 2012.

171. J. M. Epstein and R. L. Axtell. *Growing Artificial Societies: Social Science from the Bottom Up (Complex Adaptive Systems)*. The MIT Press, 1st printing edition, 1996.

172. J. M. Epstein, D. M. Goedecke, F. Yu, R. J. Morris, D. K. Wagener, and G. V. Bobashev. *PLoS ONE*, 2(5):e401, 2007.

173. ESRI GIS Dictionary. Website. http://support.esri.com/. URL http://support.esri.com/. Accessed April, 2015.

174. S. Eubank, H. Guclu, V. A. Kumar, M. V. Marathe, A. Srinivasan, Z. Toroczkai, and N. Wang. *Nature*, 429(6988):180–184, 2004.

175. European Social Simulation Association (ESSA). 2015. URL http://cfpm.org/essa/. Accessed May, 2015.

176. G. Eysenbach. *PLoS Biology*, 4(5):e157, 2006.

177. N. M. Ferguson and G. P. Garnett. *Sexually Transmitted Diseases*, 27(10):600–609, 2000.

178. J. Ferrer, J. Albuquerque, C. Prats, D. López, and J. Valls. Agent-based models in malaria elimination strategy design. In *Fourth International Symposium on Agent-Based Modeling and Simulation (ABModSim-4)*, Vienna, April 2012.

179. J. A. Filipe, E. M. Riley, C. J. Drakeley, C. J. Sutherland, and A. C. Ghani. *PLOS Computational Biology*, 3(12):e255, 2007.

180. U. Fillinger, K. Kannady, G. William, M. Vanek, S. Dongus, D. Nyika, Y. Geissbuhler, P. Chaki, N. Govella, E. Mathenge, B. Singer, H. Mshinda, S. Lindsay, M. Tanner, D. Mtasiwa, M. de Castro, and G. Killeen. *Malaria Journal*, 7(1):20, 2008.

181. U. Fillinger and S. Lindsay. *Malaria Journal*, 10(1):353, 2011.

182. U. Fillinger, B. Ndenga, A. Githeko, and S. Lindsay. *Bulletin of the World Health Organization*, 87:655–665, 2009.

183. V. A. Folcik, G. C. An, and C. G. Orosz. *Theoretical Biology and Medical Modelling*, 4:39, 2007.

184. S. Fomel and G. Hennenfent. Reproducible computational experiments using scons. In *IEEE International Conference on Acoustics, Speech, and Signal Processing*, pages 1257–1260, 2009.

185. D. Foster, C. McGregor, and S. El-Masri. A survey of agent-based intelligent decision support systems to support clinical management and research. In *Proceedings of the 2nd International Workshop on Multi-Agent Systems for Medicine, Computational Biology, and Bioinformatics*, pages 16–34, 2005.

186. B. Franz and R. Erban. Hybrid modelling of individual movement and collective behaviour. In *Dispersal, Individual Movement and Spatial Ecology*, pages 129–157. Springer, 2013.

187. J. M. Galan and L. R. Izquierdo. *Journal of Artificial Societies and Social Simulation*, 8(3):2, 2005.

188. J. M. Galán, L. R. Izquierdo, S. S. Izquierdo, J. I. Santos, R. Del Olmo, A. López-Paredes, and B. Edmonds. *Journal of Artificial Societies and Social Simulation*, 12(1):1, 2009.

189. M. Galassi, J. Davies, J. Theiler, B. Gough, G. Jungman, M. Booth, and F. Rossi. *GNU Scientific Library: Reference Manual*. Network Theory Ltd., 2003.

190. J. L. Gallup and J. D. Sachs. *The American Journal of Tropical Medicine and Hygiene*, 64(1-2 Suppl.):85–96, 2001.

191. E. Gamma, R. Helm, R. Johnson, and J. Vlissides. *Design Patterns: Elements of Reusable Object-Oriented Software*. Pearson Education, 1994.

192. M. Gardner. *Scientific American*, 223(4):120–123, 1970.

193. T. Garske, N. M. Ferguson, and A. C. Ghani. *PLoS ONE*, 8(2):e56487, 2013.

194. Y. Geissbuhler, P. Chaki, B. Emidi, N. Govella, R. Shirima, V. Mayagaya, D. Mtasiwa, H. Mshinda, U. Fillinger, S. Lindsay, K. Kannady, M. de Castro, M. Tanner, and G. Killeen. *Malaria Journal*, 6(1):126, 2007.

195. J. E. Gentile, G. J. Davis, B. S. Laurent, and S. J. Kurtz. A framework for modeling mosquito vectors. In *Summer Computer Simulation Conference (SCSC)*, July 2010.

196. J. E. Gentile, S. S. Rund, and G. R. Madey. *Malaria Journal*, 14(1):92, 2015.

197. P. W. Gething, A. P. Patil, and S. I. Hay. *PLoS Computational Biology*, 6(4):e1000724, 2010.

198. N. Gilbert. Putting the social into social simulation. In *Keynote Address to the First World Social Simulation Conference*, Kyoto, 2006.

199. N. Gilbert. *Agent-Based Models*, volume 153. Sage Publication, 2008.

200. M. T. Gillies. *Bulletin of Entomological Research*, 52(01):99–127, 1961.

201. M. Gillies and T. Wilkes. *Bulletin of Entomological Research*, 60:225–235, 1970.

202. M. T. Gillies and T. J. Wilkes. *Bulletin of Entomological Research*, 61:389–404, 1972.

203. M. Gillies and T. Wilkes. *Bulletin of Entomological Research*, 63:573–581, 1974.

204. J. E. Gimnig, A. W. Hightower, and W. A. Hawley. Application of geographic information systems to the study of the ecology of mosquitoes and mosquito-borne diseases, Chapter 4. In *Environmental Change and Malaria Risk - Global and Local Implications, Wageningen UR Frontis Series*, pages 27–39. Springer, 2005.

205. J. E. Gimnig, M. S. Kolczak, A. W. Hightower, J. M. Vulule, E. Schoute, L. Kamau, P. A. Phillips-Howard, F. O. Ter Kuile, B. L. Nahlen, and W. A. Hawley. *The American Journal of Tropical Medicine and Hygiene*, 68(90040):115–120, 2003.

206. J. E. Gimnig, M. Ombok, S. Otieno, M. G. Kaufman, J. M. Vulule, and E. D. Walker. *Journal of Medical Entomology*, 39(1):162–172, 2002.

207. E. L. Glaeser, B. I. Sacerdote, and J. A. Scheinkman. *Journal of the European Economic Association*, 1(2-3):345–353, 2003.

208. D. Goldsman. Simulation output analysis. In *Proceedings of the 24th Conference on Winter Simulation*, pages 97–103, New York, NY, 1992. ACM.

209. J. Gollub, C. A. Ball, G. Binkley, J. Demeter, D. B. Finkelstein, J. M. Hebert, T. Hernandez-Boussard, H. Jin, M. Kaloper, J. C. Matese, M. Schroeder, P. O. Brown, D. Botstein, and G. Sherlock. *Nucleic Acids Research*, 31(1):94–96, 2003.

210. B. Gompertz. *Philosophical Transactions of the Royal Society of London*, 115:513–583, 1825.

211. D. C. Goodman and J. E. Wennberg. *Journal of Public Health Management and Practice*, 5(4):1, 1999.

212. L. C. Gouagna, H. M. Ferguson, B. A. Okech, G. F. Killeen, E. W. Kabiru, J. C. Beier, J. I. Githure, and G. Yan. *Parasitology*, 128(Pt 3):235–243, 2004.

213. B. Govindasamy, S. Thompson, P. B. Duffy, K. Caldeira, and C. Delire. *Geophysical Research Letters*, 29(22):2061–2064, 2002.

214. G. P. C. Centre. Full data reanalysis, 2008. URL http://gpcc.dwd.de.

215. P. M. Graves, T. R. Burkot, A. J. Saul, R. J. Hayes, and R. Carter. *Journal of Applied Ecology*, 27:134–147, 1990.

216. B. M. Greenwood, D. A. Fidock, D. E. Kyle, S. H. Kappe, P. L. Alonso, F. H. Collins, and P. E. Duffy. *The Journal of Clinical Investigation*, 118(4):1266–1276, 2008.

217. B. T. Grenfell, B. M. Bolker, and A. Kleczkowski. *Proceedings of the Royal Society of London. Series B: Biological Sciences*, 259(1354):97–103, 1995.

218. J. T. Griffin, T. D. Hollingsworth, L. C. Okell, T. S. Churcher, M. White, W. Hinsley, T. Bousema, C. J. Drakeley, N. M. Ferguson, M.-G. Basáñez, and A. C. Ghani. *PLoS Medicine*, 7(8):e1000324, 2010.

219. V. Grimm and S. F. Railsback. *Individual-Based Modeling and Ecology*. Princeton University Press, 2013.

220. L. J. Gros. Talk to NSF Workshop on Priorities in Ethnobiology, 2002.

221. W. Gu and R. J. Novak. *Malaria Journal*, 8(1):256, 2009.

222. W. Gu and R. J. Novak. *Transactions of the Royal Society of Tropical Medicine and Hygiene*, 103(11):1105–1112, 2009.

223. K. S. Gundogdu and I. Guney. *Journal of Earth System Science*, 116(1):49–55, 2007.

224. H. V. Gupta, S. Sorooshian, and P. O. Yapo. *Journal of Hydrologic Engineering*, 4(2):135–143, 1999.

225. S. Gupta, J. Swinton, and R. M. Anderson. *Proceedings of the Royal Society of London. Series B: Biological Sciences*, 256(1347):231–238, 1994.

226. M. Haklay, D. O'Sullivan, M. Thurstain-Goodwin, and T. Schelhorn. *Environment and Planning B*, 28(3):343–359, 2001.

227. D. S. Hamermesh. *Canadian Journal of Economics/Revue Canadienne d'économique*, 40(3):715–733, 2007.

228. P. A. Hancock. *PLOS Computational Biology*, 5(10):10, 2009.

229. P. Hancock, M. Thomas, and H. Godfray. *Proceedings of the Royal Society B: Biological Sciences*, 276(1654):71–80, 2009.

230. D. Handford and A. Rogers. *Progress in Artificial Intelligence*, 1(2):173–181, 2012.

231. W. A. Hawley, F. O. Ter Kuile, R. S. Steketee, B. L. Nahlen, D. J. Terlouw, J. E. Gimnig, Y. P. Shi, J. M. Vulule, J. A. Alaii, A. W. Hightower, M. S. Kolczak, S. K. Kariuki, and P. A. Phillips-Howard. *The American Journal of Tropical Medicine and Hygiene*, 68(Suppl. 4):168–173, 2003.

232. S. I. Hay, C. A. Guerra, P. W. Gething, A. P. Patil, A. J. Tatem, A. M. Noor, C. W. Kabaria, B. H. Manh, I. R. F. Elyazar, S. Brooker, D. L. Smith, R. A. Moyeed, and R. W. Snow. *PLoS Medicine*, 6(3):e1000048, 2009.

233. S. I. Hay, J. Cox, D. J. Rogers, S. E. Randolph, D. I. Stern, G. D. Shanks, M. F. Myers, and R. W. Snow. *Nature*, 415(6874):905–909, 2002.

234. S. I. Hay, G. D. Shanks, D. I. Stern, R. W. Snow, S. E. Randolph, and D. J. Rogers. *Trends in Parasitology*, 21(2):52–53, 2005.

235. S. I. Hay, M. E. Sinka, R. M. Okara, C. W. Kabaria, P. M. Mbithi, C. C. Tago, D. Benz, P. W. Gething, R. E. Howes, A. P. Patil, W. H. Temperley, M. J. Bangs, T. Chareonviriyaphap, I. R. F. Elyazar, R. E. Harbach, J. Hemingway, S. Manguin, C. M. Mbogo, Y. Rubio-Palis, and H. C. J. Godfray. *PLoS Medicine*, 7(2):e1000209, 2010.

236. S. I. Hay and R. W. Snow. *PLoS Medicine*, 3(12):e473, 2006.

237. D. Helbing. *Social Self-Organization*. Springer, 2012.

238. D. Helbing, I. Farkas, and T. Vicsek. *Nature*, 407(6803):487–490, 2000.

239. M. A. Hernán and A. J. Wilcox. *Epidemiology*, 20(2):167–168, 2009.

240. C. Hetzel and R. M. Anderson. *Parasitology*, 113 (Pt. 1):25–38, 1996.

241. D. Higdon, M. Kennedy, J. C. Cavendish, J. A. Cafeo, and R. D. Ryne. *SIAM Journal on Scientific Computing*, 26(2):448–466, 2004.

242. A. W. Hightower, M. Ombok, R. Otieno, R. Odhiambo, A. J. Oloo, A. A. Lal, B. L. Nahlen, and W. A. Hawley. *The American Journal of Tropical Medicine and Hygiene*, 58(3):266–272, 1998.

243. R. R. Hill, R. Carl, and L. Champagne. *Journal of Simulation*, 1(1):29–38, 2006.

244. Y. Himeidan, E. Temu, E. E. Rayah, S. Munga, and E. Kweka. *Journal of Insects*, 2013:9, 2013.

245. J. C. Hogg and H. Hurd. *Parasitology*, 114(4):325–331, 1997. ISSN: 1469–8161.

246. W. M. Holmes. *Artificial Intelligence and Simulation*. Society for Computer Simulation, San Diego, CA, 1985.

247. M. Hoshen and A. Morse. *Malaria Journal*, 3(1):32, 2004.

248. R. E. Howes, F. B. Piel, A. P. Patil, O. A. Nyangiri, P. W. Gething, M. Dewi, M. M. Hogg, K. E. Battle, C. D. Padilla, J. K. Baird, et al. *PLoS Medicine*, 9(11):e1001339, 2012.

249. E. J. Hrudey. *Safe Drinking Water: Lessons from Recent Outbreaks in Affluent Nations*. IWA Publishing, 2004.

250. G. Q. Huang, J. Huang, and K.-L. Mak. *Computer-Aided Design*, 32(2):133–144, 2000.

251. Y. Huang, X. Xiang, G. Madey, and S. E. Cabaniss. *Computing in Science & Engineering*, 7(1):22–29, 2005.

252. R. Hubbard, D. E. Vetter, and E. L. Little. *Strategic Management Journal*, 19(3):243–254, 1998.

253. J. Hubble, J. Demeter, H. Jin, M. Mao, M. Nitzberg, T. B. K. Reddy, F. Wymore, Z. K. Zachariah, G. Sherlock, and C. A. Ball. *Nucleic Acids Research*, 37(Suppl. 1):D898–D901, 2009.

254. M. Hulme, J. Mitchell, W. Ingram, J. Lowe, T. Johns, M. New, and D. Viner. *Global Environmental Change*, 9(Suppl. 1:S3–S19, 1999.

255. E. Hultin. *Acta Chemica Scandinavica*, 9:1700–1710, 1955.

256. C. A. Hunt, R. C. Kennedy, S. H. Kim, and G. E. Ropella. *Wiley Interdisciplinary Reviews: Systems Biology and Medicine*, 5(4):461–480, 2013.

257. S. Imbahale, W. Mukabana, B. Orindi, A. Githeko, and W. Takken. *Journal of Tropical Medicine*, 2012:8, 2012.

258. M. O. Jackson and A. Watts. *Journal of Economic Theory*, 106(2):265–295, 2002.

259. I. Jacobson. *Object-Oriented Software Engineering: A Use Case Driven Approach*, ACM Press Series. ACM Press, 1992, ISBN: 9780201544350, https://books.google.com/books?id=A6lQAAAAMAAJ Accessed Nov, 2015.

260. G. M. Jacquez. *Journal of Geographical Systems*, 2(1):91–97, 2000. ISSN: 1435-5930.

261. K. N.-E. Jannat and B. D. Roitberg. *Journal of Vector Ecology*, 38(1):120–126, 2013.

262. M. A. Janssen and W. J. M. Martens. *Artificial Life*, 3(3):213–236, 1997.

263. B. R. Jasny, G. Chin, L. Chong, and S. Vignieri. *Science*, 334(6060):1225, 2011.

264. Java. Website. URL http://www.java.com/en/. Accessed April, 2015.

265. N. R. Jennings and S. Bussmann. *IEEE Control Systems*, 23(3):61–74, 2003.

266. F. H. Johnson and I. Lewin. *Journal of Cellular and Comparative Physiology*, 28:47–75, 1946.

267. K. Jones, G. Moon, et al. *Health, Disease and Society: An Introduction to Medical Geography continued*. Routledge & Kegan Paul Ltd., 1987.

268. H. Joseph. *College & Research Libraries News*, 73(2):83–87, 2012.

269. N. Julka, R. Srinivasan, and I. Karimi. *Computers & Chemical Engineering*, 26(12):1755–1769, 2002.

270. F. Kabbale, A. Akol, J. Kaddu, and A. Onapa. *Parasites & Vectors*, 6(1):340, 2013.

271. R. Kandwal, P. Garg, and R. Garg. *Journal of Biomedical Informatics*, 42(4):748–755, 2009.

272. E. J. Kane. *Quarterly Journal of Business and Economics*, 23(1):3–8, 1984.

273. J. W. E. Kazura. *The American Journal of Tropical Medicine and Hygiene*, 68(Suppl. 4):465–468, 2003.

274. R. Kearns and G. Moon. *Progress in Human Geography*, 26(5):605–625, 2002.

275. Kelp, a source code annotation framework. Website, 2015. URL http://kelp.sourceforge.net/. Accessed April, 2015.

276. R. C. Kennedy, K. E. Lane, S. M. N. Arifin, A. Fuentes, H. Hollocher, and G. R. Madey. *The International Journal of Intelligent Control and Systems*, 14(1):51-61, 2009.

277. M. C. Kennedy and A. O'Hagan. *Journal of the Royal Statistical Society: Series B (Statistical Methodology)*, 63(3):425–464, 2001.

278. R. C. Kennedy, X. Xiang, T. F. Cosimano, L. A. Arthurs, P. A. Maurice, G. R. Madey, and S. E. Cabaniss. Verification and validation of agent-based and equation-based simulations: a comparison. In *Agent-Directed Simulation Conference*, Huntsville, AL, April 2006.

279. R. Kennedy, X. Xiang, G. Madey, and T. Cosimano. Verification and validation of scientific and economic models. In *Proceedings of Agent*, pages 177–192. Argonne National Laboratory, 2005.

280. J. O. Kephart, J. E. Hanson, and A. R. Greenwald. *Computer Networks*, 32(6):731–752, 2000.

281. D. L. Kettenis. *Transactions of the Society for Computer Simulation*, 17(4):162–163, 2000.

282. W. J. Kettinger and C. C. Lee. *Decision Sciences*, 30(3):893–899, 1999.

283. H. M. Khormi and L. Kumar. *Journal of Food, Agriculture & Environment*, 9(2):41–49, 2011.

284. G. Killeen. *Malaria Journal*, 13(1):330, 2014.

285. G. Killeen, F. McKenzie, B. Foy, C. Schieffelin, P. Billingsley, and J. Beier. *The American Journal of Tropical Medicine and Hygiene*, 62(5):535–544, 2000.

286. G. F. Killeen, A. Ross, and T. Smith. *The American Journal of Tropical Medicine and Hygiene*, 75(Suppl. 2):38–45, 2006.

287. G. F. Killeen, A. Seyoum, and B. G. Knols. *The American Journal of Tropical Medicine and Hygiene*, 71(Suppl. 2):87–93, August 2004.

288. G. F. Killeen and T. A. Smith. *Transactions of the Royal Society of Tropical Medicine and Hygiene*, 101(9):867–880, 2007.

289. G. F. Killeen, T. A. Smith, H. M. Ferguson, H. Mshinda, S. Abdulla, C. Lengeler, and S. P. Kachur. *PLoS Medicine*, 4(7):e229, 2007.

290. T. G. Kim. *Artificial Intelligence and Simulation*. Springer, 2005.

291. K.-J. Kim and S.-B. Cho. *Artificial Life*, 12(1):153–182, 2006.

292. M. B. King and R. A. Hunt. *Journal for the Scientific Study of religion*, 14(1):13–22, 1975.

293. T. Kistemann, F. Dangendorf, and J. Schweikart. *International Journal of Hygiene and Environmental Health*, 205(3):169–181, 2002.

294. A. Kiszewski, A. Mellinger, A. Spielman, P. Malaney, S. E. Sachs, and J. Sachs. *The American Journal of Tropical Medicine and Hygiene*, 70(5):486–498, 2004.

295. U. Kitron. *Journal of Medical Entomology*, 35(4):435–445, 1998.

296. U. Kitron. *Parasitology Today*, 16(8):324–325, 2000.

297. W. Klassen. *Malaria Journal*, 8(Suppl. 2):I1, 2009.

298. D. J. Klein, M. Baym, and P. Eckhoff. *PLoS ONE*, 9(7):e103467, 2014.

299. I. Kleinschmidt, C. Schwabe, M. Shiva, J. L. Segura, V. Sima, S. J. A. Mabunda, and M. Coleman. *The American Journal of Tropical Medicine and Hygiene*, 81(3):519–524, 2009.

300. J. C. Koella. *Acta Tropica*, 49(1):1–25, 1991.

301. C. J. M. Koenraadt, S. Majambere, L. Hemerik, and W. Takken. *Entomologia Experimentalis et Applicata*, 112(2):125–134, 2004.

302. C. J. M. Koenraadt and W. Takken. *Medical and Veterinary Entomology*, 17(1):61–66, 2003.

303. N. Krieger. *Epidemiology*, 14(4):384–385, 2003.

304. S. Kurkowski, T. Camp, N. Mushell, and M. Colagrosso. A visualization and analysis tool for NS-2 wireless simulations: iNSpect. In *Proceedings of the 13th IEEE International Symposium on Modeling, Analysis, and Simulation of Computer and Telecommunication Systems*, pages 503–506, Washington, DC, 2005. IEEE Computer Society.

305. P.-C. Lai, F.-M. So, and K.-W. Chan. *Spatial Epidemiological Approaches in Disease Mapping and Analysis*. CRC Press, 2008.

306. K. E. Lane-deGraaf, R. C. Kennedy, S. N. Arifin, G. R. Madey, A. Fuentes, and H. Hollocher. *BMC Ecology*, 13(1):35, 2013.

307. A. M. Law. *Operations Research*, 31(6):983–1029, 1983.

308. D. R. Law. Scalable means more than more: a unifying definition of simulation scalability. In *Simulation Conference Proceedings*, 1998. Winter, volume 1, pages 781–788. IEEE, 1998.

309. A. M. Law. Statistical analysis of simulation output data: the practical state of the art. In *Proceedings of the 39th Conference on Winter Simulation*, pages 77–83, Piscataway, NJ, 2007. IEEE Press.

310. A. M. Law. How to build valid and credible simulation models. In Proceedings of the 40th Conference on Winter Simulation, pages 39–47, 2008.

311. B. LeBaron. *Journal of Economic Dynamics and Control*, 24(5):679–702, 2000.

312. M.-L. T. Lee, F. C. Kuo, G. Whitmore, and J. Sklar. *Proceedings of the National Academy of Sciences of the United States of America*, 97(18):9834–9839, 2000.

313. J. M. Lees. *Seismological Research Letters*, 83(5):751–752, 2012.

314. A. Le Menach, S. Takala, F. McKenzie, A. Perisse, A. Harris, A. Flahault, and D. Smith. *Malaria Journal*, 6:10, 2007.

315. T. Lewis. *Network Science: Theory and Applications*. John Wiley & Sons, 2011.

316. L. Li, L. Bian, and G. Yan. UCGIS 2006 Summer Assembly, 2006.

317. S. Lindsay, L. Parson, and C. Thomas. *Proceedings, Biological Sciences/The Royal Society*, 265:847–854, 1998.

318. LiNK Agent-based Modeling and Visualization. Website. URL http://www.nd.edu/ macaque/. Accessed April, 2015.

319. W. Liu, Y. Li, G. H. Learn, R. S. Rudicell, J. D. Robertson, B. F. Keele, J.-B. N. Ndjango, C. M. Sanz, D. B. Morgan, S. Locatelli, et al. *Nature*, 467(7314):420–425, 2010.

320. M. Luck, P. McBurney, O. Shehory, and S. Willmott. *Agent Technology: Computing as Interaction (A Roadmap for Agent Based Computing)*. AgentLink, 2005, ISBN: 085432 845 9.

321. D. A. Luke and K. A. Stamatakis. *Annual Review of Public Health*, 33:357, 2012.

322. M. Lysenko and R. M. D'Souza. *Journal of Artificial Societies and Social Simulation*, 11(4):10, 2008.

323. C. M. Macal. Agent based modeling and artificial life. In *Encyclopedia of Complexity and Systems Science*, pages 112–131. Springer, 2009.

324. C. M. Macal and M. J. North. *Journal of Simulation*, 4(3):151–162, 2010.

325. C. Macal, D. Sallach, and M. North. Emergent structures from trust relationships in supply chains. In Proceedings of the Agent 2004: Conference on Social Dynamics, pages 7–9, 2004.

326. G. Macdonald. *Proceedings of the Royal Society of Medicine*, 48(4):295–302, 1955.

327. G. Macdonald. *Bull World Health Organ*, 15(3-5):369–387, 1956.

328. G. Macdonald. *The Epidemiology and Control of Malaria*. Oxford University Press, 1957.

329. M. W. Macy and R. Willer. *Annual Review of Sociology*, 28(1):143–166, 2002, doi:10.1146/annurev.soc.28.110601.141117.

330. MadCap Software. Website, 2015. URL http://www.madcapsoftware.com/. Accessed April, 2015.

331. N. Maire, T. Smith, A. Ross, S. Owusu-Agyei, K. Dietz, and L. Molineaux. *The American Journal of Tropical Medicine and Hygiene*, 75(Suppl. 2):19–31, 2006.

332. W. M. Makeham. *Journal of the Institute of Actuaries*, 6:301–310, 1860.

333. Malaria Biology. Centers for Disease Control and Prevention (CDC). Website. URL http://www.cdc.gov/malaria/about/biology/index.html. Accessed May, 2015.

334. malERA Consultative Group on Modeling *PLoS Medicine*, 8(1):e1000403, 2011.

335. malERA Consultative Group on Vector Control. *PLoS Medicine*, 8(1):e1000401, 2011.

336. R. Malima, S. Magesa, P. Tungu, V. Mwingira, F. Magogo, W. Sudi, F. Mosha, C. Curtis, C. Maxwell, and M. Rowland. *Malaria Journal*, 7:38, 2008.

337. S. Mandal, R. Sarkar, and S. Sinha. *Malaria Journal*, 10(1):202, 2011.

338. Mapador Inc. Website, 2015. URL http://www.mapador.com/documentation.html. Accessed April, 2015.

339. Mapping Malaria Risk in Africa (MARA). Website. URL http://www.mara-database.org/. Accessed April, 2015.

340. J. M. Marshall and C. E. Taylor. *PLoS Medicine*, 6(2):e1000020, 2009.

341. P. Martens, R. S. Kovats, S. Nijhof, P. de Vries, M. T. J. Livermore, D. J. Bradley, J. Cox, and A. J. McMichael. *Global Environmental Change*, 9, Suppl. 1:S89–S107, 1999.

342. W. J. M. Martens, T. H. Jetten, J. Rotmans, and L. W. Niessen. *Global Environmental Change*, 5(3):195–209, 1995.

343. W. J. Martens, L. W. Niessen, J. Rotmans, T. H. Jetten, and A. J. McMichael. *Environmental Health Perspectives*, 103(5):458, 1995b.

344. E. Mas, A. Suppasri, F. Imamura, and S. Koshimura. *Journal of Natural Disaster Science*, 34(1):41–57, 2012.

345. M. Matsumoto and T. Nishimura. *ACM Transactions on Modeling and Computer Simulation*, 8(1):3–30, 1998.

346. R. B. Matthews, N. G. Gilbert, A. Roach, J. G. Polhill, and N. M. Gotts. *Landscape Ecology*, 22(10):1447–1459, 2007.

347. P. F. Mattingly. *The Biology of Mosquito-Borne Disease*. Allen & Unwin, 1969.

348. R. Maude, W. Pontavornpinyo, S. Saralamba, R. Aguas, S. Yeung, A. Dondorp, N. Day, N. White, and L. White. *Malaria Journal*, 8(1):31, 2009.

349. J. D. Mayer. *Social Science & Medicine*, 50(7):937–952, 2000.

350. C. M. Mbogo, J. M. Mwangangi, J. Nzovu, W. Gu, G. Yan, J. T. Gunter, C. Swalm, J. Keating, J. L. Regens, J. I. Shililu, et al. *American Journal of Tropical Medicine and Hygiene*, 68(6):734–742, 2003.

351. A. McCrae. *Annals of Tropical Medicine and Parasitology*, 77:615–625, 1983.

352. P. D. McElroy, F. O. ter Kuile, A. W. Hightower, W. A. Hawley, P. A. Phillips-Howard, A. J. Oloo, A. A. Lal, and B. L. Nahlen. *The American Journal of Tropical Medicine and Hygiene*, 64(Suppl. 1):18–27, 2001.

353. F. E. McKenzie, J. K. Baird, J. C. Beier, A. A. Lal, and W. H. Bossert. *The American Journal of Tropical Medicine and Hygiene*, 67(6):571–577, 2002.

354. F. E. McKenzie and W. H. Bossert. *Journal of Theoretical Biology*, 188(1):127–140, 1997.

355. F. E. McKenzie and W. H. Bossert. *Journal of Theoretical Biology*, 232(3):411–426, 2005.

356. F. E. McKenzie, G. F. Killeen, J. C. Beier, and W. H. Bossert. *Ecology*, 82(10):2673–2681, 2001.

357. F. E. McKenzie, R. C. Wong, and W. H. Bossert. *Simulation*, 71(4):250–261, 1998.

358. R. K. Meentemeyer, N. J. Cunniffe, A. R. Cook, J. A. Filipe, R. D. Hunter, D. M. Rizzo, and C. A. Gilligan. *Ecosphere*, 2(2):art17, 2011.

359. A. L. Melnick and D. W. Fleming. *Journal of Public Health Management and Practice*, 5(2):viii, 1999.

360. A. L. Menach, F. E. McKenzie, A. Flahault, and D. L. Smith. *Malaria Journal*, 4(1):23, 2005.

361. D. Menard, A. E. Randrianarivo-Solofoniaina, B. S. Ahmed, M. Jahevitra, L. V. Adriantsoanirina, J. R. Rasolofomanana, et al. *Emerging Infectious Diseases*, 13(11):1759–1762, 2007.

362. K. Mendis, B. J. Sina, P. Marchesini, and R. Carter. *The American Journal of Tropical Medicine and Hygiene*, 64(Suppl. 1):97–106, 2001.

363. D. Metselaar and P. van Thiel. *Tropical and Geographical Medicine*, 11:157–161, 1959.

364. L. Meyers. *Bulletin of the American Mathematical Society*, 44(1):63–86, 2007.

365. J. Midega, C. Mbogo, H. Mwnambi, M. Wilson, G. Ojwang, J. Mwangangi, J. Nzovu, J. Githure, G. Yan, and J. Beier. *Journal of Medical Entomology*, 44(6):923–929, 2007.

366. H. Min and G. Zhou. *Computers & Industrial Engineering*, 43(1–2):231–249, 2002.

367. B. Mmbando, M. Kamugisha, J. Lusingu, F. Francis, D. Ishengoma, T. Theander, M. Lemnge, and T. Scheike. *Malaria Journal*, 10(1):145, 2011.

368. J. Moffat, J. Smith, and S. Witty. *Journal of Applied Mathematics and Decision Sciences*, 2006, 2006, doi:10.1155/JAMDS/2006/54846.

369. L. Molineaux. In *Malaria: Principles and Practice of Malariology*, pages 913–998. Churchill Livingstone, Edinburgh, New York, 1988.

370. L. Molineaux, H. H. Diebner, M. Eichner, W. E. Collins, G. M. Jeffery, and K. Dietz. *Parasitology*, 122(Pt 4):379–391, 2001.

371. L. Molineaux and G. Gramiccia. World Health Organization, 1980.

372. L. Molineaux, M. Trauble, W. E. Collins, G. M. Jeffery, and K. Dietz. *Transactions of the Royal Society of Tropical Medicine and Hygiene*, 96(2):205–209, 2002.

373. B. Moonen, S. Barrett, J. Tulloch, and D. T. Jamison. *Making the Decision*, book section 1, pages 1–18. The Global Health Group: UCSF Global Health Sciences, San Francisco, CA, 2009.

374. M. Mulkay and G. N. Gilbert. *Philosophy of the Social Sciences*, 16(1):21–37, 1986.

375. G. Muller, P. Grébaut, and J.-P. Gouteux. *Comptes Rendus Biologies*, 327(1):1–11, 2004.

376. S. Munga, N. Minakawa, G. Zhou, O. Barrack, A. Githeko, and G. Yan. *Journal of Medical Entomology*, 43:221–224, 2006.

377. C. Mutero, D. Schlodder, N. Kabatereine, and R. Kramer. *Malaria Journal*, 11(1):21, 2012.

378. B. L. Nahlen, J. P. Clark, and D. Alnwick. *The American Journal of Tropical Medicine and Hygiene*, 68(Suppl. 4):1–2, 2003.

379. National Science Foundation. 2015. URL http://www.nsf.gov/. Accessed May, 2015.

380. B. A. Ndenga, J. A. Simbauni, J. P. Mbugi, A. K. Githeko, and U. Fillinger. *PLoS ONE*, 6(4):e19473, 2011.

381. R. Neghina, A. M. Neghina, I. Marincu, and I. Iacobiciu. *The American Journal of the Medical Sciences*, 340(6):492–498, 2010.

382. A. G. Nerlich, B. Schraut, S. Dittrich, T. Jelinek, and A. R. Zink. *Emerging Infectious Diseases*, 14(8):1317, 2008.

383. F. Nilsson and V. Darley. *International Journal of Operations & Production Management*, 26(12):1–24, 2006.

384. M. North and C. Macal. SwarmFest, Swarm Development Group, 2002.

385. M. J. North and C. M. Macal. *Managing Business Complexity: Discovering Strategic Solutions with Agent-Based Modeling and Simulation*. Oxford University Press, 2007.

386. M. J. North, C. M. Macal, J. S. Aubin, P. Thimmapuram, M. Bragen, J. Hahn, J. Karr, N. Brigham, M. E. Lacy, and D. Hampton. *Complexity*, 15(5):37–47, 2010.

387. D. Nute, W. D. Potter, F. Maier, J. Wang, M. Twery, H. M. Rauscher, P. Knopp, S. Thomasma, M. Dass, H. Uchiyama, et al. *Environmental Modelling & Software*, 19(9):831–843, 2004.

388. S. C. Oaks Jr., V. S. Mitchell, G. W. Pearson, and C. J. Carpenter. *Malaria: Obstacles and Opportunities*. National Academies Press, Washington, DC, 1991.

389. M. Okal, B. Francis, M. Herrera-Varela, U. Fillinger, and S. Lindsay. *Malaria Journal*, 12(1):365, 2013.

390. L. C. Okell, C. J. Drakeley, T. Bousema, C. J. Whitty, and A. C. Ghani. *PLoS Medicine*, 5(11):e226–; discussion e226, 2008.

391. F. Okumu, B. Chipwaza, E. Madumla, E. Mbeyela, G. Lingamba, J. Moore, A. Ntamatungro, D. Kavishe, and S. Moore. *Malaria Journal*, 11(1):378, 2012.

392. D. Olaru, S. Purchase, and S. Denize. Using docking/replication to verify and validate computational models. In *18th World IMACS/MODSIM Congress*, pages 4432–4438, 2009.

393. OpenABM and CoMSES. 2015. URL https://www.openabm.org/. Accessed May, 2015.

394. OpenMalaria: A simulator of malaria epidemiology and control. Website, 2015. URL http://code.google.com/p/openmalaria/. Accessed April, 2015.

395. OpenMap. Website. URL http://openmap.bbn.com/. Accessed April, 2015.

396. T. I. Ören. Assessing acceptability of simulation studies. In *Proceedings of 1980 Winter Simulation Conference*, volume 2, pages 19–22, 1980.

397. T. I. Ören. *Communications of the ACM*, 24(4):180–189, 1981.

398. T. I. Ören. Quality assurance of system design and model management for complex problems. In *Adequate Modeling of Systems*, pages 205–219. Springer, 1983.

399. T. I. Ören. Quality assurance in modelling and simulation: a taxonomy. In *Simulation and Model-Based Methodologies: An Integrative View*, pages 477–517. Springer, 1984.

400. T. I. Ören. Quality assurance in cognizant simulative design. In *Proceedings of the 18th Conference on Winter Simulation*, pages 850–852. ACM, 1986.

401. T. I. Ören. Artificial intelligence in simulation. In *Messung, Modellierung und Bewertung von Rechensystemen*, pages 375–388. Springer, 1987.

402. T. I. Ören. *Simulation*, 48(4):149–151, 1987.

403. T. I. Ören. *Transactions of the Society for Computer Simulation International*, 17(4):165–170, 2000.

404. T. Ören, M. Elzas, and G. Sheng. *ACM SIGSIM Simulation Digest*, 16(4):4–19, 1985, ISSN: 0163-6103, doi:10.1145/1102581.1102582.

405. T. I. Oren, M. S. Elzas, I. Smit, and L. G. Birta. Code of professional ethics for simulationists. In *Summer Computer Simulation Conference*, pages 434–435. Society for Computer Simulation International; 1998, 2002.

406. T. I. Ören and L. Yilmaz. *Agent-Directed Simulation and Systems Engineering*, pages 189–217, John Wiley & Sons, Inc., 2009.

407. T. I. Ören and B. P. Zeigler. *Simulation*, 32(3):69–82, 1979.

408. R. S. Ostfeld, G. E. Glass, and F. Keesing. *Trends in Ecology & Evolution*, 20(6):328–336, 2005.

409. R. Oxborough, F. Mosha, J. Matowo, R. Mndeme, E. Feston, J. Hemingway, and M. Rowland. *Annals of Tropical Medicine and Parasitology*, 102:717–727, 2008.

410. I. Oyewole, T. Awolola, C. Ibidapo, A. Oduola, O. Okwa, and J. Obansa. *Journal of Vector Borne Diseases*, 44:56–64, 2007.

411. E. Ozdenerol, G. N. Taff, and C. Akkus. *International Journal of Environmental Research and Public Health*, 10(11):5399–5432, 2013.

412. K. Paaijmans and M. Thomas. *Malaria Journal*, 10(1):183, 2011.

413. K. P. Paaijmans, S. Huijben, A. K. Githeko, and W. Takken. *Acta Tropica*, 109(2):124–130, 2009.

414. K. P. Paaijmans, M. O. Wandago, A. K. Githeko, and W. Takken. *PLoS ONE*, 2(11):e1146, 2007.

415. Pacific Asian Association for Agent-Based Approach in Social Systems Science (PAAA). 2015. URL http://www.paaa.asia/. Accessed May, 2015.

416. R. Packard. *The Making of a Tropical Disease: A Short History of Malaria.* Johns Hopkins University Press, Baltimore, MD, 2008.

417. S. Paget-McNicol, M. Gatton, I. Hastings, and A. Saul. *Parasitology*, 124(Pt 3):225–235, 2002.

418. X. Pan, C. S. Han, K. Dauber, and K. H. Law. *Ai &Society*, 22(2):113–132, 2007.

419. D. J. Pannell. *Agricultural Economics*, 16(2):139–152, 1997.

420. G. Pappas, I. J. Kiriaze, and M. E. Falagas. *International Journal of Infectious Diseases*, 12(4):347–350, 2008.

421. R. B. M. Partnership. Technical Paper - RBM/WG/2009/TP:2001, 2009.

422. H. V. D. Parunak, R. Savit, and R. L. Riolo. Agent-based modeling vs. equation-based modeling: a case study and users' guide. In *Multi-Agent Systems and Agent-Based Simulation*, pages 10–25. Springer, 1998.

423. E. N. Pavlovsky, F. K. Plous Jr., and N. D. Levine. *The American Journal of the Medical Sciences*, 252(5):161, 1966.

424. J. Pavón, M. Arroyo, S. Hassan, and C. Sansores. *Pattern Recognition Letters*, 29(8):1039–1048, 2008.

425. D. Pawlaszczyk and S. Strassburger. Scalability in distributed simulations of agent-based models. In Simulation Conference (WSC), Proceedings of the 2009 Winter, pages 1189–1200. IEEE, 2009.

426. A. J. Pel, M. C. Bliemer, and S. P. Hoogendoorn. *Transportation*, 39(1):97–123, 2012.

427. R. D. Peng. *Biostatistics*, 10(3):405–408, 2009.

428. R. D. Peng. *Science*, 334(6060):1226–1227, 2011.

429. M. A. Penny, N. Maire, A. Studer, A. Schapira, and T. A. Smith. *PLoS ONE*, 3(9):e3193, 2008.

430. L. Perez and S. Dragicevic. *International Journal of Health Geographics*, 8(1):50, 2009.

431. P. Perrot. *A to Z of Thermodynamics*. Oxford University Press, 1998.

432. D. U. Pfeiffer, T. P. Robinson, M. Stevenson, K. B. Stevens, D. J. Rogers, and A. C. A. Clements. *Spatial Analysis in Epidemiology*. Oxford University Press, 2008.

433. P. A. Phillips-Howard, B. L. Nahlen, J. A. Alaii, F. O. ter Kuile, J. E. Gimnig, D. J. Terlouw, S. P. Kachur, A. W. Hightower, A. A. Lal, E. Schoute, A. J. Oloo, and W. A. Hawley. *The American Journal of Tropical Medicine and Hygiene*, 68(Suppl. 4):3–9, 2003.

434. H. Phuc, M. Andreasen, R. Burton, C. Vass, M. Epton, G. Pape, G. Fu, K. Condon, S. Scaife, C. Donnelly, P. Coleman, H. White-Cooper, and L. Alphey. *BMC Biology*, 5(1):11, 2007.

435. F. B. Piel, A. P. Patil, R. E. Howes, O. A. Nyangiri, P. W. Gething, M. Dewi, W. H. Temperley, T. N. Williams, D. J. Weatherall, and S. I. Hay. *The Lancet*, 381(9861):142–151, 2013.

436. J. Pinikahana and R. A. Dixon. *Indian Journal of Malariology*, 30(2):51–55, 1993.

437. PLOS Computational Biology. Website, 2015. URL http://journals.plos.org/ploscompbiol/. Accessed April, 2015.

438. PLOS Computational Biology Guidelines for Authors. Website, 2015. URL http://www .ploscompbiol.org/static/guidelines.action. Accessed April, 2015.

439. W. Pongtavornpinyo, I. M. Hastings, A. Dondorp, L. J. White, R. J. Maude, S. Saralamba, N. P. Day, N. J. White, and M. F. Boni. *Evolutionary Applications*, 2(1):52–61, 2009.

440. D. J. Power and R. Sharda. *Decision Support Systems*, 43(3):1044–1061, 2007.

441. R. S. Pressman. *Software Engineering: A Practitioner's Approach*. Palgrave Macmillan, 2005.

442. L. Preziosi. *Cancer Modelling and Simulation*. CRC Press, 2003.

443. N. Protopopoff, W. Van Bortel, N. Speybroeck, J.-P. Van Geertruyden, D. Baza, U. D'Alessandro, and M. Coosemans. *PLoS ONE*, 4(11):e8022, 2009.

444. Y. Qin and H. A. Simon. *Cognitive Science*, 14(2):281–312, 1990.

445. R. The R Project. Website. URL http://www.r-project.org/. Accessed April, 2015.

446. H. Rahmandad and J. Sterman. *Management Science*, 54(5):998–1014, 2008.

447. W. Rand and U. Wilensky. North American Association for Computational Social and Organization Sciences, 2006.

448. J. C. Refsgaard, H. J. Henriksen, W. G. Harrar, H. Scholten, and A. Kassahun. *Environmental Modelling &Software*, 20(10):1201–1215, 2005.

449. J. Reibisch. *Wiss Meeresuntersuch*, 6:213–231, 1902.

450. W. K. Reisen. *Annual Review of Entomology*, 55:461–483, 2010.

451. C. Ren, C. Yang, and S. Jin. Agent-based modeling and simulation on emergency evacuation. In *Complex Sciences*, pages 1451–1461. Springer, 2009.

452. Repast. Recursive Porous Agent Simulation Toolkit. Website, 2015. URL http://repast .sourceforge.net/repast&uscore;3. Accessed April, 2015.

453. M. Resnick. StarLogo: an environment for decentralized modeling and decentralized thinking. In *Conference Companion on Human Factors in Computing Systems*, CHI '96, pages 11–12, New York, 1996. ACM.

454. C. W. Reynolds. *ACM SIGGRAPH Computer Graphics*, 21(4):25–34, 1987.

455. S. M. Rinaldi. Modeling and simulating critical infrastructures and their interdependencies. In *System Sciences, 2004. Proceedings of the 37th Annual Hawaii International Conference on*, pages 8 pp–. IEEE, 2004.

456. Roll Back Malaria (RBM). Website. URL http://www.rollbackmalaria.org/. Accessed April, 2015.

457. R. Romi, M. C. Razaiarimanga, R. Raharimanga, E. M. Rakotondraibe, L. H. Ranaivo, V. Pietra, A. Raveloson, and G. Majori. *The American Journal of Tropical Medicine and Hygiene*, 66(1):2–6, 2002.

458. G. Rosen. *A History of Public Health*. MD Publications, Inc., New York, 1958.

459. R. Ross. *The Prevention of Malaria*. John Murray, 1910.

460. A. Ross, M. Penny, N. Maire, A. Studer, I. Carneiro, D. Schellenberg, B. Greenwood, M. Tanner, and T. Smith. *PLoS ONE*, 3(7):e2661, 2008.

461. J. Rotmans. *IMAGE: An Integrated Model to Assess the Greenhouse Effect*. Developments in Cardiovascular Medicine. Kluwer Academic Print on Demand, 1990.

462. J. Rouchier, C. Cioffi-Revilla, J. G. Polhill, and K. Takadama. *Journal of Artificial Societies and Social Simulation*, 11(2):8, 2008.

463. S. Ruan, D. Xiao, and J. C. Beier. *Bulletin of Mathematical Biology*, 70(4):1098–1114, 2008.

464. J. Rumbaugh, M. Blaha, W. Premerlani, F. Eddy, W. E. Lorensen, et al. *Object-Oriented Modeling and Design*, volume 199. Prentice-Hall, Englewood Cliffs, NJ, 1991.

465. S. S. C. Rund, N. A. Bonar, M. M. Champion, J. P. Ghazi, C. M. Houk, M. T. Leming, Z. Syed, and G. E. Duffield. *Scientific Reports*, 3:2494, 2013.

466. M. J. Rytkönen. *International Journal of Circumpolar Health*, 63(1), 2004.

467. J. Sachs and P. Malaney. *Nature*, 415(6872):680–685, 2002.

468. R. Sallares. *Malaria and Rome: A History of Malaria in Ancient Italy*. Oxford University Press, 2002.

469. W. Sama, K. Dietz, and T. Smith. *Transactions of the Royal Society of Tropical Medicine and Hygiene*, 100(9):811–816, 2006.

470. W. Sama, G. Killeen, and T. Smith. *The American Journal of Tropical Medicine and Hygiene*, 70(6):625–634, 2004.

471. I. Sample. The Guardian, 2011.

472. B. D. Santer, T. M. L. Wigley, and K. E. Taylor. *Science*, 334(6060):1232–1233, 2011.

473. R. G. Sargent. Verification and validation: some approaches and paradigms for verifying and validating simulation models. In *Proceedings of the 33rd Conference on Winter Simulation*, pages 106–114, Washington, DC, 2001. IEEE Computer Society.

474. R. G. Sargent. Validation and verification of simulation models. In *Proceedings of the 2004 Winter Simulation Conference*, volume 1. IEEE, 2004.

475. G. Sarton. *A History of Science*, Volume 2, Harvard University Press, Cambridge, MA, 1952.

476. A. Saul. *Parasitology*, 117(05):405–407, 1998.

477. A. J. Saul, P. M. Graves, and B. H. Kay. *Journal of Applied Ecology*, 27:123–133, 1990.

478. T. Schelhorn, D. O'Sullivan, M. Haklay, and M. Thurstain-Goodwin. *STREETS: An Agent-Based Pedestrian Model*. Centre for Advanced Spatial Analysis UCL, 1999, http://discovery.ucl.ac.uk/267/ Accessed November, 2015.

479. T. C. Schelling. *Journal of Mathematical Sociology*, 1(2):143–186, 1971.

480. P. Schlagenhauf-Lawlor. *Travelers' Malaria*. Pmph USA Ltd Series. BC Decker, 2007.

481. S. Schlesinger, R. E. Crosbie, R. E. Gagné, G. S. Innis, C. S. Lalwani, J. Loch, R. J. Sylvester, R. D. Wright, N. Kheir, and D. Bartos. *Simulation*, 32(3):103–104, 1979.

482. B. Schneider. *The Teachers College Record*, 106(7):1471–1483, 2004.

483. R. M. Schoolfield, P. J. H. Sharpe, and C. E. Magnuson. *Journal of Theoretical Biology*, 88(4):719–731, 1981.

484. W. Schröder. *International Journal of Medical Microbiology*, 296:23–36, 2006.

485. ScreenSteps. Website, 2015. URL http://www.bluemangolearning.com/screensteps/. Accessed April, 2015.

486. J. L. Segovia-Juarez, S. Ganguli, and D. Kirschner. *Journal of Theoretical Biology*, 231(3):357–376, 2004.

487. A. F. Seila. Advanced output analysis for simulation. In Proceedings of the 24th Conference on Winter Simulation, pages 190–197, New York, 1992. ACM.

488. P. J. H. Sharpe and D. W. DeMichele. *Journal of Theoretical Biology*, 64(4):649–670, 1977.

489. W. Shen, Q. Hao, H. J. Yoon, and D. H. Norrie. *Advanced Engineering Informatics*, 20(4):415–431, 2006.

490. W. Shen and D. H. Norrie. *Knowledge and Information Systems*, 1(2):129–156, 1999.

491. A. Shendarkar, K. Vasudevan, S. Lee, and Y.-J. Son. Crowd simulation for emergency response using bdi agent based on virtual reality. In *Proceedings of the 38th Conference on Winter Simulation*, pages 545–553. Winter Simulation Conference, 2006.

492. J. Shi, A. Ren, and C. Chen. *Automation in Construction*, 18(3):338–347, 2009.

493. M. Sidman. *Tactics of Scientific Research: Evaluating Experimental Data in Psychology*. Basic Books, New York, 1960.

494. Simbios. NIH Center for Physics-Based Simulation of Biological Structures. Website. URL http://simbios.stanford.edu/. Accessed April, 2015.

495. SimTK. The Simbios biosimulation ToolKit. Website. URL https://simtk.org/home/simtk. Accessed April, 2015.

496. Simulink. Simulation and Model-Based Design. Website. URL http://www.mathworks.com/products/simulink/. Accessed April, 2015.

497. W. Smit. *A Question of Ethics*, pages 30–33. University of Wageningen, Department of Informatics, Wageningen, The Netherlands, 1999.

498. D. L. Smith, K. E. Battle, S. I. Hay, C. M. Barker, T. W. Scott, and F. E. McKenzie. *PLoS Pathogens*, 8(4):e1002588, 2012.

499. T. Smith, J. Charlwood, W. Takken, M. Tanner, and D. Spiegelhalter. *Acta Tropica*, 59:1–18, 1995.

500. D. L. Smith, S. I. Hay, A. M. Noor, and R. W. Snow. *Trends in Parasitology*, 25(11):511–516, 2009.

501. S. C. Smith, U. B. Joshi, M. Grabowsky, J. Selanikio, T. Nobiya, and T. Aapore. *The American Journal of Tropical Medicine and Hygiene*, 77(Suppl. 6):243–248, 2007.

502. T. Smith, G. F. Killeen, N. Maire, A. Ross, L. Molineaux, F. Tediosi, G. Hutton, J. Utzinger, K. Dietz, and M. Tanner. *The American Journal of Tropical Medicine and Hygiene*, 75(Suppl. 2):1–10, 2006.

503. D. L. Smith and F. E. McKenzie. *Malaria Journal*, 3:13, 2004.

504. D. L. Smith, F. E. McKenzie, R. W. Snow, and S. I. Hay. *PLoS Biology*, 5(3):e42, 2007a.

505. D. L. Smith, T. A. Smith, and S. I. Hay. *Measuring Malaria for Elimination*, book section 7, pages 108–126. The Global Health Group: UCSF Global Health Sciences, San Francisco, CA, 2009.

506. T. Smith, N. Maire, K. Dietz, G. F. Killeen, P. Vounatsou, L. Molineaux, and M. Tanner. *The American Journal of Tropical Medicine and Hygiene*, 75(Suppl. 2):11–18, 2006.

507. T. Smith, N. Maire, A. Ross, M. Penny, N. Chitnis, A. Schapira, A. Studer, B. Genton, C. Lengeler, F. Tediosi, D. De Savigny, and M. Tanner. *Parasitology*, 135(Special Issue 13):1507–1516, 2008.

508. R. W. Snow, C. A. Guerra, A. M. Noor, H. Y. Myint, and S. I. Hay. *Nature*, 434(7030):214–217, 2005.

509. F. Snowden. *The Conquest of Malaria: Italy, 1900-1962*. Yale University Press, New Haven, CT, 2006.

510. Social Sciences Computing Services, University of Chicago. Website. URL http://sscs.uchicago.edu/. Accessed April, 2015.

511. M. V. Sokolova and A. Fernández-Caballero. *Expert Systems with Applications*, 36(2):2603–2614, 2009.

512. SPSS - Statistical Package for the Social Sciences. Website. URL http://www.spss.com/. Accessed April, 2015.

513. STATPerl (Statistics with Perl). Website. URL http://sourceforge.net/projects/statperl/. Accessed April, 2015.

514. M. M. Stevenson and E. M. Riley. *Nature Reviews Immunology*, 4(3):169–180, 2004.

515. V. Stodden. The Scientific Method in Practice: Reproducibility in the Computational Sciences (February 9, 2010). MIT Sloan Research Paper No. 4773-10, 2010. Available at SSRN: http://ssrn.com/abstract=1550193 or doi:10.2139/ssrn.1550193.

516. C. J. Struchiner, M. E. Halloran, and A. Spielman. *Mathematical Biosciences*, 94(1):87–113, 1989.

517. D. Stürchler. *Travelers' Malaria*, Chapter 2. Pmph USA Ltd Series. BC Decker, 2007.

518. L. M. Styer, J. R. Carey, J. L. Wang, and T. W. Scott. *The American Journal of Tropical Medicine and Hygiene*, 76(1):111–117, 2007.

519. P. Suber. Open Access Overview, 2007.

520. T. Sueyoshi and G. R. Tadiparthi. *Decision Support Systems*, 44(2):425–446, 2008.

521. L. Sumba, K. Okoth, A. Deng, J. Githure, B. Knols, J. Beier, and A. Hassanali. *Journal of Circadian Rhythms*, 2(1):6, 2004.

522. L. A. Sumba, C. B. Ogbunugafor, A. L. Deng, and A. Hassanali. *Journal of Chemical Ecology*, 34(11):1430–1436, 2008.

523. J. M. Swaminathan, S. F. Smith, and N. M. Sadeh. *Decision Sciences*, 29(3):607–632, 1998.

524. W. Takken and B. G. Knols. *Trends in Parasitology*, 25(3):101–104, 2009.

525. S. J. E. Taylor. *Introducing Agent-based Modeling and Simulation*, book chapter 1, pages 1–10. Palgrave Macmillan, 2014.

526. S. J. E. Taylor, A. Khan, K. L. Morse, A. Tolk, L. Yilmaz, and J. Zander. Grand challenges on the theory of modeling and simulation. In *Proceedings of the Symposium on Theory of Modeling &Simulation - DEVS Integrative M&S Symposium*, DEVS 13, pages 34:1–34:8, San Diego, CA, 2013. Society for Computer Simulation International.

527. S. Tayur, R. Ganeshan, and M. Magazine. *Quantitative Models for Supply Chain Management*. Kluwer Academic Publishers, Norwell, MA, 1999.

528. F. Tediosi, G. Hutton, N. Maire, T. A. Smith, A. Ross, and M. Tanner. *The American Journal of Tropical Medicine and Hygiene*, 75(Suppl. 2):131–143, 2006.

529. F. Tediosi, N. Maire, T. Smith, G. Hutton, J. Utzinger, A. Ross, and M. Tanner. *The American Journal of Tropical Medicine and Hygiene*, 75(Suppl. 2):90–103, 2006.

530. A. Teran-Somohano, O. Dayıbaş, L. Yilmaz, and A. Smith. Toward a model-driven engineering framework for reproducible simulation experiment lifecycle management. In *Proceedings of the 2014 Winter Simulation Conference*, pages 2726–2737. IEEE Press, 2014.

531. P. Terna. *Journal of Artificial Societies and Social Simulation*, 1(2):1–12, 1998.

532. L. Tesfatsion. *Artificial Life*, 8(1):55–82, 2002.

533. J. W. Testa, K. J. Mock, C. Taylor, H. Koyuk, J. R. Coyle, and R. Waggoner. *Marine Ecology Progress Series*, 466:275, 2012.

534. The Eclipse Foundation. Website. URL http://www.eclipse.org/. Accessed April, 2015.

535. The History of Malaria, an Ancient Disease. Centers for Disease Control and Prevention (CDC). Website, 2015. URL http://www.cdc.gov/malaria/about/history/. Accessed April, 2015.

536. The Institute for Disease Modeling (IDM). Website, 2015. URL http://idmod.org//. Accessed April, 2015.

537. The Malaria Atlas Project (MAP). Website. URL http://www.map.ox.ac.uk/. Accessed April, 2015.

538. The OpenScience Project. Website. URL http://www.openscience.org/. Accessed April, 2015.

539. The Perl Programming Language. Website, 2015. URL http://www.perl.org/. Accessed April, 2015.

540. M. Theseira. *Health & Place*, 8(1):37–46, 2002.

541. J. C. Thiele, W. Kurth, and V. Grimm. *Journal of Artificial Societies and Social Simulation*, 17(3):8, 2014.

542. U. S. Tim. *Environmental Research*, 71(2):75–88, 1995.

543. H. Townson, M. Nathan, M. Zaim, P. Guillet, L. Manga, R. Bos, and M. Kindhauser. *Bulletin of the World Health Organization*, 83(12):942–947, 2005.

544. K. G. Troitzsch. Validating simulation models. In *18th European Simulation Multiconference. Networked Simulations and Simulation Networks*, pages 265–270, 2004.

545. T. Ulrichs and S. H. Kaufmann. *The Journal of Pathology*, 208(2):261–269, 2006.

546. Unified Modeling Language (UML). Resource Page. Website. URL http://www.uml.org/. Accessed April, 2015.

547. University of Notre Dame. Website, 2015. URL http://www.nd.edu/. Accessed April, 2015.

548. Vector-Borne Disease Network (VecNet). Website. URL http://www.vecnet.org/. Accessed April, 2015.

549. W. E. Walker, P. Harremoës, J. Rotmans, J. P. van der Sluijs, M. B. van Asselt, P. Janssen, and M. P. Krayer von Krauss. *Integrated Assessment*, 4(1):5–17, 2003.

550. F.-Y. Wang, K. M. Carley, D. Zeng, and W. Mao. *IEEE Intelligent Systems*, 22(2):79–83, 2007.

551. S. E. Ward and R. D. Brown. *Landscape and Urban Planning*, 66(2):91–106, 2004.

552. H. Ward, U. Goan, M. Parker, G. Kinghorn, E. Claydon, J. Weber, A. Ghani, G. Bell, and C. Ison. *International Journal of STD & AIDS*, 9(11):666–671, 1998.

553. W. H. Wen-Mei. *GPU Computing Gems Emerald Edition*. Elsevier, 2011.

554. E. Wenger and P. Eckhoff. *Malaria Journal*, 12(1):126, 2013. ISSN: 1475–2875.

555. W. Wernsdorfer, S. I. Hay, and G. D. Shanks. *Learning from History*, book section 6, pages 95–107. The Global Health Group: UCSF Global Health Sciences, San Francisco, CA, 2009.

556. A. Wesolowski, N. Eagle, A. J. Tatem, D. L. Smith, A. M. Noor, R. W. Snow, and C. O. Buckee. *Science*, 338(6104):267–270, 2012.

557. N. White. *Philosophical Transactions of the Royal Society of London. Series B: Biological Sciences*, 354:739–749, 1999.

558. M. White, J. Griffin, T. Churcher, N. Ferguson, M.-G. Basanez, and A. Ghani. *Parasites & Vectors*, 4(1):153, 2011.

559. L. White, R. Maude, W. Pongtavornpinyo, S. Saralamba, R. Aguas, T. Van Effelterre, N. Day, and N. White. *Malaria Journal*, 8(1):212, 2009. ISSN: 1475-2875.

560. *World Malaria Report: 2011*. World Health Organization (WHO), Geneva, 2011.

561. U. Wilensky. *Center for Connected Learning and Computer-Based Modeling*. Northwestern University, Evanston, IL, 1999, http://ccl.northwestern.edu/netlogo.

562. U. Wilensky and W. Rand. *Journal of Artificial Societies and Social Simulation*, 10(4):2, 2007.

563. O. Will. *Journal of Artificial Societies and Social Simulation*, 12:4, 2009.

564. O. Will and R. Hegselmann. *Journal of Artificial Societies and Social Simulation*, 11(3):3, 2008.

565. *Global Strategic Framework for Integrated Vector Management*, vol. 10, pages 1-12. World Health Organization, Geneva, 2004.

566. World Health Organisation (WHO). 2007.

567. World Health Organisation (WHO). 2009.

568. World Health Organization (WHO). Website. URL http://www.who.int/en/. Accessed April, 2015.

569. The Rainbow Tables. World Health Organization (WHO): The Rainbow Tables. Website. URL http://www.who.int/immunization/research/development/Rainbow&uscore;tables/en/. Accessed April, 2015.

570. E. Worrall and U. Fillinger. *Malaria Journal*, 10(1):338, 2011.

571. G. J. V. Wylen and R. E. Sonntag. *Fundamentals of Classical Thermodynamics*, Chapter 5.5. John Wiley & Sons, Inc., New York, 3rd edition, 1985.

572. X. Xiang, R. Kennedy, and G. Madey. Verification and validation of agent-based scientific simulation models. In *2005 Agent-Directed Simulation Symposium ADS'05*, 2005, http://www.cse.nd.edu/nom/Papers/ADS019_Xiang.pdf Accessed November, 2015.

573. J. Xu, Y. Gao, and G. Madey. A docking experiment: swarm and repast for social network modeling. *Seventh Annual Swarm Researchers Meeting (Swarm2003)*, Notre Dame, IN, 2003.

574. L. Yakob and G. Yan. *PLoS ONE*, 4(9):e6921, 2009.

575. A. Yaro, A. Dao, A. Adamou, J. Crawford, J. Ribeiro, R. Gwadz, S. Traore, and T. Lehmann. *Malaria Journal*, 5(1):19, 2006.

576. L. Yilmaz. *Computational and Mathematical Organization Theory*, 12:283-312, 2006.

577. L. Yilmaz. *Simulation*, 87(1-2):3-4, 2011.

578. L. Yilmaz. *Journal of Experimental & Theoretical Artificial Intelligence*, 24(4):457-474, 2012.

579. L. Yilmaz. Scholarly communication of reproducible modeling and simulation research using e Portfolios. In *Proceedings of the International Summer Computer Simulation Conference*, pages 241-248, Genoa, Italy, 2012. Society for Computer Simulation.

580. L. Yilmaz and T. Ören. Toward replicability-aware modeling and simulation: changing the conduct of M&S in the information age. In *Ontology, Epistemology, and Teleology for Modeling and Simulation*, pages 207-226. Springer, 2013.

581. L. Yu, S. Wang, and K. K. Lai. *European Journal of Operational Research*, 195(3):942-959, 2009.

582. Y. Zhang, editor. *Theoretical and Practical Frameworks for Agent-based Systems*. IGI Global, 2012.

583. L. Zhang, Z. Wang, J. A. Sagotsky, and T. S. Deisboeck. *Journal of Mathematical Biology*, 58(4-5):545-559, 2009.

584. X. Zheng, T. Zhong, and M. Liu. *Building and Environment*, 44(3):437–445, 2009.

585. W. Zhong and Y. Kim. Using model replication to improve the reliability of agent-based models. In *Advances in Social Computing*, pages 118–127. Springer, 2010.

586. Y. Zhou, S. M. N. Arifin, J. Gentile, S. J. Kurtz, G. J. Davis, and B. A. Wendelberger. An Agent-based Model of the *Anopheles gambiae* Mosquito Life Cycle. Unpublished, 2010.

587. Y. Zhou, S. M. N. Arifin, J. Gentile, S. J. Kurtz, G. J. Davis, and B. A. Wendelberger. An agent-based model of the *Anopheles gambiae* mosquito life cycle. In 2010 Summer Simulation Multiconference, SummerSim 2010, pages 201–208. Society for Computer Simulation International, 2010.

588. G. Zhou, S. Munga, N. Minakawa, A. K. Githeko, and G. Yan. *The American Journal of Tropical Medicine and Hygiene*, 77(1):29–35, 2007.

INDEX

Spatial Agent-Based Simulation Modeling in Public Health:
Design, Implementation, and Applications for Malaria Epidemiology, First Edition.
S. M. Niaz Arifin, Gregory R. Madey and Frank H. Collins.
© 2016 John Wiley & Sons, Inc. Published 2016 by John Wiley & Sons, Inc.

Printed and bound by CPI Group (UK) Ltd, Croydon, CR0 4YY

16/04/2025

14658521-0002